Diet, Health, and Status among the Pasión Maya

A Reappraisal of the Collapse

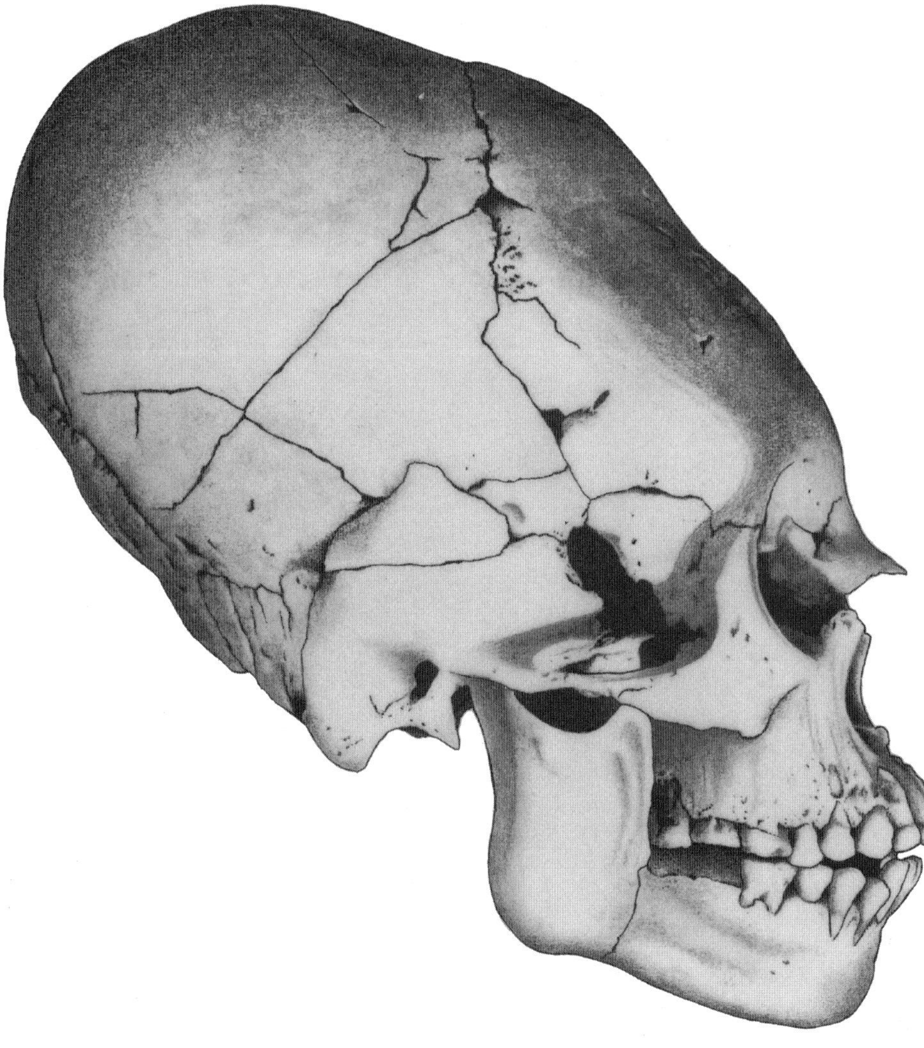

Diet, Health, and Status among the Pasión Maya

A Reappraisal of the Collapse

Lori E. Wright

Vanderbilt Institute of Mesoamerican Archaeology
Arthur Demarest, Series Editor
Volume 2

Vanderbilt University Press
Nashville

First Edition 2006

10 09 08 07 06 1 2 3 4 5

Printed on acid-free paper.
Manufactured in the United States of America
Designed by Dariel Mayer

Frontispiece: The cranium of Altar de Sacrificios Burial 60, from the Terminal Classic period. This middle adult female shows tabular oblique cranial deformation. Rendering by Luis Fernando Luin.

Library of Congress Cataloging-in-Publication Data

Wright, Lori E.
Diet, health, and status among the Pasión Maya :
a reappraisal of the collapse / Lori E. Wright.—1st ed.
p. cm.—(Vanderbilt Institute of Mesoamerican Archaeology
monograph series ; v. 2.)
Includes bibliographical references.
ISBN 0-8265-1418-9 (cloth : alk. paper)
1. Mayas—Anthropometry—Guatemala—Petexbatun, Lake. 2. Mayas—Guatemala—Petexbatun, Lake—Nutrition. 3. Mayas—Health and hygiene—Guatemala—Petexbatun, Lake. 4. Human remains (Archaeology)—Guatemala—Petexbatun, Lake. 5. Petexbatun, Lake (Guatemala)—Antiquities. I. Title. II. Series.
F1435.3.A56W75 2006
972.81—dc22 2006010319

Contents

List of Figures

List of Tables

List of Plates

Acknowledgments

For my parents

This research would not have been possible without the support, guidance, and collaboration of a long list of individuals and institutions. Vanderbilt University's Petexbatun Regional Archaeological Project, directed by Arthur Demarest, provided the culture-historical and logistical context in which the research was conducted, lots of bones, good friends, and a few colmoyotes!

In Guatemala, the Instituto de Antropología e Historia and the Ministerio de Cultura kindly granted permission for field and laboratory work with the Petexbatun Project between 1990 and 1994. I would like to extend my thanks to Lane Beck, David Pilbeam, and Viva Fisher at the Peabody Museum of Archaeology and Ethnology, Harvard University, for permission to study and sample skeletons from Altar de Sacrificios and Seibal. Kevin Johnston kindly offered the Itzan skeletal sample for inclusion in this study, along with unpublished data concerning the provenience of the burials.

This research was funded by a National Science Foundation dissertation improvement grant (BNS-9112561) and a Wenner Gren Foundation for Anthropological Research predoctoral grant (#5447), which I thankfully acknowledge. Clearly, the work would not have been possible without support and collaboration of the Petexbatun Project (which has been funded by Vanderbilt University, National Geographic Society, NEH, USAID, H. F. Guggenheim Foundation, U.S. Institute for Peace, Alimentos Kern de Guatemala, Aviateca, and the Swedish International Development Agency). During the period of research, I received support from the NSERC (Canada), the SSHRC (Canada), the University of Chicago, and the Canadian Federation of University Women.

Isotopic analysis of the archaeological human and faunal bones was carried out by Margaret Schoeninger of the University of Wisconsin, Madison, and by me at Henry Schwarcz's lab at McMaster University. Also at Madison, Jim Burton conducted the elemental analyses. The modern faunal and plant samples were analyzed isotopically and some human C/N ratios measured in Larry Tieszen's lab at Augustana College, Sioux Falls, South Dakota, with the help of Mike Chapman.

The friendship and collaboration of the archaeologists and researchers of the Petexbatun Project has been an enormous aid. Thanks for moral support, academic debate, and for finding those burials are due to a huge list of people, but especially: Oswaldo Chinchilla, Kitty Emery, Hector Escobedo, Antonia Foias, Takeshi Inomata, Nora López, Guïcho Luín, Rosalinda Mendez, Joel Palka, Teresa Robles, Estuardo Secaira, Fredy Soza, Laura Stiver, José Suasnávar, Daniela Triadan, Juan Antonio Valdés, Dirk van Tuerenhout, and Claudia Wolley. Thanks also to John and Aurora Schmidt for their hospitality at Punta de Chimino.

I thank Steve Kluskens, Eric Weidl, and Peter Kupchak for statistical counsel, though they are not to blame for any errors herein. Editorial advice and critiques from a variety of people have strengthened this work, among them Jane Buikstra, Arthur Demarest, Christine White, Steve Houston, Jim Burton, Alan Kolata, Russell Tuttle, and Henry Schwarcz.

Those who sow maize for profit
leave the earth empty of bones
because it is the bones of the
ancestors that give the maize,
and then the earth demands
bones, and the softest ones, those
of the children, pile up on top of
her, and beneath her black crust,
to feed her.

—M. A. Asturias,
Hombres de Maíz

CHAPTER 1

Biology, Culture, and the Classic Maya Collapse

Introduction

During the first millennium A.D., the Maya developed one of the world's most elaborate civilizations. Scholars have viewed these organizational, artistic, and scientific achievements as particularly impressive because the ancient Maya inhabited the hot, humid, tropical rain forest of Central America. These lowland forests have remained largely underpopulated since the earliest contact with Spanish conquistadors and are deemed inhospitable by many. Given this view, it is not surprising that environmental factors have been proposed to account for the coeval abandonment of many large Maya cities in the southern lowlands near A.D. 900. Although a variety of social and political mechanisms have been put forth, most explanations of this "collapse" include a key role for biological components, such as diet, disease, and demography, in the process of site abandonment. The Maya are described as poor environmental managers whose ever-growing population outstripped the rain forest habitat, exceeding its carrying capacity.

Such environmental models define the Maya collapse as a biological problem, and one that is amenable to testing with biological data. Physical anthropological data from ancient Maya skeletons, especially Frank Saul's (1972) landmark study of skeletal remains from Altar de Sacrificios, have been important in both the emergence, and the subsequent refinement, of these environmental explanations for the collapse (Santley et al. 1986; Saul 1972, 1973), but have seldom been used to critically evaluate such models. Advances in skeletal biology and bioarchaeology over the last two decades provide new means to evaluate environmental aspects of prehistoric adaptation using human remains (Price 1989b; Sandford 1993; Saunders and Katzenberg 1992). This monograph aims to evaluate the biological evidence from archaeological human skeletal remains that might support or contradict environmental arguments for the collapse in the Pasión region of the Southern Maya Lowlands.

Although scholars now better appreciate the complexity of Maya adaptation to the rain forest environment (Atran 1993; Fedick 1996; Flannery 1982; Harrison and Turner 1978; Killion 1992; Nations and Nigh 1980; Turner II 1983), the premise of environmental disaster is often reified to a "demonstrated fact" despite the spotty nature of the available data that support it. This tendency stands in contrast to recent trends that emphasize political factors in shaping the history of Maya occupation. The ongoing revolution in Maya hieroglyphic decipherment now allows a "conjunctive approach" to Maya studies employing this new historical data (Culbert 1991b; Fash 1988; Sharer 1978; Willey 1982), which was unavailable when environmental arguments about the collapse first became popular. These new data reveal a rich ideological tapestry of political interaction that makes possible more refined consideration of social processes over the course of Maya history (Culbert 1991a).

Human burials constitute a special type of archaeological feature that provides a unique opportunity to study the interaction of ancient biology and culture. Burials are the only type of physical remains that tie various classes of information directly to individual participants of the past. Unlike most archaeological features, which are the discarded products of human activities, burials contain the physical remains of the people themselves within a context that is constrained by especially strong ideological rules regarding social obligations and roles.

The human skeleton preserves a record of individual biology and life history. Indications of ancient illness found in skeletons can be used to reconstruct prehistoric population parameters of health and disease. Although skeletal manifestations of disease allow reconstruction of the health of individual members of a society, they are most useful on a populational level of analysis as measures of the success of a society's ecological adaptation (Buikstra and Cook 1980; Cohen and Armelagos 1984). Bone also records specific chemical characteristics of ancient diets, which can provide direct information about prehistoric foodways and ecology. Unlike archaeological measures of food and agriculture—such as paleoethnobotany or zooarchaeology—bone chemistry provides a means to examine diet at the level of the individual and thus to study individual variation and differentiation within society as a whole (Price 1989b; Sandford 1993; Schoeninger 1979a).

The archaeological context of the burial provides a link between biological and social realms. Death is perhaps the most important transition experienced by each member of a society and is afforded particular attention in the ritual and social spheres in which a given person interacted. Enacted by those whose lives are disrupted by a death, funeral rituals may explicitly reflect the social position of each person (Bloch and Parry 1982b; Chapman et al. 1981; Pearson 1999). Thus, burials provide a context rich with biological and social data that can be examined on two levels: at the level of the population and of the individual.

Here, I use archaeological human burials to study both biological and social change in the Pasión Region of the Southern Maya Lowlands, located in the Department of Peten, Guatemala. I evaluate mortuary, paleopathological, and bone chemical data for burials recovered from the sites of Altar de Sacrificios, Seibal, Dos Pilas, Aguateca, and Itzan, which span from the Preclassic through the Terminal Classic period (900 B.C. to A.D. 950). The primary emphasis of the research is on evaluating the evidence for an environmental explanation of the collapse of Classic Maya civilization in this region. Such arguments commonly propose that increasing population pressure over the span of the Classic period stretched agricultural systems to the breaking point, causing a decline in dietary quality. Subsequent malnutrition is interpreted as leading to a synergistic increase in disease and health stress, with demographic consequences that resulted in population collapse (Culbert 1988; Sanders 1962, 1963; Santley et al. 1986; Willey and Shimkin 1973).

The Pasión is a particularly good region in which to evaluate this model because it has received frequent archaeological attention that has produced several sizable skeletal samples. Moreover, the Pasión is often the subject of heated debate about the nature of the collapse, and several competing models have been proposed to account for the abandonment of sites in the region near A.D. 900 (Adams 1983; Sabloff and Willey 1967; Sharer 1977; Thompson 1970). Most of these models have invoked environmental causes as the fundamental problem underlying societal disruption, but they differ in whether and to what extent social factors are seen as the cause of these environmental problems or a result of them. Of late, the decipherment of many hieroglyphic monuments provides a new perspective on the nature of political interactions in the region (Demarest 1997; Houston 1993; Mathews and Willey 1991). These new data allow more subtle evaluation of the process of collapse and may provide social alternatives to the prevailing environmental explanations.

In this study I focus on the biological and social implications of the ecological model that are amenable to testing with skeletal data. Diet and health changes, often invoked as specific mechanisms that caused the collapse, are both admirably suited to skeletal analysis. Mortuary analysis, particularly in conjunction with paleodietary analysis, provides insight into the social factors that are elements of competing nonecological models.

Prehistoric Pasión diet is characterized here by isotopic and elemental analysis of human bone samples. The relative abundance of these isotopes and elements in bone is determined by their relative contribution to the diet of the individual. Carbon isotopic analysis is based on the differential incorporation of the stable isotopes carbon 12 and carbon 13 in plants according to two major photosynthetic pathways. Species using each pathway have distinctive carbon isotopic ratios, standardized as $\delta^{13}C$ values (Ambrose 1993; Schwarcz and Schoeninger 1991). In the Maya area, carbon isotopic ratios in archaeological bone are particularly useful for isolating the contribution of maize to the diet (White and Schwarcz 1989). Similarly, the ratio between nitrogen 14 and nitrogen 15, $\delta^{15}N$, depends on the source of nitrogen exploited by the plant. Legumes have low nitrogen isotope values while other plants that utilize soil nitrogen have slightly higher $\delta^{15}N$. These patterns are preserved throughout the food chain with characteristic fractionation between trophic levels (DeNiro 1987; Schwarcz and Schoeninger 1991; van der Merwe 1982).

Certain elements are also fractionated through the food chain and provide another means of dietary analysis. For instance, strontium and barium substitute for calcium in the crystal structure of bone mineral but are discriminated against by intestinal absorption. Hence, they are reduced in the tissues of successively higher trophic levels and are useful for distinguishing the consumption of meat and other foods with unusual elemental compositions from other dietary components (Burton et al. 1999; Price et al. 1985; Schoeninger 1979a).

I obtained bone samples from all adult Pasión skeletons that were deemed to be sufficiently well preserved and submitted them for isotopic analysis of bone collagen and elemental analysis of bone mineral. Because dietary reconstruction requires an understanding of ecosystem dynamics of both isotopes and trace elements and the Neotropical rain forest has received little study to date, I also collected a broad sample of wild and cultivated plants as well as modern and archaeological animal bones that were analyzed chemically. These data are used to reconstruct Pasión diets over time and space.

The evaluation of dietary adequacy and health status focuses on three paleopathological conditions that are frequently observed in skeletal remains. The first, porotic hyperostosis, serves as an index of nutritional quality since it is the consequence of severe iron deficiency anemia suffered during childhood (Stuart-Macadam 1987a). The second, periostosis, can be considered as a measure of infectious disease. Periostoses consist of a layer of new reactive bone deposited on original bone surfaces in response to bone infection. Often it is not possible to diagnose the infectious agent responsible for periostoses in individual skeletons, but, in some cases, diseases that may have afflicted a population can be suggested from the populational distribution of lesions (Cook 1976; Ragsdale et al. 1981). The synergistic interaction of nutrition and infection is well documented in modern peoples and has been demonstrated to account for the distribution of porotic hyperostosis and periosteal reactions in skeletal remains (Mensforth et al. 1978), so these two conditions provide a concrete means for evaluating the adequacy of ancient Pasión diets. The third condition, enamel hypoplasia, is a measure of childhood growth disruption that reflects both diet and health. Nonspecific stress during childhood produces these defects in developing teeth, which provide a unique chronological record of individual stress experience. Thus, hypoplasias can be used to examine changes in childhood illness and growth (Goodman and Rose 1990). These three conditions, documented in human skeletons, are used to examine the health consequences of Pasión subsistence strategies over time and space.

Heterogeneity in diet and health among members of a population can have a significant impact on the evaluation of population trends in skeletal research. In complex and ranked societies, social distinctions afford individual members of society with differential access to food resources (Fried 1967). As noted above, the burial context provides an avenue from which to investigate social differentiation in the ancient Pasión region. The ideological link between food—maize—and bones—as tangible ancestral remains—highlights the symbolic equation of life and death that pervades Maya art and mythology (e.g., Coggins 1988; Tedlock 1985), as does the bone/fertility theme in the mortuary practices of many societies (Bloch and Parry 1982a). The importance of food and food offerings in funerary ritual is emphasized by this symbolic relationship and raises the possibility that mortuary distinctions may mirror dietary partitioning in life, although they are bound to be distorted by cultural processes that define ritual expression. Thus, analysis of burial patterns is employed here to investigate fundamental changes in the composition of Maya society that may complicate the reconstruction of diet and health trends over time. In conjunction with dietary reconstruction, mortuary analysis provides a way to examine the economic correlates of the social hierarchy and its transformations through Maya development and denouement.

This research arose in the context of the Vanderbilt University Petexbatun Regional Archaeological Project, directed by Dr. Arthur Demarest. In order to fully evaluate the biological implications of the environmental collapse models in the context of the Petexbatun region, I expanded the study to incorporate previously studied skeletal series from the nearby Pasión sites of Altar de Sacrificios and Seibal, as well as a small number of skeletons excavated from rural Itzan by Kevin Johnston, then at Yale University. At this broader regional level, differences in diet and health between the sites become apparent, due to their differing histories of occupation. This patterning contributes to a better understanding of the biological implications of Maya settlement history for cultural survival. Aside from the specific goals of this research, I hope that the work will demonstrate the potential of the bioarchaeological approach to elucidate processes of both biological and social import to Maya prehistory.

Explaining the Classic Maya Collapse

The ancient Maya of Central America perceived time and history as proceeding in repeating cycles. Today, as reconstructions of Maya history become more detailed, students of the Maya are coming to appreciate the appropriateness of this worldview (Chase 1990; Puleston 1979; Willey 1986). Over time, Maya civilization experienced alternating periods of fluorescence and decline. The most dramatic of these "declines," labeled the "Classic Maya collapse," resulted in the virtual abandonment of large portions of the southern Maya Lowlands of Guatemala, Belize, and Honduras, and it has been a recurrent focus of archaeological enquiry. Since the collapse is the unifying theme in the monographs of this series, here I will only review arguments about the collapse that are directly relevant to the research presented in this volume.

Models proposed to explain the apparent population decline during the Terminal Classic can generally be divided between those that assign a primary role to environmental causes and those that emphasize social factors. Both of these model types have endured generations of Maya scholarship, dating back to the first explorations of Maya ruins (Adams 1973a). In truth, the environmental and social collapse models represent the extreme poles of a continuum of explanatory scenarios. Most models include both environmental and social elements, but differ in the relative priority assigned to each. In the ensuing discussion, I have elected to contrast the two extremes because they represent phenomena best evaluated with different classes of data.

Environmental Models

> The remarkable fact about the Maya
> is not that they did so much, but
> that they did it in such a place.
> —Huntington 1917:154

Environmental factors have long been important in the discussion of the collapse because of the seeming anomaly that a complex civilization developed in a humid tropical forest. Despite the presence of complex prehistoric societies in similar climes of southeast Asia, the Neotropical environment continues to be perceived as a "green hell" by many Mayanists (Drucker and Fox 1982:179). These arguments, diagrammed in Figure 1.1, are founded on assumptions about the fragility of the rain forest ecosystem, its carrying capacity, and the postulated high density of prehistoric occupation. In essence, the environmental degradation argument is Malthusian; Maya demand for food and the agricultural land to produce it was greater than the environment could provide. The Maya attempted to surpass the limits of their environment and failed (Meggers 1954). To date, the most explicit formulation of the ecological model is given by Santley, Killion, and Lycett (1986) whose arguments are recapitulated here. Santley et al. identi-

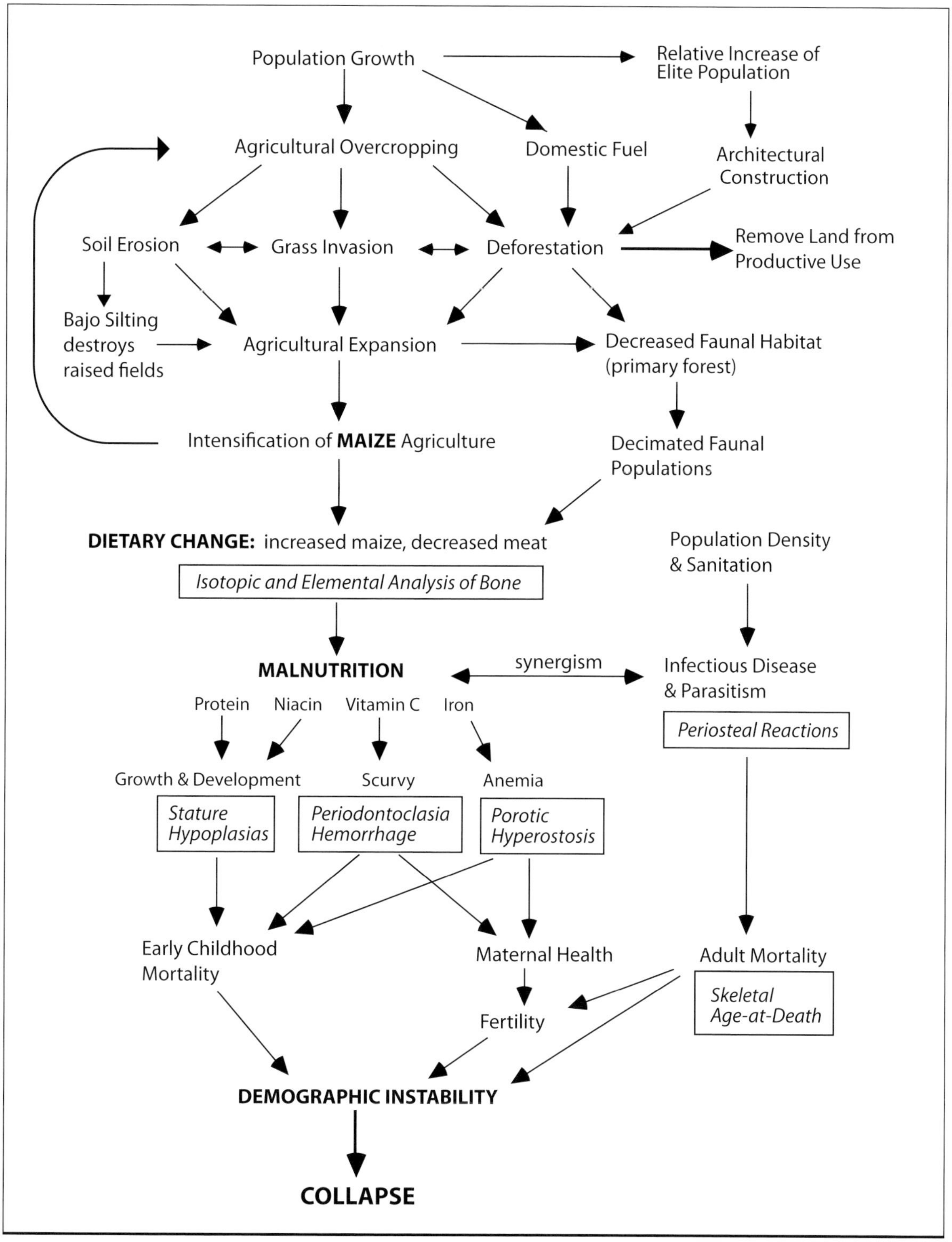

Figure 1.1. Schematic diagram of environmental arguments about the collapse

Osteological indicators that have contributed to the development of the model or that have the potential to address human biological components of the model are indicated in the boxes.

fied three causal variables in the collapse: agricultural failure, demographic instability, and the lack of macroregional resource extraction structures. Agricultural failure occurred because sufficient foods to support the large population could not be grown using sustainable multicropping techniques, and farmers were forced to intensify agriculture, causing permanent ecosystem damage. Demographic instability is argued to be a result of health stress brought on by nutritional deficiency caused by overreliance on maize as the staple food. These food shortages could not be alleviated by importing foods from neighboring regions because of the high costs of such transport (Santley et al. 1986). Many of these variables are also emphasized in discussions of the collapse by other authors (e.g., Culbert 1988; Willey and Shimkin 1973).

Agricultural aspects of the model focus on the interaction of soil exhaustion, deforestation, and erosion, and have been cited since the earliest explorations of Maya cities (Cook 1921). The soils of the Maya Lowlands are highly variable in terms of hydrology, varying from well-drained uplands to the seasonally inundated soils of swamps or *bajos* (Sanders 1977; Stevens 1964). Unlike temperate ecosystems, tropical forests concentrate most of the nutrients in biomass, and soils are relatively nutrient-poor, so significant nutrient loss can occur if forests are cut and erosion is heavy (Jordan 1984).

Based on observations of modern *milpa* agriculture, two effects of overcropping result in the removal of land from cultivation: grass invasion and erosion. Grass outcompetes both crops and forest regeneration. Morley (1946:71–72) argued that once forests were cut, grass moved in so that farming ultimately produced large artificial savannas that became uncultivable with primitive technology (see also Cook 1921). Sanders (1973:362–63) argued that the Petén Maya may have been forced to attempt grass-fallow agriculture in the final years leading up to the collapse.

Soil erosion has been linked to the destruction of uplands for *milpa* use and to silting of the wetlands. Both are implicated in the Santley et al. (1986) model. Ricketson and Ricketson (1937) called attention to terracing as evidence that erosion had been a major problem. The soil buildup observed behind terraces does provide evidence of their utility (Turner II 1983). Cooke (1931) argued that the modern *bajos* were once lakes and became silted up due to hillslope erosion caused by swidden agriculture. Rather than emphasizing arable land, he envisioned that this problem of silting affected Maya success by reducing water supplies. More recently, Harrison (1977) suggested that *bajo* silting was detrimental to intensive agriculture in raised and/or drained fields, and he noted a correlation between the distribution of *bajos* with the area of first collapse. In the *Bajo de Santa Fe* at Tikal, however, chemical analysis of soils demonstrated that the *bajos* were not originally lakes and had not silted up over time (Cowgill and Hutchinson 1963).

Data from the Central Peten lakes point to the existence of major erosion. Lacustrine sediment cores documented a thick layer of "Maya clay" deposited colluvially, which corresponds to the period of Maya occupation (Rice and Rice 1984). Yet, this sedimentation may be more attributable to architectural construction (urbanization) around the lake rather than to agriculture per se (Deevey et al. 1979). Moreover, it is difficult to extrapolate from these steeply sloped valleys to the lowlands as a whole (Turner II 1990:200).

In addition to forest degradation at the hand of agricultural expansion, deforestation would also have come about from the collection of firewood for use as domestic fuel, for the production of lime for architectural plastering, and for house construction (Abrams and Rue 1988). At Copan, domestic firewood use alone could have produced the dramatic deforestation that is suggested by pollen core data. Abrams and Rue (1988) argued that deforestation at Copan would have caused erosion of poor upland soils into the valley, diminishing soil quality in the valley, decreasing rainfall, and contributing directly to the collapse of the Copan state. It is important to note, however, that their calculations and discussion are based on the low-diversity pine forest that surrounds this site on the southern periphery of the Maya area. While similar ecotones occur in the Guatemalan highlands and the Maya mountains of Belize, it is difficult to extrapolate such calculations to the highly diverse broadleaf rain forest that covers most of the Maya area. Atran (1993:682) estimated forest clearing for domestic fuel by contemporary Peten Itza Maya to be only one or two trees per family per year, which would not have contributed to substantial deforestation.

Together, these environmental pressures are thought to have impinged upon the dietary choices available to Late Classic populations. Santley et al. (1986) argued that farmers focused on maize and beans to the exclusion of other crops and that animal protein was severely limited. Support for this idea comes from a late increase in maize pollen from Petén Lake cores; this has been interpreted as a last attempt to produce enough food (Wiseman 1985). Animal protein sources are argued to have been severely limited, in large measure because agricultural expansion would have destroyed wild faunal habitats. Santley et al. (1986:136) cited the rarity of fish bones at inland sites as evidence that they did not contribute significantly to the diet. Thus, the bulk of protein is argued to have come from maize and beans.

Santley et al. (1986:137–39) attributed several nutritional deficiencies to maize consumption. Specifically, they emphasized the low tryptophan content of maize, an amino acid precursor to niacin. Inhibition of iron and zinc absorption by phytate found in maize is also highlighted. However, cooking maize in lime water liberates the glutelin fraction of maize protein, thereby increasing the availability of tryptophan and improving the leucine/isoleucine ratio, thus alleviating the danger of pellagra, which is caused by niacin deficiency (Bressani and Scrimshaw 1958; Katz et al. 1974). Phytate occurs mainly in the pericarp of maize (Layrisse et al. 1969); removal of the pericarp is the primary goal of alkaline processing. Santley et al. noted the beneficial effects of this treatment, nonetheless they argued that niacin and iron deficiencies plagued the ancient Maya. Although there has been some speculation as to the antiquity of alkaline processing (White 1988), it seems likely that the treatment was used in Classic times, given its ubiquity in maize-based horticultural economies throughout the New World (Katz et al. 1974).

This heavy reliance on maize is posited to be a source of health and demographic instability that directly brought about depopulation, as described by Santley et al.:

> [T]he Late Classic Maya may have had considerable difficulty maintaining demographic stability. It seems likely that this instability was largely the result of a collection of nutritional deficiencies synergistically linked to a variety of parasites which collectively placed progressively greater constraints on the number of individuals surviving to reproductive age. These problems . . . were mainly a function of the high levels of basic staples consumed combined with the exceptionally low levels of meat intake (Santley et al. 1986:142–43).

Evidence for malnutrition is drawn from analyses of archaeological skeletons. Hooton (1940) presented the first data to support this idea. He observed anemic cranial lesions (then called "osteoporosis symmetrica") on the skulls from the cenote at Chichen Itza; he attributed these to nutritional deficiency and speculated that such "osteoporosis" might have caused the collapse. At Tikal, Haviland (1967; Haviland and Moholy-Nagy 1992) suggested that a deterioration in childhood health over the span of the Late Classic period caused the decline in skeletal stature that he observed in burials. Saul (1972, 1973) also described a decline in stature at Altar de Sacrificios, apparently confirming this trend. He observed enamel hypoplasias on many dentitions, which supports the interpretation of childhood health stress.

Saul's most influential contribution to the health issue was his diagnosis of nutritional deficiencies. As in Hooton's Chichen Itza skeletons, Saul (1972, 1973) identified abundant porotic hyperostosis in Altar de Sacrificios crania, which he correctly attributed to anemia. In addition, he argued that deposits of subperiosteal new bone on the limb bones of many skeletons were the result of chronic subperiosteal hemorrhages that, together with periodontal resorption and antemortem tooth loss, he interpreted as evidence for scurvy (vitamin C deficiency). This diagnosis has not been widely accepted because of the nonspecific nature of the lesions (Ortner and Putschar 1985:272–73).

Several authors have speculated about the role of infectious diseases in the collapse, especially yellow fever (Spinden 1928:148), Chagas' disease, and ascariasis (Shimkin 1973). Citing a long list of waterborne parasitic infections that are abundant in modern Guatemala, Pozo-Ledezma (1985) argued that the Maya lacked sanitary waste facilities and that human and animal wastes would have infected water supplies, producing severe public health consequences. Arguments about the wide array of tropical pathogens (Santley et al. 1986) are well founded in that tropical forests do support a high diversity of organisms; however, it is important to recognize that this large number of species is thinly spread (Janzen 1983). The characterization of tropical disease burdens as dramatically heavy is perhaps too simplistic.

Such nutritional and health stresses are postulated to have had severe consequences for prehistoric demography. Saul (1972) argued that mean age-at-death declined over the course of the Classic period at Altar de Sacrificios and raised the possibility that health stress at the hand of agricultural problems could have brought about depopulation through increased mortality. This demographic hypothesis has been integrated into subsequent archaeological models. For instance, Willey and Shimkin (1973) suggested that elevated mortality slowed the rate of population growth in Late Classic times, and, curiously, they draw attention to a low birth rate indicated by an absence of artistic "'fertility' fetishes" (Willey and Shimkin 1973:501). Santley et al. (1986:144) emphasize the demographic aspect more strongly, inferring marked demographic instability and that "parents would have had great difficulty raising children to maturity."

Frank Saul's osteological work at Altar de Sacrificios (1972, 1973) was very influential in the development of environmental collapse models, in part because it was published at a time when Mayanists began a thorough review of the collapse (Culbert 1973). However, it is important to note that Saul himself did not see health issues as direct causes of the collapse. His reservation rested on the small size of his skeletal sample; he did not attempt to statistically evaluate chronological trends in the prevalence of the paleopathological conditions that he diagnosed. Instead, he suggested that "all this is suggestive of a somewhat precarious health status that, in combination with invasions and/or internal unrest, might have resulted in the decline of the Maya, at least at Altar de Sacrificios" (Saul 1972:73).

Archaeologists have seldom heeded this reservation and apply Saul's data as documentary proof (e.g., Santley et al. 1986; Lowe 1985:92). Uncritical acceptance of this malnutrition hypothesis may be due to the "gruesome" nature of many bone lesions and the pioneering nature of Saul's study for bioarchaeology. Little comparative data on the health of other New World archaeological populations were available at the time.

The final element of the Santley et al. (1986) model is the supposed absence of "macroregional resource extraction structures," meaning state-sponsored, large-scale programs of trade in subsistence items, like those carried out by the Aztec. Santley et al. (1986) argued that this was not possible in the Maya area because transport costs would have been too high. Like Santley et al., some have seen the paucity of navigable rivers in the central lowlands as a barrier to trade (Webb 1973), but others have argued that food was regularly imported into the central Petén (Culbert 1988; Freidel 1986), a particularly densely settled area often treated as "resource poor" (Rathje 1973). To be sure, long-distance trade of salted coastal fish is known to have occurred in the Late Postclassic (Lange 1971), and there is little reason to suppose that it could not have occurred earlier.

Discussions of the collapse also include several catastrophic environmental mechanisms, such as earthquakes (MacKie 1961) and hurricanes bringing crop blights (Brewbaker 1979). Climatic theories have a long history in Maya studies (Dahlin 1983; Huntington 1917) but until recently were supported by little hard data. Recent oxygen isotope data from lake cores in the Yucatan peninsula suggest a period of slightly warmer and drier climate around the time of the collapse (Hodell et al. 1995), which could have implications for agricultural success.

Social Models

Discussions of the collapse that emphasize social factors over environmental ones can be classified into three broad groups. First, the most influential models emphasize conflict between the social classes in terms of stress put on the lower classes by excessive elite demands. Second, foreign pressure or direct invasion has frequently been suggested. Finally, a change in long-distance trade relationships is postulated to have had severe implications for Maya political economy. These elements are often combined in systemic models of the collapse that emphasize "hypercoherence" of the complex Maya sociopolitical system (*sensu* Flannery 1972) and argue that abrupt changes in any one subsystem would have catastrophic effects on the society as a whole.

The idea that conflict between the elite and nonelite sectors of Maya society was a primary cause of the collapse was popularized by J. Eric S. Thompson (1954). Thompson perceived a fundamental opposition in Maya society between the theocratic rulers and the peasant populace. In addition to ever-growing demands by priests on the peasants for labor service and surplus food taxes, Thompson argued that an ideological gulf developed between the two classes: the priests became increasingly preoccupied with exotic cults, and this shift away from agricultural concerns was viewed by the peasants as a priestly abandonment of agricultural priorities—the primary issue in their own lives—and thus precipitated a peasant revolt (Thompson 1954).

This class-conflict argument was echoed in the writings of some of Thompson's contemporaries (Altschuler 1958), but little hard evidence was marshaled to support it. Thompson drew attention to the apparently violent destruction of some monuments at Piedras Negras (Thompson 1954:89), and other instances of destruction are identified by Hamblin and Pitcher (1980:248). However, the perpetrators of these acts and their specific motivations are not reliably demonstrated. It has been suggested that stelae depicting bound figures beneath the feet of Maya rulers describe this peasant subjugation (Hamblin and Pitcher 1980:249), but the figures are now known to represent elite captives (Stuart 1985). Most crucially, the class-conflict hypothesis provides little explanation for the subsequent depopulation, unless we are to believe that Maya farmers were unable to continue cultivation without priestly guidance.

Although outright revolt is generally unsupported, the idea of social conflict remains an element in modern concepts of a two-class Maya hierarchy. Most reconstructions of Classic period sociopolitical history envision the size of the elite class expanding markedly at the expense of the commoner population. Elite demands for commoner labor are argued to have been a significant source of stress on the total economic system (Culbert 1977; Demarest 1992; Hosler et al. 1977; Sharer 1977; Willey and Shimkin 1973). Webster (1985) has investigated the potential role of labor for monumental construction and elite subsistence requirements at Copan, finding that elite demands on the populace would not have constituted a significant source of stress in their own right. His argument, however, is based upon the assumption of a very small elite body, far smaller than that envisioned for this period by many Mayanists.

External explanations of the collapse focus primarily on hypothesized foreign military invasions. Similarities between architecture at Chichen Itza and Tula led Cowgill (1964) to propose that the collapse was caused by Toltec invasion. Several subsequent archaeologists have argued that Terminal Classic incursions of Gulf Coast peoples were responsible for the collapse of the Usumacinta and Pasión regions of the western lowlands (Sabloff and Willey 1967; Thompson 1970). Thompson (1954, 1970) argued that the collapse, which followed this invasion, was in effect a peasant revolt against priests who wholeheartedly took up the new Mexican religion. Others argue that this foreign interaction was stimulated by internal events and merely exacerbated sociopolitical weaknesses inherent in the Lowland Maya system (Willey 1990). Collapse theories that are specific to the Pasión region are further discussed in greater detail below.

A final class of explanations sees foreign influences mainly in the realm of long-distance trade; these are no longer widely accepted. Rathje (1973) proposed that trade was a crucial component in both the rise and fall of the central Maya Lowlands. He characterized the central lowlands as resource deficient, particularly with respect to salt, obsidian, and volcanic stone. While the need for these basic commodities fostered the development of social complexity (an export commodity) early on, this area was unable to compete for exotic trade after the fall of Teotihuacan and thus collapsed.

More promising discussions of trade underscore the changing nature of economic interaction between cultures that is seen throughout Mesoamerica during the Late and Terminal Classic periods. Webb (1973) argued that the Terminal Classic era witnessed the development of new Mesoamerican trade networks that emphasized the exchange of secular consumption goods by professional merchants. Maya cities in the Petén were at a disadvantage in this economy because the lack of easily negotiable rivers hindered transport of these bulky goods. Moreover, the small Maya polities lacked a cohesive state policy that was needed to organize such trade.

An intriguing model put forth by Freidel (1986) emphasizes a diametrically opposite shift in trade relations. He proposes that the lowlands were a source of agricultural commodities traded throughout Mesoamerica in the Classic period and that symbiotic economic trade relationships were developed between highland and lowland areas. These relationships involved a merging of politics with economy, that is, the formation of "cartels." He argues that the Teotihuacan traits seen in Early Classic Maya art reflect such a cartel, and, after the collapse of Teotihuacan, the southern lowland ideology began to emphasize the purity of sacred bloodlines, a worldview that discouraged intermarriage with highland ethnic groups or religious syncretism. This structural impasse did not hinder cartel formation in the northern lowlands where rulership was less constrained by genealogical purity, but led to the collapse of southern lowland economies (Freidel 1986).

Trade has also been highlighted as a factor precipitating internal tensions within the Southern Maya Lowlands and contributing to systemic stress. Maya elites engaged in long-distance trade for status items such as jade and marine shells, which were displayed as symbols of their sacred purity in rituals that enhanced the charismatic power of the ruler (Demarest 1992). Internal competition between Maya polities involving the escalation of warfare may have been motivated by a desire to gain economic control over larger areas (Cowgill 1979). Demarest (1992) stresses the elite desire to control trade routes of exotic goods as a major motivation in this internal conflict. Such warfare, in turn, had direct effects on the survival of individual rulers and the polities they governed.

Many of the social mechanisms discussed above are elements commonly incorporated into systemic models of the collapse. These models emphasize the interaction of effects in the subsistence, economic, demographic, political, and ideological subsystems. Often these models are couched in the terminology of systems theory, in which perturbations in any one subsystem may have repercussions in other subsystems. Such models conceive Maya society as highly structured, with subsystems tightly woven together, a condition referred to as "hypercoherence." Hypercoherent systems are inherently unstable; even a small deviation in any subsystem can produce total system failure or collapse (Flannery 1972).

The most influential systems model was compiled by Willey and Shimkin (1973) following the collapse seminar held in 1971. Willey and Shimkin emphasize the increasing role of the elite in economic and agricultural management over time. They stress the role of elite competition in placing excessive demands on the commoners. In conjunction with decreased agricultural productivity, malnutrition and health stress led to reduction in the work capacity of commoners, further intensifying pressure on the sociopolitical system as a whole. Together with external changes in trade and foreign interaction and the inability of the elite administration to adjust to these new stresses, Lowland Maya sociopolitical organization became nonviable and collapsed. This all-inclusive or "kitchen sink" model incorporates many of the social elements discussed above but significantly retains environmental stress as an integral component of the transition.

Hosler, Sabloff, and Runge (1977) attempted to evaluate the Willey and Shimkin (1973) model mathematically. The simulation emphasizes the elements of food production, elite labor demands, and the size of the producer population, finding that the reallocation of commoners to nonagricultural production does indeed produce a systemic collapse (Hosler et al. 1977). Although such modeling can demonstrate how changes in the components of a system can produce collapse, it cannot prove how an event came about, because parameters of the model are defined by the investigator and dependent on preconceived ideas of the process involved. Similar reservations apply to the mathematical models of Lowe (1985) and Hamblin et al. (1980). While interesting as exercises, such approaches contribute no new data to study of the past.

Subsequent models also invoke ecological factors. In some cases, sociopolitical elements are preeminent and produce environmental disaster, while in others, underlying population pressure fosters elite administrative stress. Sharer (1977) follows the latter tack, suggesting that the fundamental problems of the Late Classic period were dietary stress, excessive elite demands on commoner labor, and increasing religious schism between the two classes. He posits that environmental stress produced two types of reactions in the Maya populace. The initial response was technological, with intensification of agriculture. This was followed by ideological revitalization of the nonelite populace, who attempted unsuccessfully to replace the old elite with a new hierarchy (Sharer 1977). This argument resembles Thompson's class-conflict model but retains the ecological motivation.

A more recent argument draws on new hieroglyphic evidence for political competition. With specific reference to the Pasión, Demarest (1978, 1996) has hypothesized that elite competition was transformed into a more destructive form of territorial warfare at the end of the eighth century. Expansionistic warfare led to the development of a large political hegemony under the control of Dos Pilas. Failure of the Dos Pilas dynasty to maintain control over this area resulted in its political Balkanization and escalated destructive warfare that affected the population as a whole, not solely the elite sector. Escalated warfare between neighboring sites led directly to the sociopolitical collapse of individual polities and, ultimately, large areas. Sociopolitical stress at the hand of elite competition is also proposed to have contributed to the collapse of Caracol and its hinterlands (Chase 1990).

Environmental explanations of the collapse have shown incredible tenacity in Maya scholarship and are invariably included in complex models of the collapse even by those with a preference for social or ideological mechanisms. The intellectual climate in which the ecological model emerged played a significant role in its pervasiveness in subsequent scholarship. This model arose at a time when archaeological methods were shifting toward settlement analysis (Haviland 1969, 1970b; Tourtellot III 1970; Willey et al. 1965), and new data were emerging on the huge size of prehistoric populations that had not previously been appreciated. However, there was as yet little evidence for intensive forms of agriculture. Environmental models gained force during the 1960s (Sanders 1962, 1963, 1973) and really took hold at a seminar held in 1971 (Culbert 1973), but the first confirmed reports of raised fields (Siemens and Puleston 1972) and hillslope terracing (Turner II 1974) did not appear until slightly later.

This new agrotechnology, which provided a subsistence base for the burgeoning population, was examined intensively during the 1970s and early 1980s (Flannery 1982; Harrison and Turner 1978). Yet, the ecological "contradiction" of Maya civilization held sway, perhaps because it fit comfortably in epistemological terms into the processual, cultural ecology paradigm of the day. More recent reexamination finds that we still have much to learn about the distribution and productivity of ancient Maya agrosystems (Dunning et al. 1997; Dunning and Beach 1994; Pope and Dahlin 1989). Although two forms of intensive technology have been identified, their distribution is still poorly defined. Moreover, ancient cropping systems, fallow cycles, and mulching practices are more difficult to study but have a major impact on the carrying capacity of the landscape. Characterization of ancient *milpa* agriculture as "primitive" is simplistic and underestimates the complex ecological management strategies employed in traditional farming systems (Atran 1993; Barrera et al. 1977;

Nations and Nigh 1980). The view that Maya agricultural production was sufficient to maintain large populations seems to be gaining force (Freidel and Scarborough 1982), although many still adhere to environmental factors as prime movers in the collapse (Culbert 1988). A prominent agronomist has argued that Maya population density did not reach a critical stress level, even in the Late Classic (Turner II 1990). In a review of the collapse, Culbert upheld an environmental cause but observed that "[g]iven . . . the paucity of precise data, one could construct almost any scenario of agricultural failure that suited one's fancy" (Culbert 1988:100).

CHAPTER 2

The Pasión Region

Introduction

A long history of intensive archaeological research in the Pasión region and its explicit hieroglyphic record of prehistoric political interactions provide a rich historical context from which to examine the collapse. Located in the southwestern corner of the modern Department of Petén, Guatemala, this area encompasses the drainage of the Río Pasión and its tributaries, from Alta Verapaz to a point slightly north of the confluence of the Pasión with the Salinas-Chixoy system to form the Río Usumacinta, and including the area between the Pasión and Chixoy Rivers (Mathews and Willey 1991).

Lying between 100 and 500 m in elevation, the Pasión region has a tropical climate, with a mean annual temperature of 25°C and mean annual precipitation of 2,000 mm, which falls mostly between May and December. Humidity is high throughout the year, and water seldom scarce. The topography of the region is shaped by faulting of the underlying limestone bedrock and is crossed by three graben valleys containing the Salinas, Petexbatun, and Pasión Rivers. High escarpments along the western edges of the Laguna Petexbatun and the Pasión River south of Seibal mark the faults between the uplifted horst and the graben (Dunning et al. 1997; Dunning and Beach 1994). The entire area is underlain by a karstic network of caves and underground rivers. Surface rivers are generally slow, broad, and meandering, but water levels may fluctuate by as much as 10 m annually.

The Cretaceous Neocomian-Campanian carbonate bedrock is covered by well-drained fertile rendzina soils. In contrast, the poorly drained valley soils are derived from Paleocene-Eocene marine sediments combined with highland alluvial deposits that are carried down by the Pasión and Salinas Rivers. At the confluence of the Ríos Pasión and Salinas the underlying rock is of more recent Oligocene origin, including conglomerate beds, sandstone, and clays (Vinson 1960). More detailed discussion of the region's geology and soils can be found in Dunning and Beach forthcoming in this series (see also Dunning and Beach 1994; Beach and Dunning 1995, 1997; Dunning et al. 1995, 1997, 1998).

These soils support a moist subtropical forest over much of the region. The forest is high latifoliate perennifoliate, with ceiba (*Ceiba pentandra*), mahogany (*Swietenia macrophylla*), sapodilla (*Acras zapota*), ramon (*Brosimum alicastrum*), copal (*Protium copal*), and tropical cedar (*Cedrela mexicana*) among the common canopy tree species. An abundance of palms makes up the understory, and bromeliads, orchids, and other epiphytes are common. In more poorly drained areas, the forest is transformed to *tintal bajo*, dominated by logwood (*Hematoxylum campechianum*) and palms. Secondary growth in abandoned agricultural fields (*milpas*) is a dense tangle of *Cecropia* and *Acacia* (Meave del Castillo 1990; Wagner 1964; Willey et al. 1975). The forest supports a broad diversity of reptilian, avian, and mammalian fauna. The extensive wetland system is also home to a diversity of fauna, including fish, reptiles, and water birds. More detailed descriptions of the natural history of the region can be found in Dunning (n.d.) and Emery (1997).

Dunning and Beach (1994) have documented the presence of extensive relic terracing on hillslopes in the Petexbatun region, especially near Tamarindito and north of Aguateca, which date to the Late Classic period. Although no terraces were reported during mapping operations at Seibal (Tourtellot III 1988), Dunning has observed terracing in cleared fields west of the site and believes that the technology was probably employed throughout the region (Dunning and Beach 1994). As at Seibal, terracing may go unnoticed in other heavily forested parts of the region.

Raised field agriculture, purportedly identified along the Pasión floodplain with side-looking airborne radar (Adams 1983), is unlikely throughout the Pasión watershed because of the drastic fluctuation in the water table—up to 10 m annually. This type of field has not been verified on the ground. Raised or drained fields can only function with stable water tables. Although artificial modifications of wetland environments were not undertaken in the Pasión region, low-lying areas along the rivers undoubtedly were cultivated. The fertile floodplain soils could have sustained long-term cropping without modification, since nutrients are replenished annually by rainy season floods. In uplands, *aguadas* were artificially modified with terracing that slowed soil erosion and probably allowed intensive cultivation of these localized "wetland" niches (Dunning et al. 1997; Dunning and Beach 1994).

The Pasión has been a recurrent focus of archaeological exploration and excavation, beginning with visits by Alfred Maudslay, Teobert Maler, and Sylvanus Morley near the turn of the century. Three large-scale excavation projects have been carried out: at Altar de Sacrificios (Willey 1973; Willey and Smith 1969), at Seibal (Willey 1990; Willey et al. 1975), and in the Petexbatun region (Dos Pilas, Aguateca, Tamarindito, Arroyo de Piedra, La Paciencia) (Demarest 1997, 2006). Smaller-scale research projects involving mapping and settlement studies have been carried out at Itzan (Johnston 1994) and La Amelia (Foias 1997). Exploration aimed at documenting hieroglyphic monuments has permitted detailed reconstruction of culture history (Graham 1967; Houston 1987; Houston and Matthews 1985; Mathews and Willey 1991). Further details of the history of archaeological research in the Pasión can be found in the first monograph in this series (Demarest 2006) and in a number of other sources (Houston 1993; Willey and Smith 1969; Willey et al. 1975).

Culture History of Pasión Polities

In the following pages I briefly review the culture histories of those Pasión sites that contribute to the present work. The Petexbatun material is only briefly touched on here, as it is described in detail in the other monographs of this series. Figure 2.1 illustrates the correlation between ceramic chronologies that have been defined for sites in the region which forms the basis for chronological comparisons herein.

Altar de Sacrificios

Altar is located on the south bank of the Río Pasión, near its confluence with the Salinas River. The area examined in the Peabody project is limited to the site core west of the small Arroyo San Felix and some low mounds lying further west. Group A is the larger of the two main plaza groups. The North Plaza of Group A is defined by three large range pyramids and is separated from the South Plaza by a ball court. The South Plaza is defined by a number of smaller structures. Group B, located to the west, focuses on a small patio defined by three pyramidal structures and two small courtyard groups. A third group of mounds, Group C, consists of two large connected platforms between Group B and the south plaza of Group A. Other mounds with one or more structures atop a basal platform are scattered nearby.

First occupied in the Middle Preclassic Xe phase (900–500 B.C.), Altar began as a small village of wattle-and-daub houses constructed directly on the natural ground surface. Public or monumental architecture has not been identified for this early occupation, but might have been missed in the limited excavations. A deposit of jack beans (*Canavalia ensiformis*) that probably date to this phase and ceramic spindle whorls document that agriculture was well developed, with exploitation of forest and riverine fauna indicated by the presence of deer bones and freshwater clam shells (Willey 1973).

In the subsequent San Felix phase (500–300 B.C.), the first monumental architecture was constructed. The most substantial building, Str. B-IV, reached 5 m in height, had a perishable superstructure, and was faced with mortar mixed with river

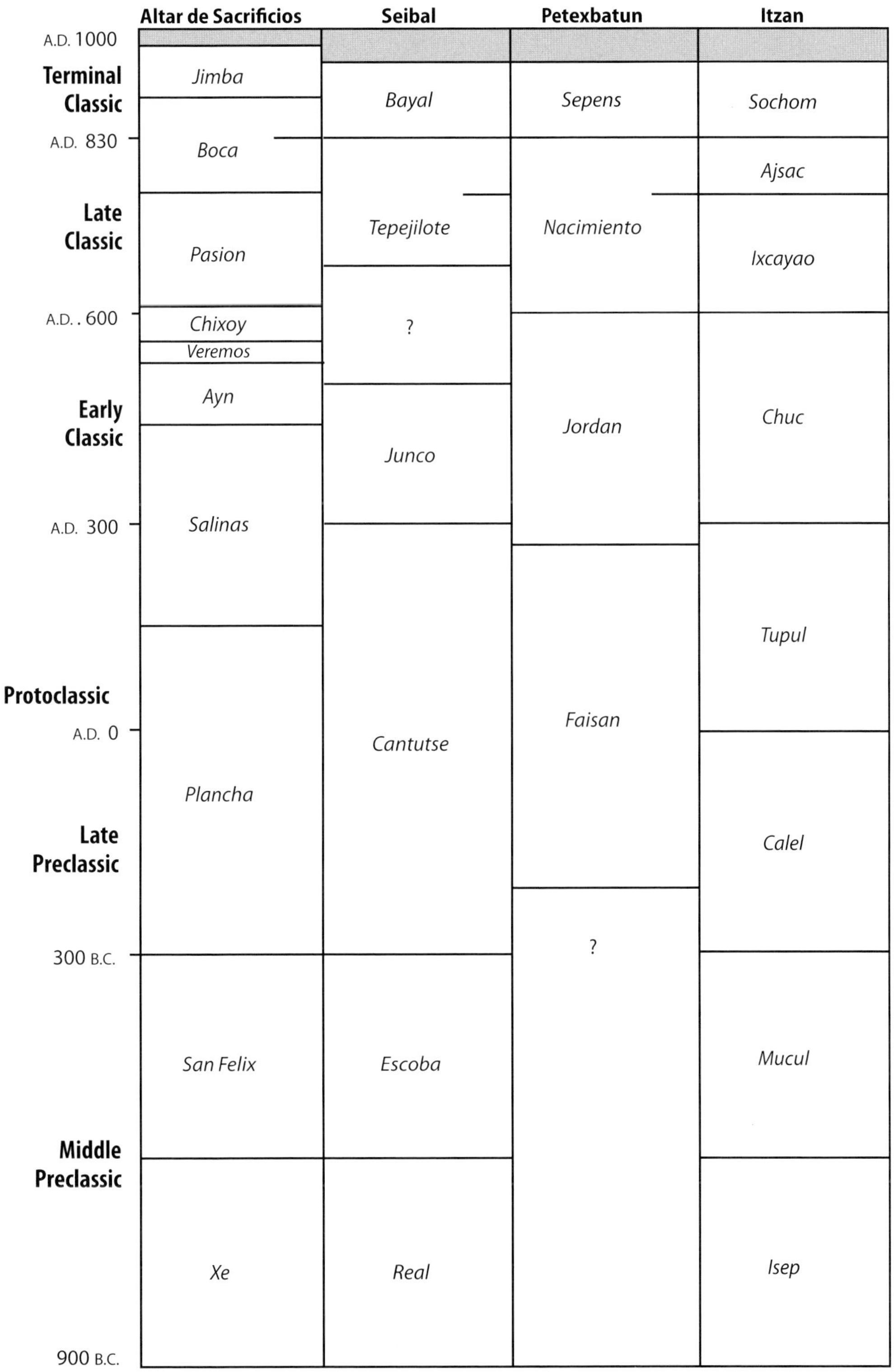

Figure 2.1. Ceramic chronologies for Pasión sites

(Adapted after Adams 1971; Sabloff 1975; Foias 1996; and Johnston 1994).

clams. In addition to obsidian, greenstone was recovered from this occupation, suggesting broader interregional contacts. The earliest maize from the region occurred in San Felix deposits and belongs to the Nal Tel race.

The early structures in Group B were enlarged during the Plancha Phase (300 B.C.–A.D. 150) by the addition of clay, clam mortar, and sandstone blocks placed along the stairways. Structure B-1, a terraced pyramid, was enlarged to 9 m in height, with a plastered and wattle-and-daub superstructure painted red. Votive caches of ceramics, obsidian, and jade were first placed in these constructions at this time. Willey (1973) argued that Plancha marked the beginnings of nonegalitarian society at Altar.

The succeeding Salinas phase (A.D. 150–450) corresponds to the Early Classic period, when the final structural modifications to Group B structures were carried out, raising Str. B-I to 13 m in height. Artifacts in graves and caches with a greater abundance of marine shells and other coastal products indicate broader trade contacts. Thereafter, in the Ayn phase (A.D. 450–600) Group B saw the addition of the first hieroglyphic monuments at the site, beginning with Stela 10, dated 9.1.0.0.0. (A.D. 455). These early monuments were carved from the same local sandstone used in the Early Classic and Preclassic construction at Altar. The final monument erected in Group B was dedicated in A.D. 524, near the end of Ayn times (Willey 1973).

A very brief phase, Veremos (A.D. 570–585), encompassed the shift in ceremonial focus to Group A, where low terraced platforms were constructed of sandstone; however, no monuments were dedicated at this time. The sculptural tradition returned in the subsequent Chixoy phase (A.D. 585–630), at which time a number of stelae were erected in the South Plaza of Group A, and many structures were enlarged. The following Pasión phase (A.D. 630–780) saw the greatest development of centralized authority and social diversity at the site. The large structures in the North Plaza underwent several enlargements; the acropolis, ball court, and other central structures were built. For both architectural construction and hieroglyphic monuments, architects shifted from the local sandstone to limestone that had to be brought into the site from an outcrop much further upstream. These changes were accompanied by an increase in domestic mound occupation.

This trend was reversed during Boca times (A.D. 780–900), although the site's population remained large. Structures A-I, A-II, and A-III received their last minimal modifications. No hieroglyphic monuments were erected at this time. However, settlement excavations outside of the main plaza indicate a vigorous community with little loss of population despite the apparent cessation of organized large-scale ritual activity.

Adams (1971) distinguished a final phase, Jimba (A.D. 900–950), from the Late Boca. He made the separation on the basis of Fine Orange and Gray paste ceramics, at the time thought to have been imported from the Gulf coast of Campeche. Neutron activation analyses demonstrate that these were local wares, and the distinction may be more functional than chronological (Sabloff 1973:121). (See below for more detailed discussion of chronological alignments between sites.) No major construction can be attributed to the Jimba phase, and occupation of house mounds appears to have been much more restricted than in the Boca Phase, a further indication that the phase may be a functional distinction instead. By A.D. 950, it seems that Altar de Sacrificios was abandoned.

The above description of Altar's history is derived from the excavation reports and summary (Adams 1971; Smith 1972; Willey 1973). New hieroglyphic data indicate that the site was important during the Early Classic period when three rulers reigned between A.D. 455 and 524. After the hiatus, one ruler held office for a considerable time (44 years), followed by three others in quick succession. Later rulers are poorly documented, and the latest monument was erected in A.D. 771 (Stela 15). Thereafter, the large Boca phase population remained at the site, but with little in the way of centralized elite authority. Unlike many neighboring sites, Altar seems to have remained independent throughout its history (Mathews and Willey 1991).

Seibal

Seibal lies at the great bend in the Río Pasión where it turns from its northward flow to drain westward and join the Usumacinta. The site sits high above the river on limestone hills of the raised horst plateau. Central Seibal is focused on two main architectural groups, A and D, located on separate hilltops and joined by Causeways I and III. At the center of the causeways joining Groups A and D, a third causeway branches to the south, leading to a curious round structure. Settlement clustered in this intervening area along Causeway II is designated as Group C. Dispersed settlement extends for several kilometers from this central architecture. Group B, designated by Morley (Morley 1938), is a small patio group with a single stela, located about 2 km south of the main center.

Like Altar, the earliest evidence for occupation at Seibal dates to the Middle Preclassic period. The Real phase at Seibal is equivalent to Xe at Altar and spanned the same period (900–600 B.C.). Refuse deposits from the Real phase were found at the base of several excavations in Group A, in association with gravel-plaster floors of low platforms. As at Altar, metates and spindle whorls indicate an agricultural economy. Faunal remains include terrestrial fauna, but a ceramic netsinker indicates that fishing was practiced.

Escoba phase ceramics pertain to the Mamom sphere and were found in many areas of the site, indicating an increase in population between 600–300 B.C. Small temple-like structures in the peripheral areas—in which limestone foundations supported a perishable superstructure—probably date to this period. Construction in Group A also began at this time, given the abundant Escoba refuse beneath later constructions, although no definite architecture can be attributed to the phase (Willey 1990).

The increasing population culminated in the Late Preclassic Cantutse phase (300 B.C.–A.D. 300), with an estimated population of 5,000 or 10,000 at Seibal. Much of the ceremonial construction in Group A probably dates to this period. Although excavations in large architecture were limited, Willey speculates that Cantutse substructures account for most of the volume of the Late and Terminal Classic structures in this group (Willey 1990:242). Groups C and D also began construction during this time, as did a large proportion of the domestic mounds surrounding these groups. The later, Protoclassic, facet of the Cantutse ceramic assemblage has been interpreted by Willey (1990:241) as representing elite wares. Together with emerging differentiation in burial accompaniments, this suggests increasing social diversity during this period (Willey 1990).

The subsequent phase, Junco (A.D. 300–500), is very poorly represented in both monumental and domestic contexts. The floors of Group A plazas were resurfaced during this phase, but little significant construction has been documented. The site was much reduced in population, and large portions of it were probably completely abandoned until around A.D. 600 or 650. This period corresponds to the hiatus of hieroglyphic monument dedication that is observed at other sites, including Altar. Unlike Altar, Seibal did not withstand whatever pressures were responsible for this hiatus, and its community functions were broadly disrupted (Willey 1990).

Seibal returned to its former prosperity during Late Classic times, the Tepejilote phase (A.D. 600–770). Tourtellot and Willey infer that this revival was occasioned by resettlement of the site by local Pasión peoples because Tepejilote ceramic and artifact assemblages are comparable to those at other Pasión sites (Willey 1990:248). Tepejilote peoples reoccupied the domestic mounds of earlier Cantutse peoples and constructed additional platforms. Group A served as the principal ritual focus of the community; its ceremonial structures were refurbished and enlarged, and stelae and hieroglyphic monuments were erected here. Group D also saw major construction, probably serving a residential function for Seibal's elite. Peripheral areas show increasing occupation in domestic patio groups and new construction of some minor centers. The archaeological indications are of a thriving community, about as large as the earlier Cantutse population, that participated in broad-scale trade and other interactions throughout the lowlands (Willey 1990). However, more recent epigraphic data suggest that Seibal played a minor political role in the region. The capture and sacrifice of Seibal's ruler Yich'ak Balam by Ruler 3 of

Dos Pilas in A.D. 735 is recorded on Seibal's hieroglyphic stairway, and it seems that Dos Pilas held political control over the site for some 60 years thereafter (Houston 1993; Houston and Matthews 1985; Mathews and Willey 1991).

After the demise of Dos Pilas and the Petexbatun sites, Seibal emerged to become the dominant political entity in the region. Terminal Classic occupation at the site is designated as the Bayal Boca phase (A.D. 830–928) and is marked by the introduction of Fine Orange and Gray paste ceramics as well as distinctive iconography in the sculptures. Originally interpreted as evidence for an invasion of Mexicanized Maya from the Gulf coast, hieroglyphic data now suggests that the site was taken over by a lord from Ucanal, named Wat'ul-Chatel, in A.D. 830 (Schele and Mathews 1998). The new ruler built a small radial temple, A-3, in the center of the South Plaza of Group A. He proclaimed both his ancestry and claim on Seibal on its stucco frieze and on stelae erected around the structure in the ensuing years. Many other structures in Group A attained their final form at this time with only minor modifications, but few other structures were built. Settlement surrounding the site center increased dramatically; most of the structures in Group C are Bayal in date, including the round Str. 79 and the Group C ball court. This increased settlement density may be due to immigration from sites being abandoned in the Petexbatun region (Tourtellot III and González 2004). This new prosperity was short-lived, however. By A.D. 928 the site center was abandoned, but radiocarbon dates on a few burials that are intrusive into Bayal levels suggest that some occupation may have lingered at the site until 1000 or 1050 A.D. (Willey 1990).

Itzan

The site of Itzan is located on a bluff above the Arroyo Itzan, a small tributary that flows into the Pasión river 6 km to the south, about 50 km west of Sayaxché by river. The site consists of a strip of settlement 300 m by 7 km long aligned northwest-southeast along the ridge top. Central Itzan consists of two main plaza areas, an acropolis, and causeways. The North Plaza is defined by range-type structures on all sides, and contains most of the known sculptural monuments from Itzan. The South Plaza gives access to the raised platform of the acropolis, via a hieroglyphic stairway on a range structure (Johnston 1994; Tourtellot III et al. 1978).

Deep tests below the South Plaza indicate that Itzan was first occupied during Early Middle Preclassic Xe times, contemporaneous with the earliest occupations at Altar and Seibal. A dense midden of the Late Middle Preclassic Mucul Mamom phase overlays the sherds, indicating that central Itzan was the focus of substantial occupation. As at Altar and Seibal, large public architecture was constructed in central Itzan during the Late Preclassic Calel Chicanel phase. Excavation in peripheral locations also produced evidence of substantial Chicanel occupation. Ceramics dating to Terminal Preclassic or Protoclassic times are also present, but Early Classic remains are rare at Itzan, indicating a decline in occupation at that time like that observed at Seibal (Johnston 1994).

Late Classic deposits of the Ixcayao Tepeu 2 phase overlie Preclassic strata with little intervening occupation at Itzan. These Late Classic ceramics are virtually identical to types represented at other Pasión sites and are found throughout the site center and hinterland. Johnston distinguishes these strata from later Ajsac Tepeu phase occupation, which correlates with the transitional phase at Seibal or the late facet of the Petexbatun Nacimiento phase. Evidence of Terminal Classic Sochom Tepeu 3 phase occupation at Itzan is limited to a surface scatter of Fine Orange and Tojil Plumbate ceramics atop a peripheral patio group, suggesting an ephemeral occupation. No Terminal Classic remains were found in the site core by Johnston (1994), although the Harvard expedition reported a single Fine Orange sherd (Tourtellot III et al. 1978). Thereafter, Itzan was apparently abandoned, until resettled by Lacandones in the 19th century (Johnston 1994).

The earliest hieroglyphic reference to Itzan is from the inscriptions of Dos Pilas, which record the marriage of an elite woman from Itzan to Dos Pilas' Ruler 1 in A.D. 652 (9.11.0.0.0). At least five rulers of Itzan are known, spanning some 180 years of the site's history. Hiatuses in this record occur between A.D. 685–741 and between A.D.

782–807, and little is known of the polity during these periods (Mathews and Willey 1991). Iconographic motifs on two stelae with eroded dates that may pertain to the later gap suggest cultural ties with elites at Piedras Negras and Yaxchilan in the central Usumacinta at this time (Johnston 1994). There is little evidence to indicate that Itzan was ever subjugated by any other polity; rather, it seems to have maintained political autonomy throughout its history. Stela 6 records the latest date at the site, 9.19.19.16.0 (A.D. 829). The proximity of this date to the onset of Terminal Classic activity at Seibal suggests that some occupation likely remained at Itzan, at least into the early years of the Terminal Classic period (Mathews and Willey 1991).

The Petexbatun Region

Details of the site locations, architectural features, and excavation findings are presented in the other volumes of this series and in Vol. 8(2) of *Ancient Mesoamerica*, to which readers are referred. Here I will only briefly describe the political history of the sites, in the context of the process of collapse and abandonment.

Sites within the Petexbatun region can be broadly grouped into those sites that were governed by the Petexbatun dynasty and those that were independent for much of their history. The Petexbatun dynasty was centered at Dos Pilas during the first part of the Late Classic period and later shifted to Aguateca for a brief period at the close of the Late Classic. Local indigenous dynasties at Tamarindito and Arroyo de Piedra predate the arrival of the Petexbatun lineage to the region, as does settlement at these sites. Although the settlement histories Punta de Chimino, Arroyo de Piedra, Tamarindito, and portions of Aguateca span from Late Preclassic times, the bulk of the occupation at each dates to the Late Classic. Terminal Classic occupations are found only at Punta de Chimino and, in a very limited way, at Dos Pilas and Tamarindito.

The rich epigraphic record for the Petexbatun dynasty allows detailed reconstruction of the political history of the region. The dynasty's emblem glyph is actually a variant of the emblem for Tikal, indicating that the Dos Pilas elite either originated there or attempted to claim descent from Tikal in order to gain a footing in the Pasión political scene (Houston and Matthews 1985). The first documented leader of Dos Pilas, Ruler 1, appears to have been involved in military contests against Tikal, indicating an antagonistic relationship between the two dynasties. Ruler 1 married a woman from Itzan, and their daughter in turn married a noble from Naranjo. Such marriages likely aided the consolidation of the dynasty within the Pasión political arena. During his reign Ruler 2, son of Ruler 1, continued in conflict with Tikal and expanded the local power base of the dynasty, enlisting the site of Aguateca as a twin capital. Inscriptions suggest that Ruler 2 supervised rituals at Tamarindito under the auspices of a local ruler, and he is posthumously described as an "overlord" on Stela 2 at nearby Arroyo de Piedra (Houston 1987, 1993; Houston and Matthews 1985). A rich burial beneath Str. L5-1 in the Main Plaza at Dos Pilas may be that of Ruler 2, since his funeral is documented on Stela 8, erected directly in front of this temple (Demarest et al. 1991).

The subsequent Ruler 3 continued this military campaign and married a woman from Cancuen (Burial DP20). Ruler 3 undertook battles against other neighboring polities, killing the ruler of Seibal and installing a branch of his own family to rule that site. The son of Ruler 3 and his Cancuen wife probably became Ruler 4, who strengthened ties with his maternal site by performing rituals there. He continued his ancestors' military campaigns, capturing lords from Akul, El Chorro, Yaxchilan, and Motul de San Jose. Ruler 4 was probably exiled after his defeat in a battle against Tamarindito, since the text on Tamarindito's Hieroglyphic Stairway 2—which records a battle dated about A.D. 760–762—is the last reference to him. Thereafter, no monuments were dedicated at Dos Pilas (Houston 1987, 1993; Houston and Mathews 1985).

The posited conflict with Tamarindito may be linked to the construction of walls encircling the major ceremonial compounds at Dos Pilas. Excavations in Str. L5-1 and the palace group illustrate the destruction of Late Classic architecture—including portions of a hieroglyphic stairway—which was quarried to provide building materials used in the construction of the walls and indicates that at least portions of the palace were abandoned at this time. The walls are distinctly defensive in character and were probably topped by a wooden palisade (Demarest et al. 1997). Within the plaza, a number of low platforms were probably constructed at the same time as the walls and appear to be foundations for wattle-and-daub domestic structures (Demarest et al. 1997; Foias 1992). Ceramics associated with these structures pertain to a late facet of the Nacimiento phase and can be securely dated to after A.D. 760. Evidently, the population of the site was greatly reduced following the dynasty's defeat.

After the defeat of Ruler 4, the dynasty appears to have retreated to Aguateca, with only a small residual occupation remaining at Dos Pilas into Terminal Classic times. This later occupation at Aguateca was also short-lived and accompanied by the threat of conflict. Like Dos Pilas, Aguateca possesses a system of defensive walls, but these are integrated more fully into the site plan, surrounding domestic as well as major ceremonial architecture. These walls were apparently constructed after the basic plan of the site had been laid out, but, in contrast to the situation at Dos Pilas, the majority of domestic groups at Aguateca continued to be occupied after the walls were constructed. In addition, eight small residential groups on the site periphery are surrounded by walls and indicate a militarized local Late Nacimiento landscape (Demarest et al. 1997; Inomata 1995, 1997; O'Mansky et al. 1995). Ceramic data indicate that both the site center and domestic settlement continued into the late facet of the Nacimiento phase (A.D. 760–830), when Dos Pilas was largely abandoned (Foias 1993; Inomata 1995). The last monuments were erected in A.D. 790 (Stelae 2 and 14, 9.18.0.0.0), but references to the dynasty appear as late as A.D. 800 at Seibal and A.D. 807 at La Amelia (Houston 1987, 1993). Despite the complex defenses, archaeological excavations reveal that the site suffered a dramatic defeat that led to its abandonment. Range structures in the avenue and plaza were abandoned with great quantities of pots, utensils, and ornaments lying on the floor and bench surfaces, and the structures' thatched roofs were burned. This finding documents that the site was abandoned precipitously while still occupied by its elite, perhaps following an enemy attack. The desperate nature of the event is suggested by the abundance and variety of intricate shell and bone ornaments that were left behind (Inomata 1995, 1997; Inomata and Stiver 1998; Inomata 2006). The absence of diagnostic Terminal Classic ceramic types at Aguateca confirms that the site was abandoned prior to A.D. 830 (Foias 1993).

The sites of Tamarindito and Arroyo de Piedra were integral players in the Late Classic history of the region. The two sites share an emblem glyph and apparently were ruled by a single dynasty, for which at least nine rulers have been identified. The two sites were subjugated beneath the rule of Ruler 2 of Dos Pilas. This control may have been secured, in part, by a royal woman from Dos Pilas who married a ruler of Arroyo de Piedra and whose heirs also ruled Arroyo. Tamarindito may have been instrumental in ousting the dynasty from Dos Pilas—probably killing Ruler 4—and also appears to have outlasted elite authority at Aguateca (Houston 1993; Houston and Mathews 1985; Mathews and Willey 1991). The last reference to Tamarindito dates to A.D. 790 on Stela 7 at Aguateca (Houston and Mathews 1985; Mathews and Willey 1991), but occupation of both Arroyo and Tamarindito appears to have outlived that at Aguateca, although population at both seems to have declined rapidly at the same time. Only a few Terminal Classic sherds were found at Arroyo (Escobedo 1997), and two peripheral groups show Terminal Classic occupation at Tamarindito (Valdés 1997).

By contrast, the fortified peninsula of Punta de Chimino remained strong well into the Terminal Classic period. Because of the eroded nature of monuments at the site, its political connections are somewhat obscure, and it may have remained independent throughout its history. Ceramics from the site indicate a strong Preclassic and Protoclassic occupation (Faisan phase 200 B.C.–A.D. 250) but little evidence of Early Classic use. The bulk of the construction, including the fortifications, appear to date to the end of the Late Classic period and continued in use through the Terminal Classic Sepens phase (A.D. 830–950). An eroded hieroglyphic panel found in the ball court is tentatively dated on stylistic grounds by Houston to some time prior to A.D. 810 (Foias 1993; Inomata et al. 1989; Wolley and Wright 1990a; Demarest and Escobedo 1997a, 1997b).

Regional Considerations for the Collapse

Since the first intensive excavations in the region, the collapse of the Pasión region has often been attributed to external influences because of the appearance of new Fine Paste ceramic types in the later occupations of Altar and Seibal, and the distinctive style of sculpture in the later monuments at Seibal. On the basis of preliminary work at Seibal and the earlier Altar de Sacrificios excavations, Sabloff and Willey (1967) proposed that the Pasión drainage was invaded by a non-Maya, probably Central Mexican culture, that set up a base at Seibal from whence they conducted raiding parties throughout the central Petén. Thompson (1970) suggested that these invaders were the Putun or Chontal Maya, a group of seafaring traders who inhabited the Gulf Coast at the time of conquest. They brought about the collapse not directly but by proletariat revolt against the new leadership. Despite dispute over the ethnic implications of the stylistic elements cited by Thompson (Graham 1973) and by Graham (Stuart 1993), skepticism about projecting colonial ethnic distributions back 700 years (Adams 1973:157), and the identification of local clays from which the distinctive Terminal Classic vessels were manufactured (Rands et al. 1982), until very recently some authors continued to identify the Putun as a foreign influence in the Pasión (Ball and Taschek 1989; Kowalski 1989; Schele and Freidel 1990:385–6).

In an analysis of burial patterns, Tourtellot (1990) argued that the Bayal population at Seibal is distinguished by other characteristics indicating an ethnic change, and he cited an increase in physical stature, new norms of cranial deformation, the cessation of dental mutilation, and shifts in orientation, body position, and location of burials as evidence of a new ethnic influx. In a synthesis of work at Seibal, Willey (1990:265) found these coeval changes too great a coincidence to dismiss the invasion hypothesis, arguing that the arrival of outside influence served to invigorate and prolong elite authority at Seibal in the face of an endemic lowland collapse phenomenon. He described the foreign presences as "responses to calls for help from the indigenous Classic Maya populations of the Pasión Valley rather than as a first wave of subjugating invaders." As mentioned above, recent work shows that a Terminal Classic Seibal ruler came from the Maya site of Ucanal (Schele and Mathews 1998), a decipherment that refocuses attention on intersite interaction within the Maya realm.

This shift toward internal Maya politics occurs at a time when advances in hieroglyphic decipherment allow appreciation of political interactions with new detail. As reviewed above, hieroglyphic inscriptions indicate increasing militarism over the Late Classic period (Stuart 1993). In the Pasión region, this is seen in the expansive tendencies of the Dos Pilas/Aguateca dynasty toward the end of the eighth century. Walls around Dos Pilas and Aguateca, and the evidence for an abrupt, traumatic end to occupation at Aguateca suggest that this warfare had become endemic by the beginning of the ninth century and that it may have been the direct cause of the abandonment of some sites. While maintenance of a high level of militarism into the Terminal Classic period is indicated by the defensive system at Punta de Chimino and by iconography at Seibal, the origins of this trend are firmly rooted in Maya culture prior to the once-posited foreign invasion. For the Petexbatun subregion, Demarest (1992, 1996, 1997, 2006) has proposed that the escalation of interpolity competition was the proximate cause of the collapse. For the Petexbatun sites, it now seems that warfare led more directly to site abandonment, as described in the volumes of this series.

Although the collapse of the Pasión region has principally been addressed by social models of conflict, environmental factors are commonly integrated into these models, often as conditions that account for the ultimate abandonment of sites. For instance, Sabloff and Willey (1967) argued that foreign invasions put additional stress on agrosystems, thereby bringing about the collapse. Twenty years later, while less convinced of the exact nature of foreign influence, Willey (1990) continued to adhere to the idea that ecological stress was involved in the transition but argued that it was in some way mediated by social changes.

The extent to which ecological factors contribute to theories of collapse clearly is dependent on our understanding of prehistoric agrotechnology and the carrying capacity of the landscape. For instance, Sharer (1977) suggested that intersite competition for access to agricultural lands and labor may have been a factor in the rise of Pasión militarism and the consequent collapse. This idea is based on the assumption that intensive agricultural techniques were not employed in the Pasión and that the productive capacity of the land was taxed by high population density. In contrast, Adams (1983) argued that the elaboration of raised-field systems in the Pasión drainage (but see Dunning and Beach 1994) produced a surge of wealth from cash crops, such as cacao and cotton. Interpreting the Petexbatun emblem glyph as evidence for domination by Tikal, he suggested that withdrawal of Tikal's control over the region led to greater competition between Pasión sites. Thus, he saw the high environmental potential of the region as a factor inducing competition and contributing to a socially motivated collapse, rather than as a limiting factor on settlement.

In summary, while there is good evidence that interpolity conflict was directly implicated in the collapse, there has been little consensus about the role that environmental processes may have played—as instigators or consequences of competition—in the decline and abandonment of the Classic Maya sites in the Pasión drainage. The research described in this volume attempts to shed some light on this issue by exploring the nature of the Pasión human condition over time as seen in the diet, the health, and the social partitioning of resources.

Sampling Strategy

In this volume I use human remains from most prehistoric mortuary features recovered by excavations at surface sites in the Pasión region of the Department of Petén, Guatemala. Although statistical analysis is limited to sites that have produced more than 10 burials, smaller burial series are mentioned when they contribute to a broader understanding of patterning in the data. Although caves served as an important locus of mortuary ritual and a large volume of human skeletal material has been recovered from caves in the Petexbatun area, this material was excluded from the current study because the skeletons cannot be precisely dated or individuated due to the secondary nature of the deposits and mixing by frequent flooding (Brady et al. 1997). The total sample consists of some 313 individuals, interred in 267 graves at nine sites: Altar de Sacrificios, Seibal, Itzan, Dos Pilas, Aguateca, Tamarindito, Punta de Chimino, Arroyo de Piedra, and La Paciencia. The majority of the features date to the Late and Terminal Classic periods, but small samples from the Preclassic and Early Classic periods are also included to provide a greater chronological perspective to the resulting patterns. Sample sizes for each site and chronological period are presented in Table 2.1.

Different subsets of burials from this sample are considered for distinct aspects of the study. Burial preservation provides the grounds for inclusion of most individuals in each part of the research. A large proportion of burials from Altar de Sacrificios were recorded in the field but deemed to be too poorly preserved to recover, and were discarded ($n = 47$) (Saul 1972; Smith 1972). Hence, the skeletal material was not available for examination or consideration in demographic, pathological, or dietary analyses. Published descriptions of the contents of these graves and accompanying photographs provide some data (Smith 1972), which I used in mortuary analyses. At Dos Pilas, cremated human material found atop Temple P5-7 could not be securely individuated because of the tiny size of bone fragments and colluvial mixing, so are likewise excluded from most aspects of this study. Otherwise, all features were included in the study as preservation permitted.

Excavation Biases

The likelihood of sampling bias is greater in the case of the Maya—who buried their dead in dispersed locations—than in cultures that interred all members in easily identified corporate cemeteries, which are the usual subject of bioarchaeological

Table 2.1. Skeletal sample sizes by site and chronological period

Site	Chronological period	Number of skeletons excavated	Number of skeletons curated
Altar de Sacrificios	Preclassic	25	21
	Early Classic	28	16
	Late Classic	37	19
	Terminal Classic	47	36
Seibal	Preclassic	8	7
	Late Classic	18	15
	Terminal Classic	30	29
Itzan	Late Classic	14	14
Dos Pilas	Late Classic	39	37
	Terminal Classic	22	22
	*(cremation M.N.I.)	(7)	(7)
Aguateca	Late Classic	21	21
Tamarindito	Preclassic	1	1
	Late Classic	14	14
Arroyo de Piedra	Late Classic	5	5
Punta de Chimino	Late Classic	3	3
La Paciencia	Late Classic	1	1
Total, all sites	Preclassic	34	29
	Early Classic	28	16
	Late Classic	152	129
	Terminal Classic	99	87
Total	All periods	313	261

* Terminal Classic cremations from Dos Pilas are excluded from totals.

investigation. The majority of Maya burials appear to be placed in domestic contexts, below the floor of houses, as was observed ethnohistorically (Tozzer 1941), but burials also occur in monumental architecture and below plaza floors. Differences in excavation strategies between projects can result in burial assemblages of markedly different character.

Over the 50-year span in which the burials examined here have been excavated, archaeological field priorities have shifted in emphasis from the ceremonial core of sites toward domestic parameters and settlement systems. Most recently, this trend is being reinforced by strict regulation of architectural excavation in Guatemala. This shift is reflected in the burial assemblages: 64% of burials excavated during the early 1960s at Altar de Sacrificios were derived from ceremonial or public contexts, with only 36% from domestic contexts; at Seibal, excavated during the late 1960s, 40% came from ceremonial contexts and 60% from domestic contexts; and 93% of burials from Dos Pilas, excavated in the early 1990s, are from domestic contexts. Because burial location may be one indicator of social status, further examination of sampling differences may be helpful in evaluating the comparability of skeletal series between sites.

The bulk of Harvard University's excavations at Altar de Sacrificios were conducted in large temple platforms of Groups A and B (Smith 1972; Willey 1973). In Group A, the Late Classic focus of the site, excavations included intensive trenching and clearing of Strs. A-I and A-III, and more restricted testing of the ball court A-V and A-II. Most of these excavations were located on the building axes. The South Plaza of Group A, however, received little attention. In Group B, excavations were focused on the small temples B-I, B-II, and B-III, with little work on the two adjoining courtyards. Excavations below plazas were placed along the axes of major structures or below stelae and altars. The architectural context of Preclassic burials recovered in these plaza pits remains largely unknown. Test pits were placed in 40 house mounds. These domestic excavations generally consisted of one or two units placed in the top of mounds. An exception to this rule was Mound 2, a basal platform supporting two small structures, which was extensively trenched, recovering 18 burials. There was no excavation of exterior domestic space, so all domestic burials were recovered from below house floors.

Harvard's major architectural excavations at Seibal were restricted to relatively smaller structures than at Altar (Willey 1990; Willey et al. 1975). In Group A, excavations were restricted to the Terminal Classic Strs. A-3 and A-13, along with the ball court, A-19. The large, presumably Late Classic temples and ceremonial platforms were untouched, with the exception of some clearing atop Str. A-14. Deep tests below the plazas of Group A investigated Preclassic strata. Group D excavations focused on deep trenches in small palaces (Str. D-12, D-26) and low mounds (Str. D-30, D-12), with only summit clearing of a small temple (D-32). Group C excavations include a small ball court (C-9) and the round Str. 79. Complementing these core excavations was an intensive program of settlement excavations that tested residential architecture in the surrounding 15.25 km^2 (Tourtellot III 1988). Although the locations of all excavation units in the peripheral program are not published, tests were placed into the summit of mounds as well as exterior patio space.

At Dos Pilas, excavations have been largely restricted to domestic contexts and mounds less than 2 m in height. The exception has been the extensive trenching of temple L5-1 and summit clearing atop temples P5-7 and L4-79. Only four burial features have come from these large structures. Domestic excavations have generally employed a probabilistic strategy that targets both subfloor and exterior space, within and beyond the patio group (Palka 1995). Structures have been selected for excavation from the central 1.5 km^2 of the site that was mapped (Houston 1987).

At Aguateca, excavation has also been limited to low structures. These have been selected to provide a sample from the various zones within the site, as defined by the concentric system of defensive walls. These excavations are spread across the central 2 km^2 area of the site that has been mapped. Burials have been recovered from excavations within domestic structures and their immediate exterior space (Inomata 1995). Because bedrock is reached about 10 cm below the present ground surface, it is unlikely that many burials would have been interred away from architecture. A subset of burials excavated from the site of Quim Chi Hilan, which is located on the escarpment edge 1.7 km north of the Aguateca site center, are also considered here. This "suburban" community can be considered part of Aguateca because of its relationship to the defensive walls that emanate from the latter center (Killion et al. 1991).

At Itzan, excavations have focused on invisible structures and small mounds damaged by road construction activities approximately 4.5 km south of the site center. A single burial was recovered from a *sacbe* or causeway, which represents the only nondomestic architecture sampled. Adjacent to the road cuts, excavations have stripped large areas of exterior space and trenched residential structures (Johnston 1994).

At Tamarindito, excavations were carried out in domestic groups at varying distances from the site center, as well as in elite palace structures (Valdés 1997). At Arroyo de Piedra, most of the excavations have been focused around the main plaza, below which some burials were found. Others are from domestic contexts nearby (Escobedo 1997). The single burial from La Paciencia is from beneath the main plaza, while the three burials from Punta de Chimino were uncovered during test-pitting operations.

In sum, the mortuary sample from each site represents a somewhat different subset of the prehistoric population. The sample from Altar contains a high proportion of burials placed in monumental architecture and lacks domestic burials from exterior space. The Preclassic samples from

Altar and Seibal are comparable in terms of context, deriving largely from monumental and subplaza contexts. Late Classic samples at all sites except Altar are predominantly of domestic origin. At Seibal, Dos Pilas, Tamarindito, and Aguateca, these domestic burials are broadly stratified across space and a variety of domestic architectural forms. The sample from Itzan is more homogeneous and best characterized as a semi-rural community. Terminal Classic series from Altar and Seibal contain similar proportions of domestic and architectural burials, but the Dos Pilas occupation at this time produced a small sample from a single domestic group.

Chronological Framework

Ceramicists have divided the long span of Pasión occupational history into phases that correspond to changes in the production and distribution of ceramic types (Figure 2.1) and correlate with shifts in the organization and success of prehistoric polities (Adams 1971; Foias 1996; Sabloff 1975). Often, these phases represent a very short time-depth, of a single century or less. Ideally, it would be best to examine mortuary, diet, and health trends using these narrow time spans as the unit of analysis, in order to gain a detailed understanding of the specific nature of bioarchaeological changes over Pasión prehistory. For the purpose of the present research, however, it is necessary to group the phases into rather longer time spans, to obtain samples of a useful size. Here, Pasión history is lumped into three broad phases: the Preclassic/Early Classic period, the Late Classic period, and the Terminal Classic period.

The earliest period spans the greatest time-depth, from approximately 900 B.C. to A.D. 600. Only burials from Altar de Sacrificios and Seibal contribute to this sample. For Altar, burials from the Xe, San Felix, and Plancha phases (900 B.C.–A.D. 150) were considered as Preclassic. Similarly, Seibal burials from the Escoba and Cantutse phases (600 B.C.–A.D. 300) were treated together. This is a long period that was characterized by dramatic evolution of social complexity but cannot be further subdivided due to the small number of burials. In fact, only a single burial dates from the earliest part of the occupation (Altar Burial 135); most postdate 600 B.C. Early Classic burials from the Salinas, Ayn, and Veremos phases (A.D.150–600) at Altar were grouped with the Preclassic burials for paleopathological analyses due to their very small numbers. At Altar, the Early Classic occupation seems to arise directly from the preceding occupation and may represent neither a substantial increase in population nor a shift in land use practices, which would have the greatest bearing on disease processes. In contrast to Seibal, which was minimally unoccupied during the Early Classic, Altar seems to have successfully managed the transition from the Preclassic. The pathological data from the Early Classic skeletons (only Altar) are from too small a sample to merit much attention on their own, so grouping these data with the Preclassic data seemed a better solution than either omitting them or grouping them with the Late Classic period, which saw much greater changes in social stratification, population density, and interpolity interaction. However, the Early Classic was considered separately from the Preclassic for mortuary, demographic, and dietary analyses, allowing some consideration of the processes affecting this occupation in its own right.

At each site, the Late Classic can be fairly easily defined as beginning around A.D. 600. However, the end of the period is somewhat more difficult to pinpoint. Both Sabloff (1975) and Foias (1996) place the end of the Late Classic period at A.D. 830, with the onset of the Terminal Classic heralded by the appearance of Tres Naciones and Altar fine paste ceramics in the Bayal phase at Seibal and the Sepens phase in the Petexbatun area. These ceramic changes are well correlated with political shifts documented epigraphically. Here, I follow the same division. In the Petexbatun, a small sample of burials from the Sepens phase are available only from Dos Pilas; the bulk of burials date squarely to the Late Classic Nacimiento phase (early facet). For Seibal, only burials identified as Bayal were treated as Terminal Classic. Tepejilote and transitional burials were assigned to the Late Classic horizon. The entire burial sample from Itzan dates to the Late Classic period.

For Altar de Sacrificios the chronology is more complex. Adams defined the Boca phase as spanning the years from A.D. 771–900 and subdivided it into early and late facets (Adams 1971, 1973b). The ceramic assemblage of the late facet contains some Fine Orange wares that Adams attributed to early trade pieces. He argued that the succeeding Jimba phase almost exclusively contained fine wares. Sabloff (1973:121) has argued that this separation is artificial since Adams (1971:106) admits his inability to isolate a pure Jimba deposit at Altar. Instead, Sabloff would consider the late-facet Boca and Jimba together, as functional distinctions within a single phase assemblage, as seen in the Bayal ceramics of Seibal. Here, I follow this interpretation, so that the chronological division between Late and Terminal Classic periods at Altar can be brought in line with the other sites. Burials from the Pasión and early facet of the Boca phase are considered as Late Classic in date. Only five burials designated as Boca phase can be attributed to the late facet because of the presence of Fine Orange ceramics or other diagnostic late facet modes, and these I lump with burials designated as Boca/Jimba or Jimba in the Terminal Classic period.

CHAPTER 3

Demographic Framework

Introduction

At the base of any analysis of burial remains is the need for accurate identification of the skeletal material contained in the graves. Demographic characteristics must be known in order to consider mortuary patterning across age and sex categories, and to provide demographic control for intersample comparison of disease loads and dietary consumption. Furthermore, the demographic structure of a skeletal series itself provides an indication of the processes affecting a population. The age distribution of deaths in a population is largely shaped by fertility rate (Johansson and Horowitz 1986; Sattenspiel and Harpending 1983). Because acute malnutrition is correlated with low fertility in modern populations (Bongaarts and Delgado 1977; Spielmann 1989), the possible effects of changing subsistence practices and infection rates on fertility are relevant to the Maya collapse. Furthermore, changes in fertility appear to have played a key role in other demographic transitions (Buikstra et al. 1986; Johansson and Horowitz 1986). Mortality and cultural factors such as migration or social patterns of interment also influence the resultant distribution, so paleodemographic analysis requires careful consideration of processes potentially affecting the population under study.

Methodology

The estimation of age-at-death and sex from skeletal remains provides a greater challenge to the Maya osteologist than to those working in less humid areas. The suboptimal preservation of Maya skeletal materials hinders the application of many osteological techniques that involve observation of delicate skeletal structures and requires a diverse strategy for data collection.

A secure estimate of sex was possible for 30% of the adult skeletons using the sexually dimorphic form of the cranium and pelvis (Bass 1987; Buikstra and Ubelaker 1994; Steele and Bramblett 1988). In diagnosing sex from the cranium, I emphasized the form of the mastoid process, supraorbital ridges, and nuchal lines, but also considered the mental area and gonial angles of the mandible when present. Pelvic remains were generally poorly preserved but examined to assess the breadth of the sciatic notch, form of the preauricular area, and pubic shape (Phenice 1969).

In order to evaluate the sex of more fragmentary skeletons, I developed a series of discriminant functions using a combination of skeletal and dental measurements (Ditch and Rose 1972; Giles 1964; Giles 1970; van Vark and Schaafsma 1992). I recorded a set of 31 measurements from all adult skeletons as preservation permitted and collected buccolingual crown measurements for all available teeth. I considered skeletons that could be visually sexed using cranial and pelvic features to be of known sex and used these to define discriminant functions for application to more fragmentary remains. For skeletal measurements, data from the left and right sides of the body were averaged, to minimize the effects of activity-related asymmetrical robusticity (Ruff 1992; Ruff and Hayes 1983). For dental measurements, preferential use of the left antimere simplified the data manipulations, since dental asymmetry is random and fluctuating (Noss et al. 1983). From the skeletal measurements collected, I used only those for which a significant difference was detected between males and females of "known" sex (1-tail t-test, $p < 0.01$) and for which the number of measurable sexed skeletons was greater than ten. The 22 skeletal measurements considered for use are defined in Appendix A.

Discriminant functions were calculated with SPSS/PC+, using the stepwise procedure that minimizes Wilks' Lambda as the variable selection rule (Norusis 1988). Because of the large number of missing values, a number of functions had to be calculated using different combinations of variables in order to estimate sex for as many skeletons as possible. The 23 skeletal and 7 dental discriminant functions used are presented in Table 3.1, ranked in order of quality by eigenvalue and canonical correlation (Norusis 1988; Tatsuoka 1971). Each of the skeletal functions was associated with a value of chi-square that was significant at the 0.0005 level of confidence. The dental functions performed less well, but were accepted with a value of chi-square that was significant at $p < 0.05$. A much larger number of functions were calculated than are listed in Table 3.1, but many were rejected as inadequate. The classification of each unsexed skeleton by a given function was accepted only when the posterior probability, $P(G_i/D)$, of that case was greater than 0.70. In most instances, a skeleton was classified to the same sex using several functions. A few conflicting classifications were resolved by selecting the result with the higher posterior probability (Tatsuoka 1971) in consideration with the relative rank of the function (Table 3.1).

I estimated age-at-death using a variety of skeletal markers of development and degeneration. For the majority of subadults, I estimated age from the state of dental development and eruption, following the standards of Ubelaker (1978) for North American Indians, which are similar to eruption patterns in the Maya (Steggerda and Hill 1942). For those few subadult skeletons from which teeth were not recovered, the state of epiphyseal fusion and skeletal maturation (MacKay n.d.; Steele and Bramblett 1988) were used to estimate age-at-death.

For adults, I used a variety of techniques according to the preservation of useful skeletal structures. Pubic symphyseal morphology was examined using the Suchey-Brooks system casts (Katz and Suchey 1986; Suchey et al. 1988; Suchey et al. 1979), but is available for observation in only ten individuals. I scored the closure of ectocranial sutures according to the system of Meindl and Lovejoy (1985). Generally, the vault sutures were employed, owing to the absence of several lateral-anterior sites. Three seriations of auricular surface morphology (Lovejoy et al. 1985) were constructed using iliac bones from the Petexbatun, Altar de Sacrificios, and Seibal skeletal samples. Black and white photographs of the specimens were then used to link the independent series into a single seriation of 43 individuals.

In addition to the macroscopic techniques described above, I selected first mandibular premolar roots from 21 individuals from Dos Pilas for cemental annulation age estimation (Charles et al. 1986; Condon et al. 1986). The roots were decalcified in 10% formic acid and 5% formaldehyde, embedded in Paraplast Plus, sectioned to 7 μm, affixed to slides, and stained with Toluidine blue O stain. Areas of cementum showing clear annuli were photographed at 132X using Kodak Technical Pan film, and annuli counted from the negatives projected as slides. Age-at-death was calculated by adding the mean annulus count for two observers to 10.5 years, the approximate age of eruption of the tooth (Demirjian and Levesque 1980; Steggerda and Hill 1942). Further details of the methods of specimen preparation can be found in Wright (1989). Unfortunately, only nine premolars produced suitable areas for photomicrography, because of poor preservation of the cementum.

Approximately 44.6% of the adult skeletons could be aged using the above techniques, leaving a large number of skeletons aged only as "adult." Accordingly, these individuals were aged by their position in a seriation of dental attrition relative to the more accurately aged individuals. I graphically recorded the extent of dental attrition—enamel facets, exposed dentine, and pulp cavities—on a standardized drawing for each skeleton. The drawings were then seriated in order of increasing attrition. I divided the attrition series into four age groups according to the distribution of skeletons for which age had been estimated by other crite-

Table 3.1. Skeletal and dental discriminant functions used in sex estimation

DF	Variables included	Number of males	Number of females	Percent correct	Eigenvalue	Canonical correlation
1	timaxap, tinfcir, timincir	16	11	96.30	4.3632	.9020
2	timaxap, tinfcirc	17	12	96.55	4.0709	.8960
3	humincir, tibmaxap, femidapw	16	13	96.55	3.9375	.8930
4	ulmaxcr, radcirc	21	15	100.00	3.0161	.8666
5	humincir, tibmaxap	16	14	96.67	3.5701	.8838
6	femaxhead	12	13	96.00	3.3766	.8784
7	ulmaxcr, femidcir	17	17	94.12	2.7964	.8583
8	timaxap	19	15	94.12	2.5407	.8471
9	mastoid, humincir	16	15	93.55	2.2485	.8320
10	timincir	20	16	88.88	2.0637	.8207
11	mastoid, femidcir	18	15	93.94	2.0066	.8169
12	ulmaxcr	23	17	90.00	1.7023	.7937
13	humincir, huminsh	22	21	88.37	1.7439	.7972
14	humincir	24	23	89.36	1.6112	.7855
15	huminsh	26	22	87.50	1.4690	.7713
16	mastoid	25	16	87.80	1.1852	.7365
17	clavcirc	14	12	84.62	1.1845	.7364
18	mastoid, mandboht	17	10	85.19	1.1388	.7297
19	femidapw, femidcir	25	23	85.42	1.1287	.7282
20	femidapw	26	22	84.00	0.9997	.7071
21	radcir	23	20	86.05	0.9166	.6915
22	femidcir	25	23	83.33	1.0011	.7073
23	mandboht	25	11	77.78	0.4351	.5506
24	UI1, UP3, UC	23	13	79.49	0.6098	.6155
25	UC, UP3	37	12	70.37	0.3069	.4846
26	UI2, UC	28	14	69.05	0.3040	.4828
27	UM1, UC	29	10	75.00	0.2826	.4694
28	LP3, LM1	28	12	62.75	0.1731	.3842
29	UC	43	17	68.33	0.1495	.3606
30	LC	35	18	56.60	0.0814	.2743

The following are indicated: the variables included in the function, the number of males and females of "known" sex on which the function is based, the percent of "known" sex skeletons correctly classified, and the eigenvalue and canonical correlation of each function.

ria. Age categories were defined as follows: infant, 0–5 years; child, 6–11 years; teenage, 12–19 years; young adult, 20–34 years; middle adult, 35–50 years; old adult, >50 years. Finer subdivision of the adult age is not feasible given the small number of independently aged skeletons and the nature of attrition.

To investigate the implications of the resulting demographic data, the age distributions are plotted as histograms for each site and chronological period, using the age categories defined above. Adults that could not be assigned to a specific age class are treated as a separate category rather than arbitrarily apportioning them among the adult age classes as is commonly done in paleodemography. The latter approach does not contribute any new information to the age distribution but may obscure real patterning, as the unaged skeletons may not derive evenly from the different age classes. The Terminal Classic samples from Seibal and Dos Pilas (Figures 3.1 and 3.2) are dominated by skeletons from a single unusual deposit each. Seibal Burial 4 contained at least 11 disarticulated individuals. The published burial description gives few details (Tourtellot III 1990:90–1), but burning and breakage of some bones suggests some unusual perimortem processing of the bodies. In another unusual deposit, 16 decapitated crania were recovered from the patio midden of Group L4-3 at Dos Pilas. Accordingly, the contribution of these contexts to the sample profiles is indicated by distinctive shading.

I visually compare the death profiles to distributions adjusted to the same age categories for skeletal series from Copan; Teotihuacan; the Libben Site, Ohio; and modern data for the Yanomamo and Guatemala (Milner et al. 1989) (Figure 3.3). The age-at-death distribution for the Late Classic population from Copan, Honduras, was generated from Table 4.6 in Whittington (1989). The distribution for the Late period (A.D. 550–700) burial population from the Tlajinga 33 compound from Teotihuacan, Mexico, was compiled from Table 8 of Storey (1985). For the Libben Site, Ohio, the distribution of deaths was reconstructed from the abridged life table for that site (Lovejoy et al. 1977). A distribution with high fertility and mortality similar to that of the modern Yanomamo was generated using the Coale and Demeny (Coale and Demeny 1983) Model West tables, with a gross reproductive rate of 3.0 and life expectancy at birth of 20 years. An estimate of modern, preantibiotic Guatemalan deaths was derived from the d_x values of a life table calculated by Arriaga (1968) from 1893 census data. The 1893 census data was chosen over more recent data, which show a dramatic increase in life expectancy due to the demographic transition (Chackiel et al. 1985; Early 1982). Given the small size of the Pasión samples, a cautious approach is required for interpretation of the death profiles.

Results

Table 3.2 lists the sex ratio statistics of the samples. Age-at-death distributions of the 223 skeletons examined are presented in Figures 3.1 and 3.2 for each of the sites and time periods represented. Detailed age and sex data for each skeleton are in Appendix B.

The Pasión samples show a consistent bias toward greater representation by male skeletons (Tables 3.1 and 3.2). Weiss (1972) observed that this is a common characteristic of skeletal samples and attributed it to a bias in skeletal sexing techniques. Yet, males are less accurately sexed than are females, on the basis of both the cranium and pelvis in well-preserved material (Meindl et al. 1985a). The accuracy and bias of sexing techniques could be very different, though, in fragmentary remains. However, a significant proportion of Pasión skeletons could not be sexed.

This proportion is greatest for the samples from Altar de Sacrificios and may reflect either the poor preservation or spotty collection of skeletal elements from that site. Differential preservation of robust male skeletons might also contribute to the bias. If predominantly female, the indeterminate skeletons are sufficiently abundant to correct for this bias in most samples.

It is possible that this male sex bias is partly real. Nations (1979a) documented biased child sex ratios in modern Lacandon Maya villages. He argued that child spacing is optimized by infanticide and neglect of children of the unpreferred sex, resulting in unbalanced sex ratios. For the Lacandon, the direction of this bias is keyed to postmarital residence patterns, in that male children are preferred in patrilocal villages while female children are preferred in matrilocal villages. If the Classic Maya operated largely under a predominantly patrilocal system (Haviland 1970a), an analogous pattern of child preference might account for the overabundance of adult male skeletons. Postmarital residence patterns might also affect choice of burial location between the sexes and contribute to sampling bias.

In addition to the total sex bias, the age distribution of sexed skeletons is illustrated in Figures 3.1 and 3.2. In the samples from Late Classic

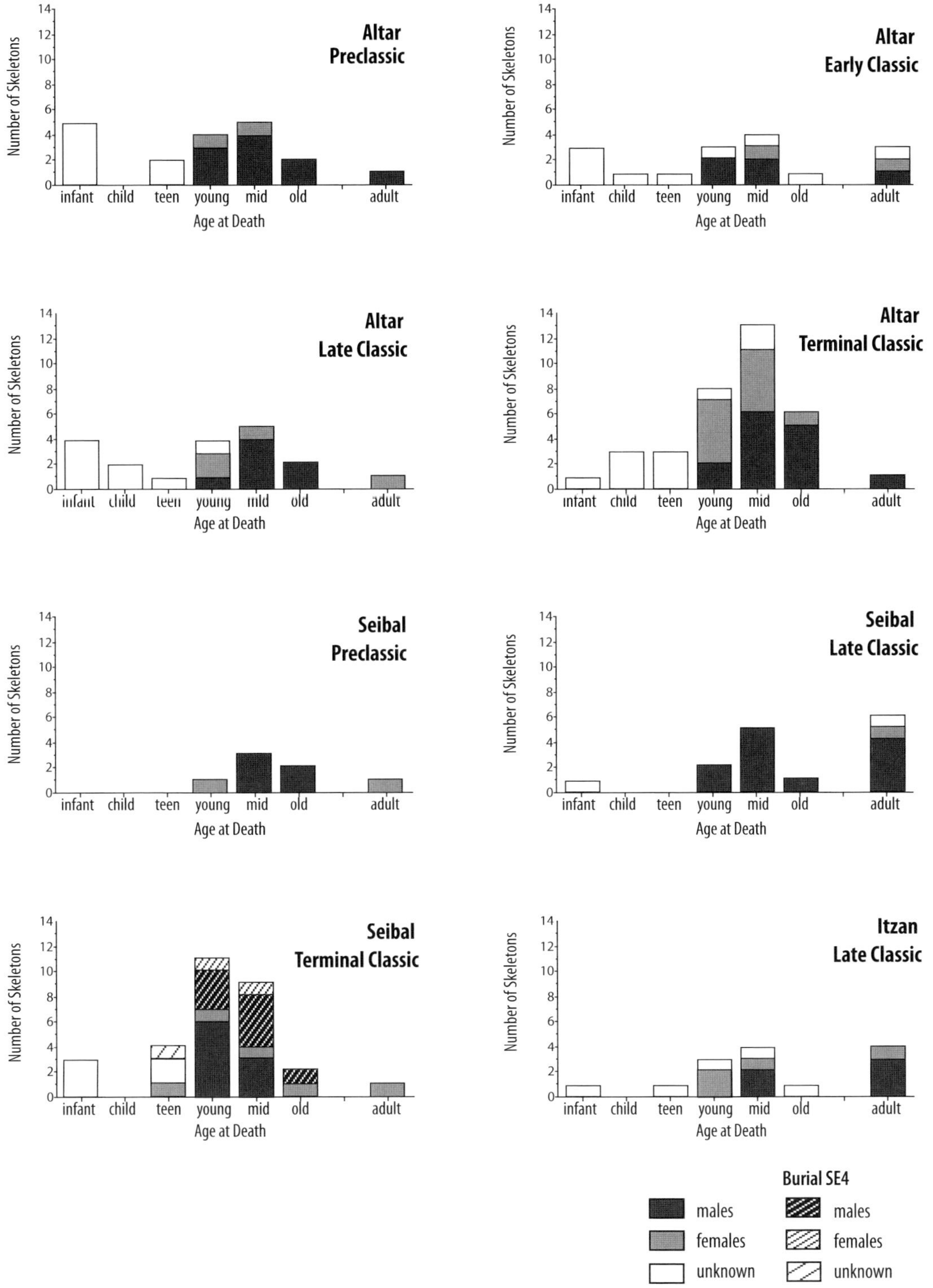

Figure 3.1. Death profiles for skeletal samples from Altar de Sacrificios, Seibal, and Itzán, by chronological period

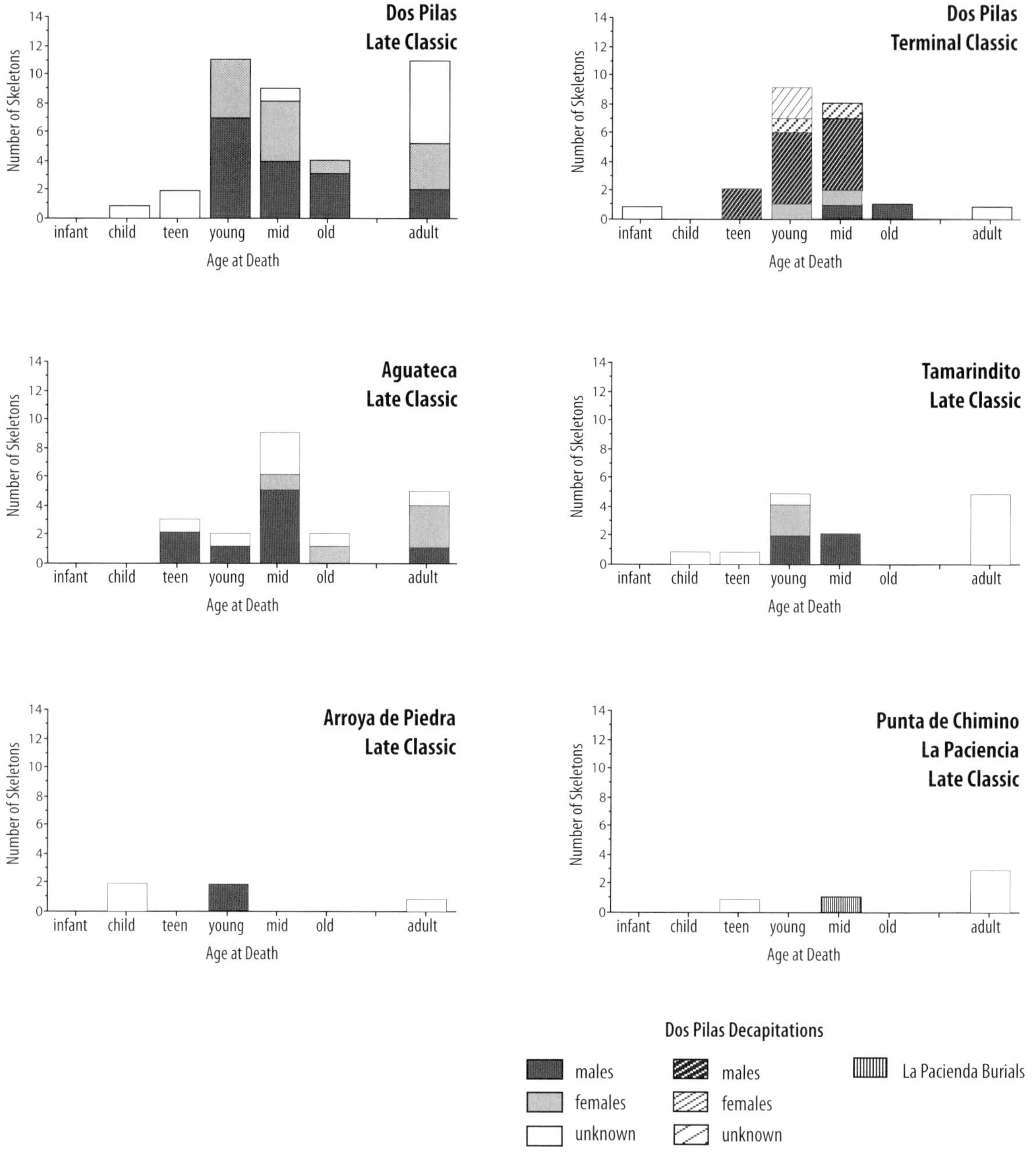

Figure 3.2. Death profiles for skeletal samples from Petexbatun Regional Archaeological Project excavations at Dos Pilas, Aguateca, Tamarindito, Arroyo de Piedra, and Punta de Chimino, by chronological period

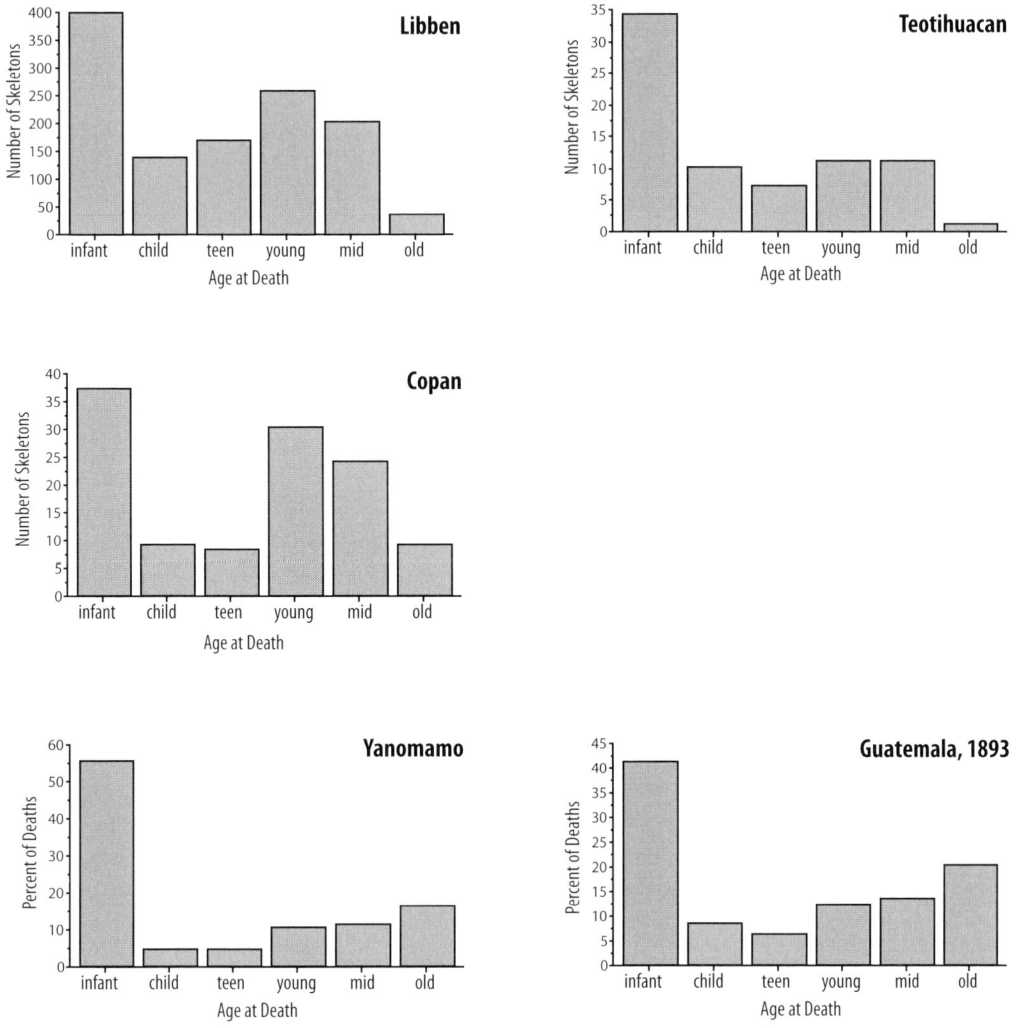

Figure 3.3. Death profiles for comparative series from the Libben Site, Teotihuacan, Copan, a simulated Yanomamo profile, and the 1893 Guatemalan census

Altar, Itzan, Dos Pilas, and Terminal Classic Altar, females account for a sizeable proportion of younger adult deaths, but males dominate among older deaths. Although it is tempting to interpret this in terms of younger mortality of childbearing females, it might also be an artifact of the increasing robusticity of the female cranium with age (Meindl et al. 1985a). This might lead to the misclassification of some older females as males, as cranial estimates provide the bulk of morphological sex assessments.

The sex ratio is highest in samples from the Preclassic and Terminal Classic periods and from Seibal. In the Preclassic period, a male bias could reflect the differential placement of male burials and an emphasis on axial excavation of monumental architecture to reach hidden Preclassic structures. The effect of mortuary bias is clearly shown in the Terminal Classic samples from Seibal and Dos Pilas, where a single unusual deposit at each site with a high sex ratio—Seibal Burial 4 and the decapitations from Dos Pilas Group L4-3—contributes excessively to the male bias of the total sample (Table 3.2). Interestingly, Seibal consistently shows a high ratio in all periods. The possibility that skeletons in the Seibal population

Table 3.2. Adult sex ratios in Pasión skeletal samples

Site	Period	Number of males	Number of females	Number of adults	Sex Ratio (M/F)
Altar	Preclassic	10	3	8	3.3
Altar	Early Classic	5	3	8	1.7
Altar	Late Classic	7	4	8	1.8
Altar	Terminal Classic	14	11	10	1.3
Seibal	Preclassic	5	2	0	2.5
Seibal	Late Classic	12	1	2	12.0
Seibal	Terminal Classic/all	17	7	5	2.4
Seibal	Terminal/Burial 4	8	2	1	4.4
Seibal	Terminal/Burial 4 excluded	9	5	0	1.8
Dos Pilas	Late Classic	16	12	7	1.3
Dos Pilas	Terminal Classic/all	14	4	4	3.5
Dos Pilas	Terminal/decapitations	12	2	2	6.0
Dos Pilas	Terminal/decapitations excluded	2	2	1	1.0
Aguateca	Late Classic	7	5	6	1.4
Tamarindito	Late Classsic	4	2	6	2.0
Itzan	Late Classic	5	4	3	1.2

have been misclassified as male because of a larger body size can be rejected because t-tests comparing skeletal dimensions between Seibal and the other sites are nonsignificant ($p > 0.05$) for all measures except maximum femoral head diameter ($t = 2.87$, d.f. = 34, $p = 0.007$), which was not used in isolation to sex any Seibal skeletons and is a particularly dimorphic measure. The predominance of males at Seibal is probably due to a combination of mortuary and excavation biases.

Turning to age-at-death, the most obvious characteristic of each sample is the virtual absence of skeletons in the infant and child age classes, unlike the two modern distributions. Infant underenumeration is a common characteristic of prehistoric skeletal series, which was recognized by early paleodemographers (Angel 1969; Moore et al. 1975; Weiss 1973). The delicate bones of small children suffer greater damage by soil microorganisms and postinterment processes that lead to bone decay than do durable adult bones (Gordon and Buikstra 1981). Often only enamel caps of subadult teeth may remain.

Infant underenumeration is more severe in the Pasión series than at either Copan or Teotihuacan (Figure 3.3). The latter sites are located in more arid environments than the southwestern Petén, which may account for this difference. However, archaeological recovery may also be a factor. Fill deposits were not screened in all Pasión excavations, so infant burials reduced to dental fragments might not have been identified if not signaled by accompanying mortuary features such as grave walls or artifacts. At Copan, some fill deposits were regularly screened, which may contribute to the higher infant recovery success (Storey 1992a). Within the Pasión series, the greater abundance of infants from Altar de Sacrificios might be accounted for by soil and hydrological differences between this locality and the other Pasión sites. Ceremonial construction at Altar includes the use of sandstone and *almeja* clam mortar (Smith 1972), which are absent from the other sites. Furthermore, the location of the site on the floodplain of the Pasión River may provide more consistent soil humidity than at the better-drained sites.

Differential mortuary practices are probably also a significant factor in the low recovery of subadult remains. Young children may have been afforded a funerary treatment that is archaeologically invisible and excludes them from the skeletal sample. Infants might have been buried away from domestic groups and monumental architecture, where the majority of adult remains are encountered, or their corpses treated in some other manner that did not facilitate preservation. Investigations of cave deposits in the Petexbatun region indicate that children are a large component of skeletal remains in caves (Brady et al. 1991; Brady et al. 1997), but these are generally older children and adolescents and cannot account entirely for the paucity of infants and younger children at surface sites. The likelihood of sampling error is greater in the case of the Maya—whose funerary practices distributed burials across a variety of architectural forms and locations—than in cultures that interred all members in easily identified corporate cemeteries, which are the usual subject of paleodemographic investigation.

Differential mortuary behavior is less compelling as an explanation for the unusual patterning in adult age-at-death distributions, though it cannot be discounted. In all Pasión samples the old adult age class is consistently small, but should be the largest according to modern demographic analogy. In the samples from Early Classic Altar and from Late Classic Itzan, Seibal, and Dos Pilas, the paucity of old adults might be hidden in the large number of adults that could not be assigned to an age class. Old adults who suffered severe antemortem tooth loss could not be aged by attrition seriation and may contribute disproportionately to the "adult" class. Yet, the elderly are also underrepresented in samples with few unaged adults.

Many aging techniques tend to underage the skeleton, particularly in the older age ranges, a bias that could be responsible for the rarity of elderly skeletons that occurs in some skeletal distributions (Acsadi and Nemeskeri 1970; Jackes 1992). Of the techniques used to age the Pasión series, a negative bias, or tendency to underage, has been reported for the pubic symphysis (Meindl et al. 1985b), auricular surface (Lovejoy et al., 1985), and dental attrition (Molleson and Cohen 1990). However, some skeletal populations show a realistically large elderly class (e.g., the Oneota series of Milner et al. [1989]), suggesting that the magnitude of this bias cannot fully account for the pattern. Preservation biases against elderly skeletons who had suffered from osteoporosis is also possible, but it is most likely in the case of Altar de Sacrificios where a large number of poorly preserved skeletons were not collected (Saul 1972). Poor preservation is an unlikely explanation for underenumeration of adults because virtually all adult burials are accompanied by mortuary features that permit the identification of a grave even in a few instances of complete skeletal decay.

This pattern is also seen in the skeletal series from Copan, Teotihuacan, and the Libben Site (Figure 3.3). Despite its large size, the Libben series has been criticized as demographically unrealistic. The Libben life table implies an implausible age structure in the living population, with only two generations living at a given time and a high rate of orphanage (Howell 1982). For Teotihuacan, Storey (1985) argues that the paucity of older skeletons is due to high mortality in the stressful urban environment. For Copan, Whittington (1989) suggests that the population might not be stable; hence, the distribution of deaths could have little correspondence to the living population.

The application of demographic techniques to interpret the vital characteristics of a skeletal sample relies on the assumption that the population is at least stable (of constant growth rate) if not stationary (of constant size). For archaeological assemblages this assumption is often justified by the assertion that stability is approached in cemetery samples that span several generations (Sattenspiel and Harpending 1983; Weiss 1973). In addition to stability, demographic closure is necessary for a death profile to reflect vital rates. That is, all members of the population must die within their natal population. Substantial nonreciprocal migration could mask the pattern of internal demography in a death sample (Weiss 1973:10). Finally, heterogeneity of vital rates between subgroups of a single population (e.g., social classes) may confound the nature of the overall series (Vaupel and Yashin 1985; Wood et al. 1992). This is particularly relevant to comparisons between series in which sampling differences may be large.

In the case of Copan, the sample spans chronological horizons for which a constant rate of growth cannot be assumed. Survival analysis of temporally restricted subsamples indicates lower fertility rates during the Coner phase than in the earlier Acbi phase (Whittington 1989, 1991). This chronological heterogeneity in the larger sample may mean that the resulting profile indicates little about the population in general. The assumption of closure may also be violated in the archaeological populations considered here. At both Teotihuacan and Copan the late period fertility is insufficient to account for the growth documented archaeologically, and immigration from the surrounding areas has been proposed (Storey 1985; Whittington 1991).

Although the small size of the Pasión skeletal samples limits their interpretive value, they consistently resemble the three archaeological series and differ from the modern distributions. This probably indicates that they derive from nonstable, open, and/or extremely heterogeneous populations. Reconstructions of Pasión population history indicate alternating periods of growth—Preclassic and Late Classic—and decline—Early and Terminal Classic—but stability cannot be assumed over the duration of each period. In addition, site populations were probably not closed. Dos Pilas was perhaps settled by elites from the central Petén (Houston and Matthews 1985) but may have drawn the bulk of its population from other local sites, as is suggested by architectural styles (Valdés and Suasnávar 1991). It was largely abandoned near A.D. 760, and most of its populace presumably fled to Aguateca. Similarly, the growth of Seibal during the Terminal Classic period appears to be the result of immigration (Willey 1990), perhaps largely from the Petexbatun region (Demarest 1997:220; Demarest and Escobedo 1998; Demarest 2006). Moreover, sampling differences between sites may also have introduced heterogeneity of status.

In spite of these caveats, two patterns are apparent in the distributions of Pasión deaths. In the majority of samples the middle adult class is represented by the greatest number of skeletons. However, in the Late Classic samples from Dos Pilas and Altar and the Terminal Classic sample from Seibal, young adults predominate. These three samples represent the last periods of fluorescence at their respective sites, which appear to have been accompanied by increased militarism.

Milner et al. (1989) have illustrated that victims of violent deaths contribute differentially to a peak in young adults in prehistoric Oneota deaths, which otherwise match a Yanomamo-like distribution. This pattern is not exactly replicated in the Terminal Classic Dos Pilas and Seibal samples where the occupants of unusual mortuary features, who may be interpreted as victims of violence, are not disproportionately young adults. Yet, the possibility that war casualties were returned to their home site for domestic burial cannot be excluded.

Unfortunately, the extent to which instability, migration, warfare, archaeological sampling, and small sample size are responsible for the structure of Pasión sex ratios and death distributions cannot be evaluated from these data alone. In view of these problems, it does not seem wise to interpret the data in terms of fertility differentials. Age-specific morbidity as revealed through paleopathological analysis may provide some clues to the nature of Pasión mortality.

CHAPTER 4
Social Dimensions of Pasión Burial Ritual

Mortuary practices have been a recurrent focus of archaeological studies aimed at reconstructing the nature of ancient social systems throughout the world (Brown 1971b; Carr 1995; Chapman et al. 1981; Morris 1992; O'Shea 1984; O'Shea 1996; Pearson 1999; Tainter 1978). Despite early demonstration of the value of mortuary data for social reconstruction (Rathje 1970, 1973), burial data have seldom been studied systematically in the Maya area, and a coherent approach to the implications of Maya funeral practices is lacking (Becker 1988:117; Coggins 1988:64). Here, I use mortuary data to characterize status distinctions that might bear upon social patterns of dietary consumption among subpopulations of the prehistoric Pasión region. I take a fundamentally processual perspective in terms of analytic methodology, but my interpretation benefits by evaluation of the results in a historical context of Maya mortuary symbolism and death ritual as perceived through ethnohistoric, epigraphic, and iconographic studies.

Mortuary Analysis and Social Structure

Archaeological mortuary theory is grounded in the premise that the principles governing ancient social structure are captured in archaeologically recoverable remnants of funeral rituals. This view is based on early anthropological conceptions of the funeral as a collective representation of death (Hertz 1907) and a rite of passage (Van Gennep 1909). Early proponents of the processual school argued that mortuary features constituted a direct representation of the structure of the societies that produced them. Borrowing Goodenough's (1965) concept of the social persona, Saxe (1970) and Binford (1971) viewed burial attributes as symbols of social identities or roles that together constitute the social persona of an individual and are deemed appropriate for expression in funeral ritual. The proposition that the structure of the society is represented by the manner in which attribute sets covary across the disposal domain was tested and generally supported by ethnographic data from a range of societies (Binford 1971; Saxe 1970). Societies composed of more formally structured roles (greater complexity) were found to produce a more highly structured mortuary domain, characterized by a high redundancy of attribute sets (Brown 1971a; Saxe 1970).

Vertical social distinctions have been identified on the basis of two principles: the identification of rank differences in energy expenditure and the differential distribution of symbols of authority. Tainter (1975, 1978) hypothesized that the breadth of social roles recognized in mortuary ritual (i.e., vertical distinctions) is reflected in the amount of energy expended in the funeral. This energy expenditure might be played out in the size (labor cost) of the interment facility or in the duration and complexity of funeral rituals. In contrast, Peebles and Kus (1977) suggest that a superordinate (vertical) dimension is signified by symbols of social office. Braun (1979) has operationalized this idea by examining the covariation of grave goods in relation to their appearance in refuse deposits. This approach has been implicit in the examination of long-distance trade goods as status markers in prehistoric Europe (Champion 1982; Shennan 1982a, 1982b).

The use of broad ethnographic generalizations for the interpretation of prehistoric social structure has been attacked by postprocessual archaeologists arguing for a contextual interpretation of mortuary remains (Hodder 1982, 1989; Shanks and Tilley 1982). In essence, these critiques focus on the undeniable fact that mortuary rituals are enacted by living members of a society, not by the deceased (Bloch 1977:286; Goody 1962:29; Hodder 1982; Lévi-Strauss 1976:320; Ucko 1969). Although some processual studies recognize this fact (e.g., Braun 1979:68), the structural principles of the mortuary domains are often taken as faithfully representing those of the society at large. Instead, death presents an opportunity to rewrite the social role of the deceased. Mortuary ritual may be employed to manipulate the perception of social structure or to reaffirm a dominant elite ideology, be it one of social differentiation or collectiveness (Bloch 1977; Cannon 1989; Hodder 1982; Humphreys 1981).

These criticisms have particular relevance to the identification of vertical status distinctions. Although the energy-expenditure principle has been gainfully employed to identify social ranking (Buikstra 1976; Goldstein 1980; Tainter 1975, 1978), differences in energy expenditure might not necessarily relate to social differentiation (Barrett 1990; Braun 1981; Shanks and Tilley 1982). Symbolic approaches to ranking may be firmly grounded when elites are legitimized by lineal descent from the dead. Yet, symbols may be manipulated and subject to trends of fashion, resulting in false social differences in diachronic burial samples (Bradley 1988; Cannon 1989).

Postprocessual critiques do not negate the general social patterns illustrated in ethnographic funeral data, but they emphasize a need for care in the interpretation of mortuary problems. For instance, Carr (1995) has shown that many attributes of mortuary behavior have ideational correlates as often as social ones. An important contribution of these critiques is the call for consideration of the historical context of a particular study. As symbols are defined in terms of their specific historical context at any given time (Hodder 1987, 1992), evaluation of mortuary data from a historical perspective may remove some of the difficulties in applying cross-cultural generalizations.

Maya Funerals and Death Symbolism

Unlike many prehistoric societies, the wealth of ethnohistoric, epigraphic, and iconographic materials from the ancient Maya provides a context from which to interpret Maya burial remains. Unfortunately, much of this data sheds light exclusively on the elite, who were the focus of prehistoric artistic and literary preoccupations. Yet, ethnohistoric data illustrate a variety of mortuary correlates of status that may have pertained in the prehispanic era.

In the Yucatan peninsula and the Guatemalan highlands, modern Maya peoples conduct a basically Catholic ceremony, with some remnants of prehispanic practice. Yucatec shamen (*h'men*), rather than priests, often preside over the actual burial (Rodríguez Lazcano 1991). Gourd cups (*jícaras*), money, food, and clothing are deposited in the grave throughout the Maya area (Guiteras-Holmes 1961; McGee 1990; Rodríguez Lazcano 1991; Ruz Lhuillier 1968). Among the Tzotzil, grave accompaniments vary by sex; for instance, spindles are placed only with women (Guiteras-Holmes 1961:141). Likewise, sex-specific artifacts are placed with Lacandon men and women in Chiapas (McGee 1990; Ruz Lhuillier 1968:67). In Yucatan, prestige is demonstrated by the high cost of food and drink provisions for a well-attended wake (Rodríguez Lazcano 1991:12).

Sixteenth-century chronicles provide evidence for social mortuary differentiation in both Yucatan and Guatemala on the basis of grave "wealth," grave location, energy expenditure, and symbols of social office. In the Pokoman highlands, Fuentes y Guzman (1932:266) described the burial of a Southern Pokom lord as follows:

> As soon as he was dead, the first thing that keepers and gentlemen of his chamber did was to hand over the body . . . and they bathed it and purified it with decoctions of aromatic herbs and flowers, without using other ceremony or unguent to preserve the body from decay. . . . They dress him afterwards in rich and figured clothes, in the style that he wore in life, *with the same insignia which he wore reigning*; and in this manner, they place him on a platform above figured tapestries of beautiful colors. . . . There was a large guard of lords and

principal men, through 2 days. There was weeping of his women in turn, wailing over the corpse. And in this time all sorts of people were permitted to enter and see him.
At the entrance of night, at the close of the 2 days, they cleared away the palace and in the quiet of night they go forth with the corpse to the place of burial, assisted in this by a great number of lords and principal men and followed by a great concourse of people of the pueblo.

The sons of the lords with great finery went before; they carried on their shoulders mantles and mats with gold, silver, crystal and other stones, and plumes of the quetzal, parrot, macaws and other birds, and foods of maize and meat, and not a little fuel, to enter with the dead man, because they said it was important that nothing be lacking in the other life for a great lord. . . . In this way a great procession was formed with many of their priests, who were those who placed him in the tomb. . . . After ceremonies and words of farewell by the priests, they place him in the tomb [making offerings to their great god *Exbalamquen* (who would take care of him)]. They had prepared a great olla of earthenware. . . . and this was placed in the hole which was very large. They placed within it the corpse and the jewels and the plumes; the rest they placed round about the urn, and they covered it with a flagstone and promptly filled in the pit with earth. *Above it they raised a little mound, more or less high according to the status of the dead man* and this is made of stone and mud. . . . (Translation in Miles 1957:749, emphasis added, phrase in brackets omitted by Miles, my translation).

This description illustrates the range of funerary accompaniments included with royal burials and specifies that symbols of rulership were interred as worn in life. The height of the burial monument varied as predicted by the energy expenditure principle.

A northern Pokom burial witnessed by Las Casas (1909:629–31) differs somewhat in form, but illustrates many of the same principles of social differentiation:

When he stops breathing they immediately dispatched messengers to all the towns subject to him and to those other lords that they had as friends making known to them the death and that they waited to bury him until such and such a day. . . . They dressed him in the best clothes and richest blankets that he had, adorning him with certain jewels of gold and stones that he had left and set aside, so that they buried these with him, because the rest, being already come near death, he had divided among his sons and wife, and brothers and relatives. They placed a dais where they seated him, for thus he was to be buried. For the day of burial all came who had been called; and from the friendly lords came the lord or brother of the lord or other person of authority and brought a slave (male or female, or both) and clothes and some pieces of gold to adorn the body of the dead man, each according to his mind, consoling the living and showing the weight and grief that all his servants and friends had had at the death.

All the things that everyone had brought were put together and they placed them over those he already had, and thus, well dressed, with many folded mantles and decorated with his jewels, they placed him in a box made of stones or wood, with a cover, in which he was carried seated cross-legged. This box they placed in the tomb, which was a grave or hole made in the top of a mountain or on the mountain heights. Then, placing the lord within, they killed the male and female slaves that they had to go to serve. *With the men laborers they placed their gear and implements for farming and with the hunters, for hunting their bows and arrows, and so with the rest. With the women were the stones for grinding maize, pots for cooking and preparing food, the vessels for drinking, plates and bowls.* The lord placed in the tomb, *his face toward the south* (*held by them as more fortunate than the north*) they put around him all the dead servants. Afterward they filled the hole or tomb with earth . . . above the tomb they made an altar a cubit high, of lime and stone well whitened, on which they commonly burned incense and offered other sacrifices (Translation in Miles 1957:749–50, emphasis added).

Importantly, this passage describes sexual differentiation in grave goods and indicates that the compass orientation of the skeleton was ritually meaningful. Las Casas further noted that social participation in funerals—breadth of community disruption—varied with the status of the deceased (*sensu* Tainter 1978).

> All the said ceremonies were common to all, great and small . . . each one according to his estate, and that which the friendly lords did for other lords when they died, the same did the relatives or those of his family for a dead man, and thus they bring garments and jewels, each one according to his ability (Translation in Miles 1957:750).

Moreover, these passages emphasize that burial goods were often gifts from both the local and neighboring communities, and do not represent personal wealth per se.

In the Quiche capital of Utatlan, social status also determined the location of burial, as described by Tomás López Medel:

> [M]agistrates and administrators of the republic . . . watched for the public good, and when they died they buried them in the houses of the cabildos and ayuntamientos in that very spot where they were accustomed to sit and to administer justice and to vote and execute those notable works which they did in the republic. This was the most sovereign glory which could be given to a man among them (Tozzer 1941:227).

This spatial component of mortuary differentiation is also described by Bishop Diego de Landa for the Yucatec Maya (and is reiterated by Herrera in Tozzer 1941:220), who indicates that differential burial location was further emphasized by distinctive modes of corpse handling and disposal between social classes:

> They buried them inside or in the rear of their houses, casting into the grave with them some of their idols, and if he was a priest, some of his books. And if he was a sorcerer, they buried with him some of his stones for witchcraft and instruments of his profession. Usually they abandoned the house and left it deserted after the burials, except when there were a great many persons in it so that they with their society lost some of the fear which remained on them of account of the death. As for the nobles and persons of high esteem, they burned their bodies and placed their ashes in great urns, and they built temples above them . . . when they were of very high rank, they enclosed their ashes in statues of pottery made hollow. The rest of the people of position made for their fathers wooden statues of which the back of the head was left hollow, and they then burned a part of the body and placed its ashes there, and plugged it up; afterwards they stripped off the dead body the skin of the back of the head and stuck it over this place and they buried the rest as they were wont to do (Tozzer 1941:129–31).

Each of these testimonies documents a common variety of grave accompaniments. Although care should be taken in interpreting the distribution of grave goods as direct indicators of wealth as couched by Spanish observers, neither should all elements described in these accounts be taken as symbols of hierarchical status, although some clearly are. Replete with symbolic associations, the precious stones—jade—and red shells—*Spondylus*—were also used as currency and exchanged by Postclassic traders (Tozzer 1941:95–96), so may not have been limited to elite use.

Epigraphic data from the Prehispanic era provide some direct, albeit limited, information about funerary practices. Hieroglyphic expressions have been deciphered that signify "death" and "to bury," but generally occur in contexts that simply record the death and burial of isolated Maya royalty. The most lavish Maya burial yet excavated was that of Pacal, a king of Palenque whose identity is confirmed by hieroglyphic inscriptions on the sculptured stone sarcophagus that contained his bones (Lounsbury 1974; Ruz Lhuillier 1973). At Tikal, the skeleton in Burial 116 most likely belonged to Hasaw Chan K'awil (Ruler A), whose death is described on a pair of carved bones contained in the grave (Coe 1990:609; Jones 1977). Such interpretations require caution, however, as arguments linking known individuals to contemporaneous tombs are somewhat circular, and texts associated with a grave may be funeral gifts or heirlooms (Houston 1989:8). Among the burials considered in the present study, three graves have been tentatively identified as royal personages on the basis of hieroglyphic death inscriptions on carved monuments associated with structures containing the graves: Tamarindito ruler Chanal Balam (TA6), Dos Pilas Ruler 2 (DP30) and the Woman of Cancuen (DP20). However, these identifications are somewhat less secure as the texts were not directly located in the graves (Demarest et al. 1991; Valdés 1997; Wolley and Wright 1990b). Each of these graves contains an abundance of goods including polychrome ceramic vessels, jade, and shell artifacts, and are housed in well-constructed tombs or crypts, below elaborate monumental architecture. Although these data do not provide a basis for interpreting the broad range of mortuary behavior encountered archaeologically, they do illustrate the nature of burial attributes associated with the uppermost stratum of Classic Maya society.

Reconstructions of prehispanic funerary ideology and interpretations of the symbolic meaning of grave goods have often been based on the origin myths recounted in a 16th-century Quiche Maya text, the Popol Vuh (Tedlock 1985). The manuscript recounts the descent of the hero twins—Hunahpu and Xbalanque—into the mythical underworld of Xibalba. This underworld is entered through a cave and is rank with disease and the odor of rotting corpses. There, the twins faced a series of challenges to defeat the nine lords of death. In the final test, they cut each other to pieces, are resurrected, and trick the Xibalban lords into volunteering for the trick but do not bring them back to life. The twins escape and rise to become the sun and moon (Tedlock 1985). Schele and Miller (1986) suggest that the myth describes the journey followed by Maya rulers at death. Like the twins, rulers fall to the underworld upon their death, combat the lords of death, and are reborn as deified celestial ancestors.

On the basis of funerary ceramic and sculptural images and associated hieroglyphic texts, the Classic period underworld is thought to have differed somewhat from that of the Quiche Xibalba. Principally, it is characterized by marine associations and may have been similar to the primordial sea before the first sunrise as recounted in the opening pages of the Popol Vuh (Coggins 1988; Hellmuth 1987). For instance, in the grave of Tikal's Hasaw Chan K'awil, mentioned earlier, the carved bones show canoes carrying underworld deities, with a glyphic text proclaiming that "Ruler A canoed 4 katuns to his passing" (Schele and Miller 1986:270). A marine element is also found in the grave goods. For instance, marine shells are logical accompaniments for a deceased individual bound for the watery underworld.

Coe (1973, 1975) suggested that burial ceramics depicted the hero twins and that the funeral rite was described in the ceramic texts. Decipherments of these glyphs reveals that the vessels were not produced solely for funerary disposal but are also utilitarian (Houston et al. 1989). The majority of ceramic vessels were probably placed in graves holding foods such as tamales (Taube 1989), *atole* (Houston et al. 1989) or cacao (Stuart 1988b), just as food is placed in Maya graves today (Guiteras-Holmes 1961; McGee 1990; Rodríguez Lazcano 1991). Others may have served as receptacles for sacrificial blood, let to ensure rebirth of the deceased (Coggins 1988).

Ethnohistoric chronicles also reveal the symbolic meaning of some prehispanic grave accompaniments. A symbolic association between jade artifacts and maize has a long history in Mesoamerica. This relationship is expressed by Landa's observation:

> Once dead, they put them in a shroud, filling their mouths with ground maize, which is their food and drink, which they call koyem, and with it they placed some of the stones which they use for money, so that they should not be without something to eat in the other life (Tozzer 1941:129).

These stones have been interpreted as jade, following Tozzer and subsequent archaeologists. This practice is also depicted by Sahagún for the Aztec (Sahagún 1950–1963:Bk. 3, Fig. 15). Furst (1995) shows that this practice was related to the Aztec concept of the soul, or *yolia*. During excavation, however, it is rarely possible to ascertain whether a jade bead found in a grave had been located in the mouth or worn as a pendant. As maize provided the foundation of Maya agriculture, the use of jade in graves calls to mind the rebirth theme in the tale of the hero twins and in funerary iconography.

Landa also describes the use of "little saws" (Tozzer 1941:191) as instruments of ritual genital bloodletting. These implements are undoubtedly the stingray tail barbs that are found in the pelvic region of some burials. Royal bloodletting is depicted in Classic period sculpture and ceramic art (Stuart 1984, 1988a). Iconographic discussions emphasize the ideological role of royal bloodletting in maintaining the agricultural and dynastic cycles (Joralemon 1974; Schele and Miller 1986).

Pyrite mirrors found in graves may well be symbols of rulership since the ruler was referred to as "the mirror of the community" (*u nen cab*) in Late Postclassic Yucatan. On ceramic vessels, portraits of rulers gazing into mirrors may be intended to reflect their royal descent (Coe 1988; Schele and Miller 1983). However, Coggins (1988) suggests that mirrors were used in ritual fire drilling in order to light a new fire to restart the annual agricultural cycle. Further, she argues that perforated ceramic plates also may have been used in fire-drilling ritual, an intriguing alternative—given the absence of scorching—to Coe's idea that plates were "killed" to allow the soul to escape through a plate covering the cranium. For the Aztec, the *tonalli* soul is implanted in a body by fire (Furst 1995), so such explanations may not necessarily be mutually exclusive.

Given this iconographic database, it appears that many burial attributes functioned symbolically to ensure the rebirth of the deceased. Although many of the images are prehispanic, their interpretation is based on colonial period beliefs, projected back in time. Inherently, symbolic meaning is defined in the context of a prior meaning (Hodder 1992), but archaeological reconstruction of symbolic processes necessarily proceeds in the opposite direction, from the recent to the distant past, so it is difficult to evaluate ideological history. Additionally, most iconographic data refers directly to the uppermost stratum of Maya society, and the symbolic implications of less elaborate features are less certain. We can assume that all social strata shared common religious beliefs, but the expectations on death could have varied dramatically among social strata. Burial data may provide a means to examine changes in the structure and symbolism of Maya funerals.

In the following pages, I apply analytic approaches to the identification of social differentiation among burials to the Pasión data. The goal of this analysis is to identify dimensions of social variability within the burial samples and to classify the burials into broadly comparable social groups. Then I use this classification to evaluate the possibility of status-specific consumption. Additionally, mortuary correlates of social status may illustrate changes in the social hierarchy over time and provide an avenue to investigate social processes that may have been implicated in the demise of Pasión Maya society.

I employ principal factoring to examine the interrelationship of mortuary attributes. If burial-program structure is somehow related to social divisions, then a high redundancy of attributes should be found. I use cluster analysis to classify burials into groups sharing common attributes. I examine the composition and social implications of the resulting clusters in light of the funerary symbolism outlined above, in order to better define the nature of social distinctions illustrated by Pasión funeral rituals.

Methods

Virtually all mortuary features encountered by excavations in the region are included in the analysis, but only those burials from sites that yielded eight or more skeletons are treated statistically. Only preliminary field estimates for age-at-death and sex are available for a few skeletons from Altar de Sacrificios that were discarded in the field or otherwise unavailable for study; otherwise, demographic data follows that of Chapter 3. Mortuary data are from the published burial descriptions for Altar de Sacrificios (Smith 1972) and Seibal (Tourtellot III 1990). Data for Itzan and the Petexbatun sites are taken from the burial excavation forms and field notes of the Yale Itzan Project and the Vanderbilt Petexbatun Regional Archaeological Project, respectively. When mentioned individually, burials are designated by a two-letter term for the site followed by the burial number, for example, DP20.

Definition of Mortuary Variables

I examined variability in burial form using formal attributes described in ethnohistoric and iconographic sources as socially or ritually meaningful. Mortuary attributes were chosen to maximize the variety of data considered while minimizing the redundancy of information conveyed. Given the broad variety of grave goods, grave morphology, skeletal positions, and contexts in which Maya burials occur, some arbitrary decisions had to be made. While the adequate representation of variability in burial patterns requires using a sufficient variety of variables, the number of variables must be manageable and should represent a significant number of positive occurrences.

Burial variables were defined within the following attribute classes: structural association, grave morphology, skeletal position, and grave furniture (Table 4.1). Although many studies have restricted analysis to grave goods, the use of spatial variables and body position can have a significant effect on the patterns detected and allows consideration of burials with few or no grave goods (Brown 1987; Goldstein 1980).

Traditionally, Mayanists have identified the status of a skeleton, in part, from its architectural context and location in public or private space. Here, the classification adopted emphasizes a distinction between monumental and domestic architecture and between burials placed within buildings and those in exterior space. A more elaborate typology might be devised, but uncertainty as to the function of many architectural forms and the aforementioned desire to keep the number of variables to a minimum support the use of a simplistic typology.

A grave is defined as the facility that was prepared to receive the human remains in the ground. Classifications of Maya graves typically have been specific to the forms encountered in a single site, but Welsh (1988:16–8) has attempted to synthesize a single typology from the literature. The classification used here was condensed from typologies defined by Smith (1972:212) for Altar de Sacrificios; those defined by Tourtellot (1990:85) for Seibal; and the types defined by Welsh (1988) that were identified in excavations by the Petexbatun Project and Itzan Project.

Under the heading of "Skeletal Position" I also consider the extent of articulation of the skeleton and the orientation of the skeleton within the grave. Such a classification might be endless because of the broad variety in skeletal position exhibited by Pasión burials, but is condensed to a brief list of attributes defined in Table 4.1.

A broad variety of burial furniture occurs in Pasión burials, including both local and foreign materials. I designated grave good variables on the basis of material and form. In order to provide a classification that would be applicable over the span of Maya occupation, I defined ceramic attributes on the basis of vessel form, rather than type or ware, which are temporally restricted. To avoid redundancy in scoring both vessel forms present and the number of vessels, I scored vessel quantity only once, to indicate burials with six or more vessels, which would otherwise be indiscernible from burials with fewer vessels but with a broad variety of forms. Many burials show four or five vessels, but very few show six or more, so this seems a useful cut-off. Artifactual accompaniments include a variety of local and imported goods. Local goods include worked and unworked bone, chert, and polished and ground-stone implements. Imported goods include jade or greenstone beads and artifacts, *Spondylus* beads and valves, other marine shell, stingray spines, hematite, and obsidian. Specific quantities of these exotic goods may have symbolic meaning (Moholy-Nagy 1985), but the rarity of these artifacts in Pasión burials precludes more detailed evaluation.

The presence of grave goods was scored, but their relative location in the grave was not. Although the symbolic meaning of an artifact may be contingent upon its placement (Pader 1982), to score location would be redundant with the presence/absence scoring. Furthermore, locational data for these attributes are not consistently recorded for all sites.

As one goal of the analysis was to identify individual skeletons for dietary comparison, analysis was conducted at the level of the individual skeleton rather than the grave. Skeletons interred in multiple burials are so designated with the "single skeleton" variable (absence). I scored all grave goods in a multiple burial as present for each individual, as it is difficult to define associations between grave goods and individual skeletons securely. This will result in some artificial leveling of grave good distributions between individuals in such burials, but is preferable to arbitrarily assigning a differential distribution.

I scored each variable as present or absent for

Table 4.1. Attributes used in statistical analysis of mortuary patterns

Structural association	
residential	in a low mound, either single or part of a domestic group, excluding palace groups
patio	below exterior space associated with a domestic group or mound, either within the center of the group or behind the structures
ceremonial	within a large temple, ceremonial platform, or palace structure, usually in the elite core of the site, and not associated with domestic architecture
plaza	below an exterior floor associated with monumental architecture, such as a main plaza, causeway, ball court alley, etc.
axial	along the major axis of the structure or directly beneath the center of an enclosed patio or plaza
Skeletal position	
articulated	essentially all of the skeleton is present and articulated, with no obvious postmortem manipulation (dismemberment or secondary disposal). Skeletons that were evidently interred complete but disturbed by later intrusive construction are also included here.
legs only	only the lower half of the skeleton is included, may include hips; absence of the upper body cannot be accounted for by postdepositional disturbance (see articulated).
thorax, no legs	only the upper half of the skeleton is included, usually with cranium and arms; absence of legs cannot be accounted for by postdepositional disturbance (see articulated).
no cranium	otherwise fully articulated skeletons in which the cranium has been removed; absence of cranium cannot be accounted for by unintentional postdepositional disturbance
cranium only	only the cranium was interred, may be either secondary deposition or primary decapitated.*
single skeleton	grave contains only one individual; multiple burial is indicated by absence of single skeleton
extended	skeleton lies on back, legs fully extended but may be crossed at ankles, arms may be crossed over chest or extended.
flexed on back	legs and arms are flexed over supine thorax
flexed on left	flexed arms and legs, skeleton lying on its left side
flexed on right	flexed arms and legs, skeleton lying on its right side
flexed prone	flexed arms and legs are beneath face down thorax
seated	tightly flexed arms and legs against vertical thorax
*head to north***	head lies to north on line drawn through head and hips
head to south	head lies to south on line drawn through head and hips
head to east	head lies to east on line drawn through head and hips
head to west	head lies to west on line drawn through head and hips
Grave morphology	
simple	an interment in construction fill with no special grave preparation. They are often thought to have been placed during building construction as no pit outlines are visible, but also include intrusive pit burials for which the nature of the fill and mound surface precludes observation of pit outlines (Welsh 1988:16; Tourtellot 1990:85).
pit	an unlined, intrusive hole with its outline defined by a difference between soil contained in the pit and the surrounding fill or by a damaged floor above the burial (Welsh 1988; Tourtellot 1990; but includes some graves defined as "cist" by Smith 1972).
slab	the body was placed on a stone slab that was intentionally placed as flooring for the grave (Tourtellot 1990). Also included here is Welsh's (1988) "ceiling slab" type, in which the body is placed on the capstone slabs of a pre-existing burial (only DP40).
cap	an unlined pit with stone slabs placed directly on the skeleton and not resting on the walls of the pit, defined after Tourtellot (1990) and somewhat akin to Welsh's (1988) "partial cist." Tourtellot's (1990) "cap-slab" type is also included here, in which the skeleton is both placed on and covered by slabs.

capped pit — an unlined pit with capstones that cover the top of the pit and rest on its sidewalls but not directly on the skeleton (Welsh 1988; Tourtellot 1990:"pit crypt").

cist — a crude ring of unshaped stones or rough, vertically placed slabs surrounding the skeleton, which is *not* covered by capstones (Welsh 1988; Tourtellot 1990:"cist").

head cist — unshaped stones or rough slabs placed around and/or over the cranial end of the skeleton only (Welsh 1988; Tourtellot 1990:"head crypt").

simple crypt — vertically placed slabs or a few courses of horizontally placed slabs completely surround the skeleton, which is covered by capstones that rest on these grave walls (Welsh 1988; Smith 1972:"crypt"; Tourtellot 1990:"crypt").

elaborate crypt — a much larger air-filled chamber with walls of dressed stone slabs horizontally placed in courses and roofed with wooden beams, large dressed capstones, or a rough corbelled vault (Welsh 1988; Smith 1972:"crypt"; Tourtellot 1990:"crypt").

urn — the skeletal remains are held within a ceramic vessel, e.g., a jar, or between two plates or bowls set lip to lip.

Grave Furniture

jar — a vessel with restricted neck and flaring rim

plate — a flat vessel with sides slightly raised; often has feet

vase — a cylindrical vessel with height greater than diameter

bowl — a rounded serving vessel with height less than orifice diameter

≥ 6 ceramic vessels — six or more vessels accompany the skeleton

ceramic figurine — anthropomorphic or zoomorphic figurine or ocarina

ceramic artifact — other ceramic artifacts, e.g., sherd discs, drums, beads, adornos, etc.

worked bone — bone artifacts that have been carved, polished, or otherwise modified

unworked bone — unworked nonhuman bone elements

stingray spine — tail-barb of a stingray

jade bead — perforate jade or other greenstone, worn as a pendant

other jade artifacts — nonbead greenstone artifacts, e.g., ear flares, plaques, mosaic pieces

Spondylus *beads* — perforate beads fashioned from shell of *Spondylus americanus*

Spondylus *valve* — entire valves of *Spondylus americanus* , worked or unworked

nacreous shell — the inner "mother of pearl" coating from a bivalve, freshwater or marine

other worked shell — worked shell of other species, e.g., *Marginella, Oliva, Strombus,* or freshwater shells

unworked shell — unworked shell of species other than *Spondylus*

hematite mirror — hematite mosaic pieces that formed a mirror or a slate back to which the reflective surface was affixed

red pigment — cinnabar or red ochre coating the skeleton, furniture, or grave structure

chert tool — chipped-stone implements or eccentrics included as grave furniture, excluding flakes in structure fill exterior to the grave structure itself

obsidian — blades or other tools of obsidian included as grave furniture

polished stone — nonsiliceous stone artifacts, e.g., ear flares, spindle whorls, axes, etc.

ground stone — coarse stone implements, e.g., manos, metates, "donut" stones

---

* Secondary and primary crania clearly indicate very different mortuary behavior but are difficult to separate archaeologically because of poor preservation or incomplete recovery of associated vertebrae; hence, they are pooled together here.

** For orientations between the cardinal directions, some arbitrary rules were adopted. In flexed burials the cardinal direction to which the skull was facing was selected, according to whether it lay on the left or right side. In supine or prone positions, orientation was restricted to N or S, whichever was closest. For seated burials, head orientation was recorded as the direction the body faced.

a given skeleton, or as "missing" if its condition was unknown. Some of the variables are mutually exclusive, so the binary scoring method introduces some inherent redundancies into the analysis. Redundant variables account for greater differentiation between principal factors and terminal clusters. To resolve this problem, these variables might be collapsed into a single binary state, but this would entail an unjustified simplification of the variability under investigation. The redundant variables are structural association, grave morphology, and skeletal position. The assumption that the location of a burial or nature of its facility is a relatively more useful indicator of social status than are grave goods may be valid to a degree, as these are reflections of energy invested in the interment (Tainter 1975, 1981; cf. Braun 1981). As noted above, this has been a common assumption in Maya archaeology. Keeping this bias in mind when interpreting the results of multivariate classification should alleviate the problem somewhat.

Univariate Analysis

To obtain a general understanding of variable patterning, I first subject the data to a series of univariate comparisons. Initially, the occurrence of each variable is examined in relation to site and chronological period using the Yates-corrected chi-square statistic upon the total mortuary sample from the Pasión Region, with significant differences accepted at $p < 0.05$. The occurrence of more abundant variables is then examined in relation to age and sex by chronological period for each site. Sample sizes are too small to allow separation by narrow age groups, so age comparisons consider only the distinction between subadults (<12 years) and adults (>12 years). This division was drawn with adolescence rather than skeletal maturity, because this is an age when biological changes of sexual maturity are often accompanied by changes in social role, that is, occupation or marriage. Mortuary correlates of age and sex can not be evaluated for many samples due to the rarity of females (SELC) or children (SELC, DP, AG, IT). Significance of age and sex patterning is tested with the Fisher Exact test. Given the small sample sizes, I accepted a differential distribution with $p < 0.10$, recognizing the lower reliability of this significance level.

Multivariate Analysis

According to the recommendations of Brown (1987) and O'Shea (1984), I use two forms of multivariate analysis to study the data. First, R-mode principal factoring (an iterative form of principal components analysis [Krzanowski 1988]) is applied to examine interactions between variables in the burial sample of each site for each time period. This technique reveals interrelationships in the distribution of variables that may correspond to social personae recognized in mortuary ritual (Braun 1979). It provides a means to examine the nature of social groups in each sample and differences between them. Second, Q-mode cluster analysis is used to isolate groups of comparable burials in each sample. The resulting burial clusters form the basis of intersite and chronological dietary comparisons in Chapter 7.

Principal factoring employed only those attributes present for at least 5% of graves, following O'Shea (1984:66). In some samples, this means that attributes represented only once are included, while in others, attributes are only considered if present in at least two burials. This criterion allows maximal information to be extracted from small samples while preventing the number of variables considered in larger samples from becoming unwieldy. The analysis is conducted upon a matrix of phi coefficients (φ) generated with pairwise deletion of missing values for the included variables and extracted principal factors with eigenvalues greater than 1. The factors are rotated according to the varimax orthogonal solution to maximize the variance explained by the factors. The weighting of variables on each factor is examined to define the nature of patterning in each sample and then compared between samples. I compare eigenvalue falloff curves between samples to evaluate the relative importance of variable associations (O'Shea 1984).

Cluster analysis is performed to identify clusters of burials exhibiting similar attributes (Q-mode). As in the principal factor analysis, only variables present for 5% of graves are considered. Euclidean distance is used as the measure upon which clusters are divided (Hodson 1970). A matching coefficient that excludes negative matches (e.g., Quilter 1989; Tainter 1975) is not used because the absence of certain variables signifies an alternate state (Braun 1981), such as multiple burial indicated by the absence of single burial. The use of many mortuary symbols may be governed by social rules akin to sumptuary laws. Hence, the absence of a burial attribute may convey as much social information as its presence, and use of a matching coefficient would undermine this information.

I chose polythetic agglomerative cluster analysis using the complete linkage method (farthest neighbor) as the algorithm for cluster definition. In contrast to monothetic divisive analysis, polythetic agglomerative methods give equal weight to all attributes, thereby minimizing the bias imposed by partial redundancy among variables (Braun 1981; Brown 1987). The complete linkage method ensures maximum homogeneity within and maximum difference between clusters (Tainter 1975:5). Single- or average-linkage cluster algorithms would reveal more subtle differences in the burial differentiation but would not serve the goal of defining broadly comparable categories between samples. The cutoff point for cluster definition is chosen arbitrarily at 0.60. Selection of a higher level (e.g., 0.70) would result in only one or two clusters per sample, while a lower level (0.50) would produce almost twice as many clusters. Resulting clusters are evaluated in light of the dimensions of variable association revealed by the principal factor analysis.

Results

Univariate Analysis

Contingency table analysis of the distribution of burial variables by site and chronological period reveals significant differences for a number of variables (Table 4.2). Unfortunately, many rare artifacts cannot be evaluated because of low expected frequencies. Most variables show chronological tendencies that also contribute to a number of the intersite differences, in conjunction with sampling differences and discrepancy in the occupational span of various sites.

For instance, disarticulated burials are most common in the Terminal Classic, largely because of the multiple disarticulated burial SE4 at Seibal and the deposit of decapitated crania in Dos Pilas Group L4-3, which account for a large portion of the M.N.I. in each respective sample. Similarly, multiple burial is most common in the Terminal Classic at Seibal, owing to the same deposit.

Chronological patterning in skeletal position is evident for extended skeletons that account for many Preclassic burials and for the "flexed on the right side" position that was more common during all Classic period phases. The "flexed on the left side" position is found principally at Altar, where it was used in all periods. Orientation shows chronological patterning, with the "head to the east" orientation predominant during the Terminal Classic. Orientation to the west is frequent in the Early Classic period, represented only by the sample from Altar, but also occurs in other periods. Also common at Altar is the "head to the south orientation," which is emphasized in the Preclassic sample.

Grave form shows both site and chronological differences. For instance, simple crypts are virtually restricted to Dos Pilas, Itzan, and Aguateca, and to the Late Classic period. Simple graves predominate in the Early Classic Altar sample. In contrast, pit graves have their highest frequency in the Terminal Classic period. A second peak in the Preclassic owes to the prevalence of other types during the Late Classic, in part, and to the detection and definition of the type. A high occurrence of intrusive pits corroborates changes in the location of burial focus during the Terminal Classic. The prevalence of pits in the Preclassic samples may reflect the greater visibility of intrusive features in Preclassic monumental architecture in contrast to Late Classic residential architecture.

Ceramic assemblages also vary chronologically, with greater representation of bowls in Early Classic graves giving way to plates and vases in Late Classic times; plates and vases are particularly common in graves at Dos Pilas, Itzan, and Aguateca. Terminal Classic graves show few ves-

Table 4.2. Chi-square comparisons of variable occurrence by site and chronological period, for all samples pooled

Variable	Site	Period	Variable	Site	Period
articulated	**38.67**	**12.13**	plate	**25.09**	**31.01**
legs only			vase	**12.91**	**8.85**
thorax only			bowl	**24.25**	**18.28**
cranium removed			> 5 vessels		
cranium only	**61.38**	**23.95**	figurine		
single skeleton	**10.48**	**12.79**	ceramic artifact		
extended	0.86	**10.40**	worked bone		
flexed on back	**12.65**		unworked bone		
flexed on left side	**15.32**	4.69	stingray spine		
flexed on right side	**10.14**	**9.44**	jade bead	10.87	**11.86**
flexed prone			other jade		
seated			*Spondylus* bead		
head to north	**32.21**	**17.71**	*Spondylus* valve		
head to south	**15.70**	**11.37**	nacreous shell		
head to east	**13.16**	**10.76**	other worked shell		
head to west	10.09	**28.09**	unworked shell		
simple	**75.23**	**21.54**	hematite		
pit	**34.30**	**35.88**	red pigment		
slab			chert		
cap			obsidian		
capped pit			polished stone		
uncapped cist			ground stone		
head cist			residential	**34.84**	**44.47**
simple crypt	**95.07**	**50.64**	ceremonial	**94.60**	**43.34**
elaborate crypt			patio	**62.02**	**13.13**
urn			plaza	**15.63**	6.17
jar			axial	8.41	**19.69**

Values in **bold** indicate significance at the $p < 0.05$ level of confidence.

sels of any form. Jade beads are evenly distributed among sites but clearly decrease in circulation over time, with only a single Terminal Classic grave containing jade.

Residential burials are rare in the Terminal Classic period when ceremonial burials were common at Altar and Seibal. This pattern may partly be a result of sampling bias toward ceremonial complexes at these sites. Burials beneath residential patios occur only in the Late and Terminal Classic Periods, but this may be an artifact of excavation bias, as patios were not sampled at Altar, which is the location of most early graves. At Seibal, the patio locus is more common for Late than Terminal Classic burials, so it is probable that the temporal pattern is partly real. The prevalence of axial burials decreases over time, reflecting excavation bias; stratigraphic excavations have generally been placed on the axes of structures, while horizontal excavations that encounter nonaxial burials have generally been shallow, sampling only later constructions.

Table 4.3. Fisher Exact probabilities for age-at-death and sex comparisons for selected variables by sample

	Adult Sex										Age at Death				
Variable	**ASPC**	**ASEC**	**ASLC**	**ASTC**	**SETC**	**DPLC**	**DPTC**	**AGLC**	**ITLC**	**TALC**	**ASPC**	**ASEC**	**ASLC**	**ASTC**	**SETC**
articulated	.12	-	**.10**	1.00	.39	1.00	.53	-	1.00	.43	.45	1.00	.64	1.00	.27
cranium	-	-	.51	-	-	1.00	.53	-	1.00	.43	-	-	1.00	1.00	-
single	.38	-	.33	1.00	.70	-	1.00	1.00	-	1.00	**.01**	-	**.02**	.13	.61
extended	1.00	.44	.58	.29	1.00	.33	-	1.00	.17	1.00	1.00	.62	.58	1.00	.54
flexed on back	1.00	.17	.58	**.05**	-	-	.28	-	-	-	1.00	1.00	1.00	1.00	-
flexed on left	1.00	.17	1.00	1.00	1.00	-	1.00	.27	-	1.00	1.00	.55	.64	1.00	1.00
flexed on right	-	.17	1.00	.24	1.00	.26	.49	.59	.21	1.00	-	1.00	.54	.65	.29
head to north	1.00	.52	.52	**.01**	1.00	.65	**.07**	.35	1.00	1.00	1.00	.64	**.06**	.31	1.00
head to south	.63	.44	1.00	1.00	-	1.00	-	1.00	.44	1.00	.57	1.00	.56	.57	-
head to east	1.00	1.00	.33	**.02**	1.00	1.00	1.00	.46	-	1.00	1.00	1.00	.63	.19	1.00
head to west	1.00	.52	1.00	-	.32	-	-	1.00	1.00	-	1.00	1.00	.36	.14	**.04**
simple	1.00	.40	.33	.71	1.00	**.06**	.28	-	1.00	1 00	**.06**	1.00	.16	1.00	**.08**
pit	.38	-	1.00	.69	.41	-	-	-	.50	-	**.01**	1.00	1.00	1.00	**.10**
capped pit	-	-	-	-	1.00	1.00	-	.50	.17	-	-	-	-	-	1.00
simple crypt	-	-	-	-	1.00	.40	-	.35	1.00	1 00	-	-	-	-	1.00
plate	1.00	.40	.61	.23	.34	.40	-	**.08**	.52	49	1.00	.61	.69	.57	.56
vase	-	1.00	.56	1.00	1.00	.64	-	.15	.50	49	.24	.50	.55	1.00	1.00
bowl	.30	.20	.33	1.00	.70	.64	-	.24	1.00	1 00	.66	.17	.13	1.00	1.00
jade bead	.31	.50	1.00	-	.32	.60	-	-	.50	43	.28	1.00	.30	-	1.00
residential	1.00	1.00	.60	1.00	.21	1.00	1.00	.23	.44	1.00	.18	**.03**	.71	.57	1.00
ceremonial	1.00	.47	.60	1.00	.71	1.00	-	.23	-	1.00	**.07**	**.07**	.71	1.00	.13
plaza	1.00	.40	-	.49	1.00	-	-	-	-	1.00	1.00	.50	-	.32	.36
axial	1.00	.40	.51	1.00	.39	.62	-	**.01**	-	1.00	.50	1.00	1.00	1.00	.27
patio	-	-	-	-	**.08**	.17	1.00	-	.44	1.00	-	-	-	-	.17

Values of $p \leq 0.10$ are indicated in **bold**.

Relatively few significant differences are detected in variable distributions with respect to age and sex (Table 4.3). Given the large number of comparisons, many of the observed differences could well be due to Type I error, but some interesting patterns may be real. Age associations of mortuary variables could be examined for only a few samples due to the extreme subadult underenumeration. In the Preclassic sample from Altar, subadults are significantly associated with multiple burial, pit graves, and ceremonial architecture. The Early Classic children continue to be disproportionately interred in ceremonial architecture, while adults are associated with domestic architecture. Late Classic subadults were also commonly buried in multiple burials and show a "head to north orientation" not used for adults. Although no Terminal Classic age patterns are evident at Altar, Seibal subadults are disproportionately buried facing west or in simple graves.

Sexual differences in mortuary attributes are more revealing. At Altar, no sexual correlations are apparent—except for a disproportionate number of males among Late Classic disarticulated skeletons—until the Terminal Classic when the sexes were distinguished by skeletal position—males tend to be flexed on the back, females flexed on the right—and orientation—males headed to north, females to east. At Terminal Classic Seibal, no sexual differences are apparent, although female skeletons are more abundant in patio interments. No sexual distinctions are apparent in the small Itzan sample. In contrast, the Petexbatun sites do show Late Classic sexual distinctions. At Dos Pilas, females are more abundant in simple graves. At Aguateca, males are associated with vases and graves in axial locations.

The chronological patterns in skeletal position, orientation, and grave form described above indicate some stylistic changes over time and perhaps changes in the symbolic referents of specific attributes and/or rules governing their use. Changes in the location and furniture of Terminal Classic graves suggest a change in the structure of mortuary rules during the final occupations of some sites. A smaller proportion of graves were furnished with ceramic vessels and jade beads over time, which may indicate increasingly narrow definitions of social identities or a reduction in the relative size of that social segment (see also Rathje 1970). In fact, Terminal Classic burials are impoverished in all exotic grave goods—jade, *Spondylus*, stingrays, and shell—perhaps implying interruption of trade routes at this time.

The implications of age and sex correlation trends are difficult to evaluate. It is probably telling that the two largest samples (Altar Terminal Classic, Dos Pilas Late Classic) show the greatest number of sexual distinctions. Absence of sexual correlates from others may be a consequence of sample size. Yet, it is interesting to note that the identified Late Classic sex differences focus on grave form and artifacts while the Terminal Classic sex differences focus on skeletal position and orientation. This might indicate a change in the nature of sex roles in the final occupation of the region.

Multivariate Analysis

Principal factoring isolated between 4 and 12 factors with eigenvalues greater than 1 in each sample. Rotated factor matrices are presented in Tables 4.4 to 4.15, and eigenvalue falloff curves for chronological and intersite comparisons are in Figure 4.1. Three basic patterns of variable loading were identified in the samples. Five samples are characterized by a first principal factor (PF1) on which many variables show strong positive loadings, known as a grouped pattern. The remaining factors are characterized by a mixture of small grouped variable loadings and bipolar variable loadings (strong positive and negative loadings). These samples show exponentially shaped eigenvalue falloff curves. The second pattern is similar but lacks the strongly grouped PF1 and shows a more linear eigenvalue fall-off curve. The final pattern contains some grouped and bipolar factors, but a number of factors show specific loadings (a single strong loading, either positive or negative). Mortuary correlates of pattern 1 are a highly structured redundant set of burial attributes that covary to define mortuary groups. The large number of redundant attributes on PF1 set off this group as a superordinate dimension of status (Braun 1979; Peebles and Kus 1977). Pattern 2 indicates a highly structured mortuary domain,

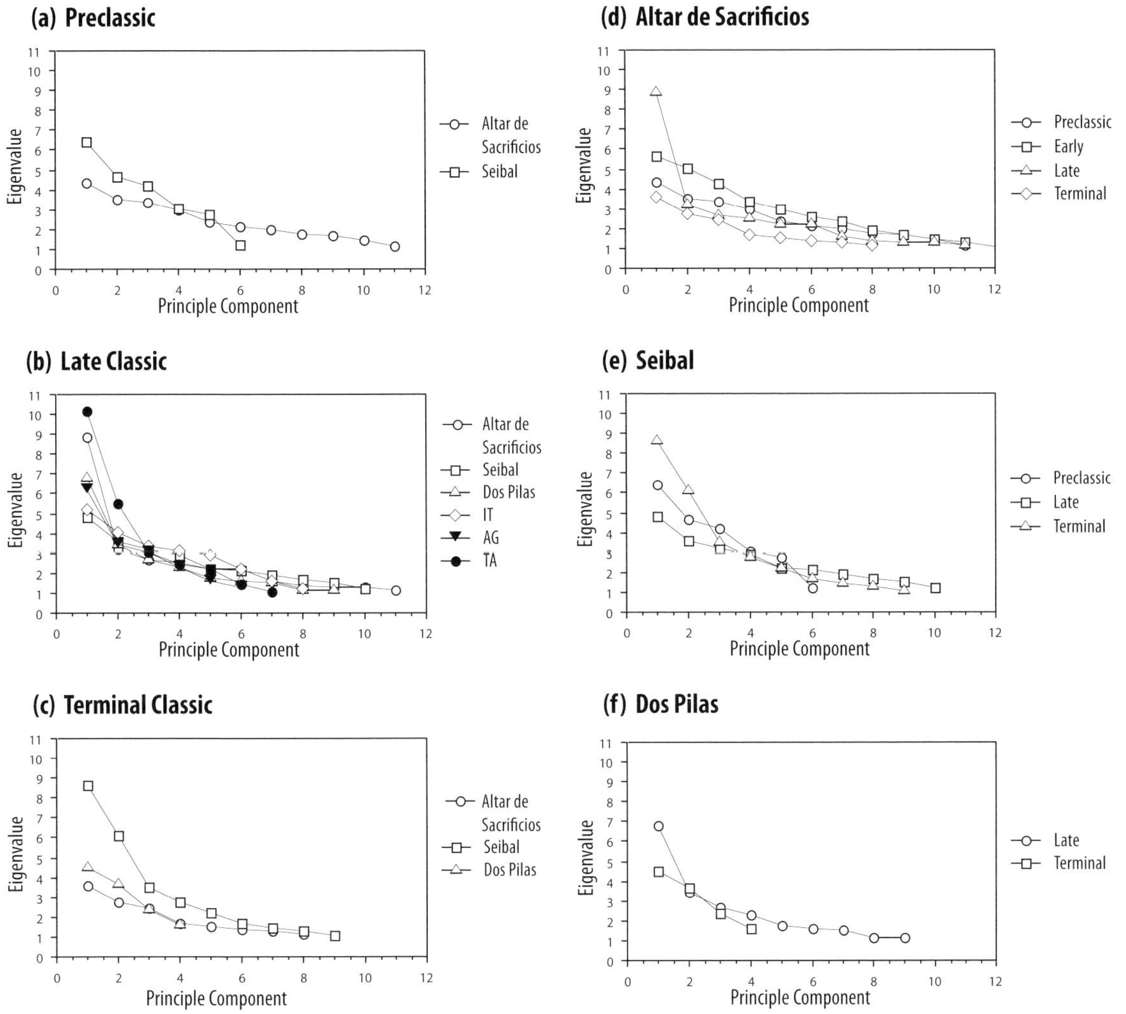

Figure 4.1. Eigenvalue falloff curves for comparisons between sites and chronological periods

but one that lacks a distinct superordinate dimension. Pattern 3 indicates slight grouping of some burial attributes, but overall an unstructured mortuary domain where archaeologically recoverable funerary ritual is not governed by strict rules.

The Preclassic samples from Altar and Seibal conform to the second pattern (Figure 4.1a). Variable loadings in both samples are distributed evenly, with bipolar loadings or a few grouped variables on most factors. For instance, in the Altar sample, PF1 demonstrates an association between articulated, single, and simple graves (Table 4.4). PF2 and PF3 contrast burial location, while PF4 and PF5 demonstrate covariation of several artifacts, skeletal positions, and orientations. Principal factor distinctions in the Seibal sample are similar in nature (Table 4.5), but the variables combine differently in the two samples, indicating site-specific differences in the use of mortuary symbols. The eigenvalue falloff curves show a gradual decrease in importance from the first factor to succeeding ones in a basically linear manner (Figure 4.1a). At Altar, the first factor does not account for much more variation than succeeding factors do. The curve for Seibal is steeper, but also linear. Given the small size of this sample, how-

Table 4.4. Varimax rotated factor matrix for Preclassic Altar de Sacrificios burials

Variable	PF1	PF2	PF3	PF4	PF5	PF6	PF7	PF8	PF9	PF10	PF11
articulated	**.676**	.213	-.111	.130	.116	.551	.067	.074	.282	.077	.012
no cranium	.063	.103	.101	-.126	.028	**-.871**	-.075	-.053	-.066	-.102	-.096
single	**.910**	-.133	-.090	.104	.034	-.112	.127	.069	-.176	.080	.144
extended	.154	.117	-.002	-.416	.473	-.069	.114	.184	.186	.027	-.633
flexed on back	.224	-.125	.181	**.788**	-.365	.071	-.131	-.105	-.065	-.178	-.107
flexed on left	.131	.069	-.276	-.029	.010	-.061	-.003	-.034	.132	.097	**.884**
head to north	.108	.076	**-.954**	-.086	-.107	.060	-.065	-.049	-.097	-.100	.018
head to south	.102	.193	.295	-.315	**.561**	-.136	-.308	.218	.278	-.414	.094
head to east	.299	-.061	.261	-.174	**-.569**	.210	**.569**	-.121	-.006	-.045	-.200
head to west	.126	.027	.049	**.693**	.031	-.058	-.108	-.081	-.075	.650	-.000
simple	**.760**	-.080	-.077	-.279	-.076	-.081	-.352	.096	-.325	.165	-.050
pit	**-.910**	.133	.090	-.104	-.034	.112	-.127	-.069	.176	-.080	-.144
cist	-.020	.152	.060	**.812**	.122	.114	.069	-.000	-.059	-.019	.011
elaborate	.025	.155	.023	-.026	.016	-.059	**.915**	-.008	-.029	-.060	-.076
jar	.201	-.030	.104	-.132	-.113	.046	-.019	-.042	.045	**.920**	.117
plate	.049	-.084	.012	.005	.046	-.020	-.029	**.972**	-.022	-.060	-.085
vase	-.221	.265	.031	-.022	.022	.041	-.128	-.012	**.760**	-.049	-.184
bowl	-.293	-.044	.364	-.096	.284	**.454**	.303	-.216	-.373	.055	-.123
worked bone	**-.804**	-.380	.043	-.058	-.147	-.056	-.010	-.042	-.276	-.009	.076
unworked bone	.146	.315	.208	-.204	-.002	.174	-.175	.041	-.167	.050	**.691**
jade bead	.169	-.152	.085	.318	**.604**	.119	.407	.328	-.152	.117	-.246
other jade	.173	-.239	.114	-.083	**.599**	.093	-.028	-.182	-.118	-.173	-.089
unworked shell	.049	-.084	.012	.005	.046	-.020	-.029	**.972**	-.022	-.060	-.085
red pigment	.086	.251	.073	-.027	-.005	**-.726**	.520	-.048	-.047	.218	.038
chert	-.014	-.229	.075	-.164	-.079	.087	.064	-.042	**.888**	.059	.116
polished stone	.185	-.074	.229	-.293	-.113	.224	.020	**.651**	.028	.069	.257
residential	-.026	**-.921**	.224	-.024	.092	.099	-.099	.152	.006	.038	-.123
ceremonial	-.027	**.896**	.315	.069	-.046	-.127	.118	-.130	.039	.012	.111
plazas	.100	.042	**-.952**	-.081	-.090	.050	-.044	-.037	-.083	-.097	.015
axial	-.067	.446	**.774**	.056	-.188	-.047	-.019	.124	-.164	-.193	-.156

Heavy loadings are indicated in bold. Together, the components account for 89.4% of the variance.

ever, it is unwise to extrapolate comparisons between the samples.

In the Early Classic Altar sample, the factor matrix illustrates the first pattern outlined above (Table 4.6). Heavy loadings on PF1 occur for eastern orientation, worked bone, stingray spines, *Spondylus* valves, and hematite. Symbolic associations can be posited for several of these attributes. Stingray spines indicate bloodletting, as well as marine associations, which are also inherent in *Spondylus* valves. Hematite mirror fragments may symbolize rulership. This factor has a higher eigenvalue than that of the Preclassic PF1, steepening the curve somewhat (Figure 4.1d). Subsequent factors are smaller and grouped, indicating association between several variables. For PF2 through PF5, grouped variables include each a position or orientation, grave type, and some grave goods. The final factors, PF6 through PF12, are bipolar or specific, indicating mutually exclusive variable

Table 4.5. Varimax rotated factor matrix for Preclassic Seibal burials

Variable	PF1	PF2	PF3	PF4	PF5	PF6
articulated	.234	-.258	-.061	**.900**	.236	-.091
thorax	-.234	.258	.061	**-.900**	-.236	.091
extended	-.331	-.153	.447	-.084	-.279	**-.727**
flexed on back	-.196	-.047	**-.819**	.413	-.201	.170
flexed on left	.683	.119	.121	.054	**.703**	.055
head to north	-.383	-.162	**.812**	.080	.243	.292
head to south	**.990**	.099	.025	.029	-.044	-.015
head to east	-.281	.100	**-.856**	-.102	-.221	-.291
simple	.143	**.928**	.240	-.164	.136	.019
slab	-.070	**-.797**	.444	.082	-.199	-.215
simple crypt	-.117	-.417	**-.759**	.133	.021	.190
jar	**.990**	.099	.025	.029	-.044	-.015
plate	-.190	.143	.300	-.341	.547	**.654**
vase	**.990**	.099	.025	.029	-.044	-.015
bowl	.683	.119	.121	.054	**.703**	.055
unworked bone	-.152	.130	.260	-.489	-.249	**.768**
jade bead	-.097	.057	.133	.042	**.966**	.088
worked shell	-.273	.323	.400	.403	**.623**	-.085
ground stone	-.070	**-.797**	.444	.082	-.199	-.215
residential	.388	.326	.158	**-.733**	.405	.127
ceremonial	-.305	.550	.058	**.682**	-.331	-.127
plaza	-.143	**-.928**	-.240	.164	-.136	-.019
axial	.194	**.791**	.124	-.175	-.538	-.043

Heavy loadings are indicated in bold. Together, the factors account for 96.9% of the variance.

distributions and coding redundancies. This result is consistent with the emergence of a superordinate social dimension in the Early Classic that had not been recognized in the Preclassic mortuary program. The emergence of a distinctive cluster of "elite" burial traits that may signify rulership has also been noted for Early Classic tombs at Rio Azul and Tikal in the northeastern Petén (Hall 1989). The hieroglyphic writing system used to legitimize rulership also emerged during this period and corroborates the new mortuary development.

The Late Classic Altar sample shows many of the characteristics of the preceding period, with PF1 a strong grouped factor (Table 4.7, Figure 4.1b,d). As in the Early Classic sample, *Spondylus* valves and worked bone load highly on PF1, while eastern orientation shows a positive loading but loads more highly on other factors. A number of other exotic artifacts (jade, shell, and obsidian) and a superabundance of ceramic vessels also load on this factor. PF6 is also a grouped factor, indicating an association between plates, vases, jade beads, and chert. The remaining factors are grouped or bipolar, emphasizing location, articulation, position, and orientation of skeletons. In contrast to the earlier samples, the eigenvalue curve is more exponential than linear in form, with PF1 explaining much more of the variation than other factors (Figure 4.1b,d). Thus, PF1 is more strictly defined than its Early Classic counterpart, suggesting a more rigid definition of elite stratum symbols.

A very similar pattern is indicated for Late

Table 4.6. Varimax rotated factor matrix for Early Classic Altar de Sacrificios burials

Variable	PF1	PF2	PF3	PF4	PF5	PF6	PF7	PF8	PF9	PF10	PF11	PF12
articulated	.044	.027	.007	.062	.068	**.951**	.043	.016	-.03	-.058	-.019	.002
no cranium	-.041	-.025	-.034	-.054	-.053	**-.945**	-.025	-.004	.011	.062	.013	-.006
extended	.334	-.278	-.144	.355	.011	**-.482**	.076	-.228	-.200	-.037	.207	-.339
flexed on back	-.048	**.793**	.002	.013	-.112	.037	.110	-.064	.007	.069	.054	.266
flexed on left	-.139	-.154	-.121	-.186	.296	.216	.068	-.034	**.822**	.180	.052	-.041
flexed on right	-.126	-.104	-.179	-.185	-.173	.260	-.162	.366	**-.578**	.214	-.344	-.007
flexed prone	-.095	.002	-.040	-.009	-.021	.039	-.059	-.028	-.004	**-.840**	-.022	.172
head to north	-.156	**.417**	-.166	-.168	-.279	.286	.013	-.238	-.329	.348	.298	.369
head to south	-.070	-.208	-.064	-.006	**.722**	-.003	.496	-.059	-.073	.088	.038	.038
head to east	**.704**	-.158	-.059	.665	-.066	.030	-.078	-.030	.037	-.014	.040	-.003
head to west	-.201	-.146	-.173	-.192	-.076	-.307	-.215	.291	.340	**-.400**	-.357	**-.400**
simple	.040	.224	-.447	-.457	.099	-.065	.143	**-.483**	.100	-.104	**.456**	.029
pit	-.014	-.062	-.041	-.023	-.075	.063	-.050	-.064	-.088	.078	**-.932**	-.066
cist	-.021	-.192	-.039	**.950**	-.038	.020	-.115	-.007	.019	.050	.020	.037
head cist	-.021	-.029	-.054	-.019	-.039	.019	-.023	**.976**	-.096	.036	.035	-.042
urn	-.018	-.135	**.978**	-.046	-.038	.011	-.084	.004	-.008	.033	.022	.024
jar	-.018	-.017	-.047	-.021	-.076	.032	-.092	-.051	.035	-.007	.068	**.699**
plate	-.075	-.053	-.133	**.418**	-.194	.190	-.347	-.174	.023	.255	.280	**-.375**
vase	-.025	**.825**	.053	.131	-.072	.065	.109	-.046	.020	.001	.080	-.248
bowl	-.294	.045	.135	.092	.108	-.096	.163	.161	.180	**.683**	-.193	.380
worked bone	**.993**	-.032	-.017	-.026	-.018	.006	.041	-.008	.005	-.037	.005	-.014
unworked bone	-.018	-.135	**.978**	-.046	-.038	.011	-.084	.004	-.008	.033	.022	.024
stingray	**.713**	-.024	-.026	-.025	.649	.043	-.004	-.002	.085	.030	.011	.070
jade bead	.434	-.075	-.077	-.089	**.551**	.066	-.165	-.151	-.314	.121	.173	-.190
other jade	.542	.296	.048	.130	.039	-.034	**.697**	-.047	-.115	.009	-.009	-.083
Spondylus bead	-.011	-.006	-.017	-.013	**.925**	.057	-.039	.007	.085	.078	.009	.102
Spondylus valve	**.993**	-.032	-.017	-.026	-.018	.006	.041	-.008	.005	-.037	.005	-.014
worked shell	-.086	.232	.027	.086	-.057	.056	**.883**	-.071	.081	.122	.064	-.030
unworked shell	-.031	.437	.080	**.840**	-.032	.022	.205	-.003	.001	.029	-.022	-.035
hematite	**.993**	-.032	-.017	-.026	-.018	.006	.041	-.008	.005	-.037	.005	-.014
red pigment	-.039	.469	**.816**	.118	-.022	.026	.240	.008	-.059	.015	-.021	-.058
obsidian	-.039	.469	**.816**	.118	-.022	.026	.240	.008	-.059	.015	-.021	-.058
polished stone	-.067	-.031	-.044	-.090	**.735**	.037	-.122	-.029	.231	-.077	.012	-.231
ground stone	-.031	.437	.080	**.840**	-.032	.022	.205	-.003	.001	.029	-.022	-.035
residential	-.195	.429	-.223	.181	.144	-.206	**-.415**	-.244	.045	**.467**	-.217	.208
ceremonial	.222	-.382	-.134	-.160	-.121	.199	**.476**	-.138	.006	-.517	.210	-.204
plaza	-.028	-.118	.666	-.047	-.055	.027	-.077	**.706**	-.075	.049	.040	-.014
axial	.263	.252	-.247	.257	-.115	-.234	-.239	-.213	**.660**	.069	.032	.220

Heavy loadings are indicated in bold. Together, the components account for 88.9% of the variance.

Table 4.7. Varimax rotated factor matrix for Late Classic Altar de Sacrificios burials

Variable	PF1	PF2	PF3	PF4	PF5	PF6	PF7	PF8	PF9	PF10
articulated	.122	-.061	.115	.034	**.797**	-.054	-.446	-.139	.139	-.184
legs only	-.018	.278	-.271	-.014	-.127	-.061	**.778**	.077	-.102	.147
cranium only	-.058	-.191	.231	.002	**-.812**	-.159	-.105	.127	-.062	.205
single	.101	.126	-.038	.140	-.162	.092	-.086	-.052	-.084	**.825**
extended	.385	.017	**.536**	-.060	.321	.270	-.103	.348	-.405	-.144
flexed on back	-.100	-.021	.128	.166	.067	-.115	-.063	.105	**.899**	-.134
flexed on left	-.191	.053	**-.846**	-.011	.128	-.012	.225	.182	-.208	.058
flexed on right	-.067	.194	.112	-.104	.072	-.056	-.107	**-.910**	-.091	.091
head to north	-.183	.322	**.451**	-.404	.362	-.057	-.160	-.022	-.024	.399
head to south	-.100	-.013	.033	-.095	.017	-.073	**.860**	.092	.072	-.380
head to east	.309	-.106	**-.595**	.057	.190	.248	-.475	.340	-.017	-.084
head to west	-.075	.014	.141	.581	.023	-.096	-.053	**-.682**	.021	-.054
simple	-.097	.024	.024	**-.708**	.118	-.556	.138	.117	.036	-.102
cap	-.001	.188	-.064	**.827**	.196	-.113	-.036	.080	.204	.133
plate	.212	-.172	.115	-.244	.314	**.600**	.123	.005	.041	-.324
vase	.557	-.165	-.076	.016	-.000	**.766**	-.068	.042	-.045	.080
bowl	.226	-.260	.027	.214	**.695**	-.017	.011	.287	-.194	.325
≥ 6 vessels	**.967**	-.093	.033	-.017	.029	.189	-.012	.009	-.008	.012
ceramic artifact	**.839**	.040	.073	.013	.059	.073	-.139	.148	-.158	-.060
worked bone	**.553**	.028	.034	-.294	.211	-.106	-.007	-.273	.059	.330
jade bead	.463	-.071	.092	-.022	.096	**.767**	-.076	.119	-.128	.112
other jade	**.967**	-.093	.033	-.017	.029	.189	-.012	.009	-.008	.012
Spondylus valve	**.967**	-.093	.033	-.017	.029	.189	-.012	.009	-.008	.012
worked shell	**.967**	-.093	.033	-.017	.029	.189	-.012	.009	-.008	.012
red pigment	**.967**	-.093	.033	-.017	.029	.189	-.012	.009	-.008	.012
chert	.189	-.130	-.084	.106	-.048	**.904**	-.082	.070	-.066	.045
obsidian	.821	.006	-.127	.293	.112	.084	-.074	.112	-.060	.054
residential	-.109	**.962**	-.009	.098	.003	-.156	.059	-.067	-.060	.027
ceremonial	.109	**-.962**	.009	-.098	-.003	.156	-.059	.067	.060	-.027
axial	-.084	**.654**	.072	-.122	-.004	-.018	.262	-.171	.423	.278

Heavy loadings are indicated in bold. Together, the components account for 88.6% of the variance.

Table 4.8. Varimax rotated factor matrix for Late Classic Dos Pilas burials

Variable	PF1	PF2	PF3	PF4	PF5	PF6	PF7	PF8	PF9
articulated	.094	.150	.14	**-.733**	-.539	.056	.110	-.041	.029
no cranium	-.068	-.012	-.053	-.017	**.849**	.094	-.034	-.130	-.070
cranium only	-.097	.006	.359	**.825**	-.110	.069	-.079	-.122	-.119
extended	.229	-.212	-.269	-.200	.195	**.768**	.025	.054	.166
flexed on right	-.108	.304	.082	-.167	-.115	**-.847**	.028	-.222	.063
head to north	-.211	**-.846**	-.146	-.091	.109	.107	.131	-.201	.138
head to south	-.076	.015	.185	-.088	-.072	.102	.101	**.888**	.001
head to east	.155	**.864**	-.077	-.217	.044	-.150	-.181	-.268	.068
simple	-.134	.377	-.31	.244	-.209	-.125	**-.691**	.005	.049
cap	-.050	-.123	**.867**	-.008	-.028	.032	-.238	.070	-.080
simple	-.334	-.121	-.209	-.225	-.062	.063	**.813**	-.056	.016
elaborate	**.985**	-.008	-.013	.021	-.019	.106	.019	-.020	.019
jar	-.069	-.265	.155	.028	**.582**	-.080	-.040	.497	-.149
plate	.172	-.148	-.167	-.112	-.008	.217	.350	.030	**.584**
vase	**.513**	-.385	.111	-.095	-.177	-.051	.271	-.045	.348
bowl	.265	-.038	-.192	.289	-.145	.002	**.737**	.267	-.085
≥ 6 vessels	**.952**	-.089	-.031	.033	-.084	.061	.012	-.015	-.060
worked bone	**.594**	.147	-.14	.075	-.000	-.276	-.171	.043	.034
stingray	.493	.092	-.104	**.754**	-.019	.018	-.013	.001	.047
jade bead	**.747**	.238	-.016	-.085	.265	.279	.169	-.154	-.039
other jade	**.985**	-.008	-.013	.021	-.019	.106	.019	-.020	.019
Spondylus valve	**.985**	-.008	-.013	.021	-.019	.106	.019	-.020	.019
worked shell	.561	.134	-.066	.108	**.609**	.119	.093	.007	.187
obsidian	-.045	.089	**.873**	.091	-.010	-.099	.073	.181	-.008
residential	**-.625**	-.240	.037	-.088	-.050	-.176	.165	-.033	-.531
axial	.109	.252	.325	.093	-.179	**.676**	.204	-.193	-.031
patio	-.099	-.026	-.006	-.016	-.061	-.109	-.164	-.058	**.835**

Heavy loadings are indicated in bold. Together, the factors account for 83.4% of the variance.

Classic Dos Pilas (Table 4.8). In this sample, PF1 shares heavy loadings with variables that compose PF1 at Altar and also has a high eigenvalue, giving the curve an exponential shape (Figure 4.1b,f). Subsequent factors show small groups of variables and bipolar contrasts. The PF1 variables in this sample occur in two graves that have been identified as members of the Dos Pilas ruling dynasty on the basis of associated glyphic monuments. These are burial DP30, thought to be Ruler 2 (Plate 4.1), and DP20, the "Woman of Cancuen." Accordingly, the factor may be taken to define symbols of rulership.

Similarly, at Tamarindito, PF1 has a very high eigenvalue (Figure 4.1b, Table 4.9). This factor shows heavy loadings of the same variables that load on PF1 at Altar and Dos Pilas. As at Dos Pilas, these variables are found at Tamarindito in

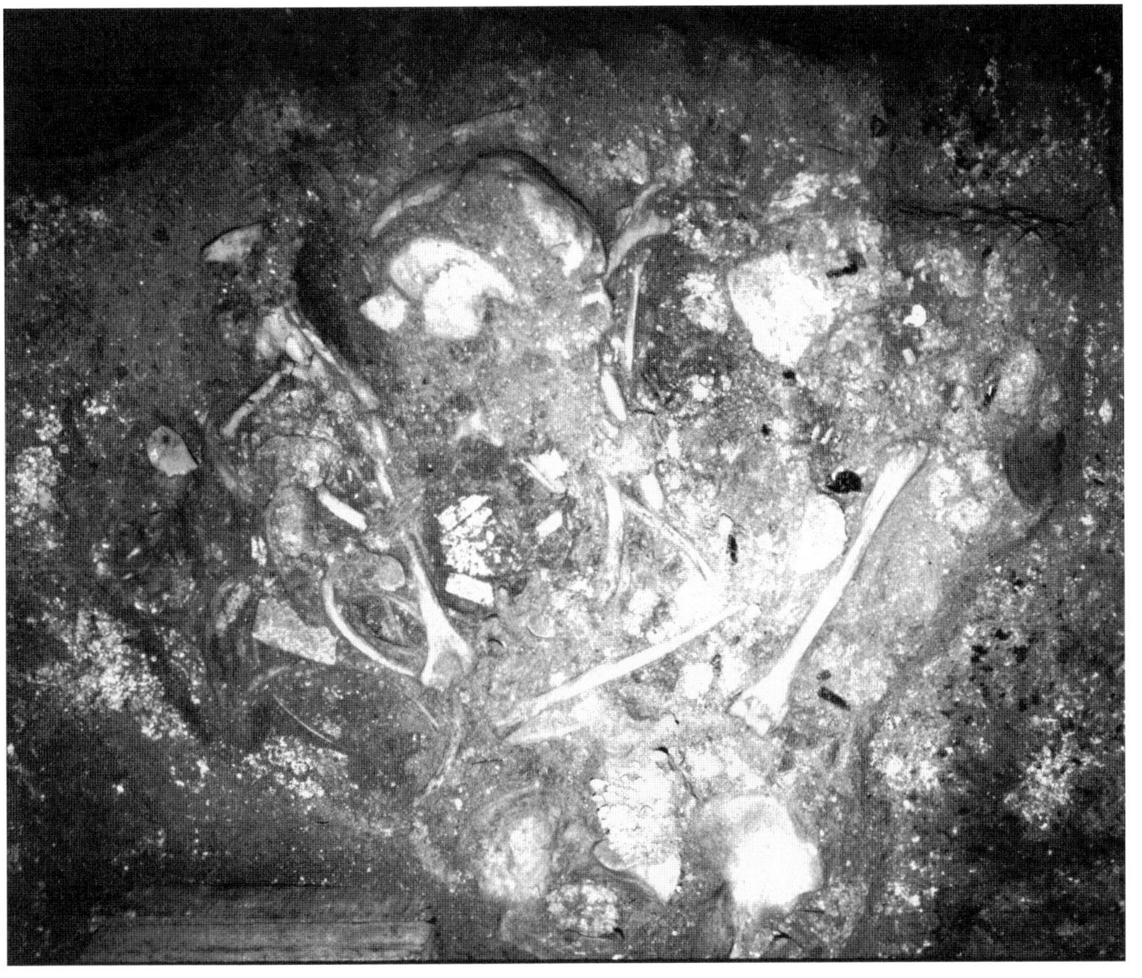

Plate 4.1. Cranial half of the skeleton from DP30, thought to be Ruler 2 of Dos Pilas. A dense accumulation of jade and shell ornaments cover the chest region.

burial TA6, suspected to be that of the ruler "Chanal Balam." The remaining factors at Tamarindito are grouped and bipolar.

This pattern is not found in the sample from Seibal (Table 4.10) in which PF1 is not preeminent, the eigenvalue curve is flatter (Figure 4.1b,e), and the factors show grouped or bipolar patterns among grave types, locations, positions, and accompaniments. The samples from Aguateca and Itzan likewise lack a grouped preeminent PF1 (Figure 4.1b) and are characterized by comparable grouped and bipolar factors (Tables 4.11 and 4.12). The absence of a superordinate dimension from these samples should not be taken to mean that an elite stratum was absent from the sites, for ruling dynasties are documented in monumental sculpture at each site. Sampling bias is clearly to blame at Aguateca and Itzan because excavation has emphasized domestic platforms where royal graves are unlikely to occur. At Seibal, absence of this dimension can be attributed to decided undersampling of Group B, which was the Late Classic ceremonial focus. However, Tourtellot (1988) has argued that the occupation was very small at this time, so may not have been able to command control of trade for PF1 superordinate symbols,

Table 4.9. Varimax rotated factor matrix for Late Classic Seibal burials

Variable	PF1	PF2	PF3	PF4	PF5	PF6	PF7	PF8	PF9	PF10
articulated	.239	**.544**	-.078	.248	.128	.416	.053	.082	.349	.030
cranium only	.091	.103	-.054	-.031	-.044	-.058	**.959**	-.048	-.087	.003
extended	-.061	.184	**.913**	-.018	-.021	.043	-.031	-.048	-.009	-.016
flexed on back	-.329	.113	-.189	**.689**	-.181	-.004	-.187	-.273	-.252	.061
flexed on left	.322	**-.841**	.046	-.147	-.080	.328	-.077	-.062	.077	-.066
flexed on right	.090	**.597**	-.226	-.298	.278	-.136	-.231	.370	.268	.011
head to north	-.063	.043	.392	.341	-.207	-.193	-.210	.398	**-.450**	-.379
head to south	-.111	.033	-.057	-.051	**.986**	-.035	-.037	-.026	-.059	-.014
head to east	.227	-.100	-.145	-.161	-.116	-.145	-.110	-.166	**.858**	-.093
head to west	-.016	.108	-.148	-.073	-.134	**.649**	-.174	-.179	-.250	.586
simple	**-.622**	.080	.247	-.242	-.333	-.351	-.232	-.398	.139	-.032
pit	-.022	-.095	-.058	-.086	-.056	.624	**.749**	-.032	-.102	-.030
cap	**.892**	-.053	-.182	-.117	-.064	.005	-.249	-.014	-.012	.089
capped pit	-.144	.048	-.066	-.050	-.070	-.025	-.040	**.921**	-.050	.009
cist	-.097	.036	-.050	-.048	**.985**	-.033	-.032	-.025	-.058	-.014
head cist	.010	-.033	-.009	**.955**	-.004	-.047	.003	.040	-.030	-.046
plate	.386	**.658**	.296	-.238	-.150	-.086	.300	-.123	-.044	.025
vase	**.577**	.013	-.062	-.051	-.035	-.037	.480	-.009	.022	.526
bowl	.241	.317	.312	.289	.339	-.069	-.205	**.375**	.373	-.337
worked bone	.368	.237	-.062	-.086	-.039	-.004	-.116	.066	-.177	**.788**
jade bead	-.121	-.233	-.027	-.086	-.034	**.912**	.068	.005	-.053	-.044
other jade	.448	.395	-.135	-.123	-.073	.036	-.205	.023	-.330	**-.603**
unworked shell	-.240	.116	-.060	-.050	-.069	-.035	-.065	.073	**.676**	-.033
residential	**.887**	.127	-.158	-.156	-.103	-.067	.237	-.109	.098	.036
ceremonial	.010	-.033	-.009	**.955**	-.004	-.047	.003	.040	-.030	-.046
plaza	-.076	-.259	**.864**	-.126	-.082	-.172	-.065	-.020	-.213	-.050
axial	.547	.453	.324	-.095	-.141	.070	-.316	-.233	-.036	.170
patio	**-.794**	.061	-.395	-.212	.153	.194	-.185	.096	.056	.021

Heavy loadings are indicated in bold. Together, the components account for 89.8% of the variance.

particularly during the period when it was under the control of Dos Pilas.

Among Terminal Classic samples, only Seibal burials show pattern 1 (Table 4.13, Figure 4.1c,e). Here, PF1 is characterized by heavy loadings of seated position, capped pit, jar, six or more vessels, worked bone, jade beads, worked shell, and polished stone. The remaining factors indicate covariation among small groups of variables. This pattern shares much in common with Late Classic samples from Altar and Dos Pilas but differs from contemporary burials at the same sites. Although differing in the nature of attributes that load highly, the presence of this superordinate dimension is consistent with the archaeologically documented maintenance of political authority into the final phase of Seibal occupation.

For Terminal Classic Altar burials, the variables that contributed to the Late Classic PF1 are notably absent, and PF1 indicates covariation

Table 4.10. Varimax rotated factor matrix for Late Classic Aguateca burials

Variable	PF1	PF2	PF3	PF4	PF5	PF6	PF7	PF8
single	**.779**	.035	.079	-.557	.023	-.077	.043	.154
extended	.289	-.172	-.197	-.135	**.785**	.167	-.130	-.178
flexed on left	.302	-.177	.332	.023	-.349	**-.635**	.013	.386
flexed on right	**-.635**	.384	-.044	.110	-.456	.327	.031	-.283
head to north	-.158	.166	-.415	-.409	**.657**	-.151	.022	.300
head to south	.016	-.035	**.857**	-.113	-.184	.119	.006	.063
head to east	.045	-.077	-.107	**.837**	-.218	.215	-.028	-.159
head to west	.185	-.118	-.116	-.236	**-.609**	-.062	-.032	-.363
simple	.023	-.055	-.062	-.015	-.071	.037	**.979**	.047
cap	.060	-.073	-.104	.125	-.114	.110	-.079	**-.895**
capped pit	.049	-.028	**.909**	.009	.031	-.116	-.032	.043
cist	**-.936**	-.060	-.091	-.097	.009	.064	-.095	.162
head cist	-.015	-.012	-.097	-.068	-.006	**-.907**	-.035	-.015
simple crypt	.513	.108	-.195	-.286	.076	.357	-.297	**.526**
plate	**.664**	.114	.148	.129	-.007	.377	-.400	.353
vase	.170	-.115	**.553**	-.011	.542	.046	-.022	.037
bowl	**.621**	.130	-.425	.136	.128	.272	-.337	.315
figurine	.059	**.985**	-.048	-.070	-.022	.045	-.018	.049
worked shell	.059	**.985**	-.048	-.070	-.022	.045	-.018	.049
unworked shell	-.020	.028	-.036	**.867**	.072	-.106	.004	-.009
chert	.021	**.749**	-.075	.583	-.002	-.006	-.03	.051
residential	**.936**	.060	.091	.097	-.009	-.064	.095	-.162
axial	.180	.361	.357	**.515**	.110	.041	.452	.068

Heavy loadings are indicated in bold. Together, the factors account for 87.4% of the variance.

among bowls, worked bone, and axial locations in residences (Table 4.14). Factor 2 is also grouped, documenting covariation of seated burials facing north and with plates. Instead, the matrix matches pattern 3, with a linear eigenvalue fall-off curve. Most factors are specific or bipolar, but incorporate coding redundancies, thus indicate minimal structure in the mortuary program. Because sampling recovered many Terminal Classic burials in monumental architecture, absence of the superordinate dimension cannot be easily attributed to sampling error. Recall that excavation and epigraphic evidence indicates that this occupation followed the collapse of elite authority at the site. These mortuary data suggest a breakdown or simplification of rules governing funerary ritual among the remnant population in conjunction with that collapse.

The small Terminal Classic sample from Dos Pilas shows similar bipolarity, with PF1 composed of attributes found only in a single subadult burial (Table 4.15). Eigenvalue falloff curves for these two samples are gradual, resembling the Preclassic curves more closely than either the Seibal sample or other Late Classic sites (Figure 4.1c,f). This sample is small and limited to a single domestic group, which undoubtedly explains the narrow definition of variable groupings and paucity of factors.

In addition to the emergence and disappearance of a superordinate dimension, these results also illustrate spatial and temporal changes in

Table 4.11. Varimax rotated factor matrix for Late Classic Itzan burials

Variable	PF1	PF2	PF3	PF4	PF5	PF6	PF7	PF8
articulated	-.223	**.933**	.152	-.139	.067	.003	-.131	.142
cranium only	.214	**-.931**	-.143	.131	-.058	-.127	.117	-.150
extended	-.369	.202	-.133	.180	**.813**	-.108	-.322	.027
flexed on right	.129	.505	.300	-.106	**-.803**	-.100	.184	.059
head to north	.240	**.821**	-.478	.069	.085	-.058	.031	-.056
head to south	**-.924**	-.115	-.025	.070	.083	.053	-.071	.146
head to west	.075	-.032	**.855**	-.385	-.076	.074	-.112	.061
simple	.078	-.540	-.097	.104	-.041	-.049	.105	**-.798**
pit	**-.823**	.081	-.063	.097	-.074	-.071	-.119	-.067
cap	.075	-.027	.043	**-.939**	.074	-.005	-.077	.024
capped pit	.209	.259	.508	.258	**.639**	-.145	.300	.032
cist	.182	.131	-.125	.204	.126	-.072	**-.833**	-.054
simple crypt	.298	-.033	-.315	.250	**-.638**	.218	.279	.513
plate	.370	-.199	-.143	-.399	**.573**	.350	.203	.401
vase	.155	.218	-.095	.146	**.648**	-.122	.294	.060
bowl	.425	-.101	.026	.111	.145	.136	**.753**	-.101
worked bone	.046	.047	-.040	.088	-.066	**.991**	.069	.028
unworked bone	**-.588**	-.578	-.104	.127	.073	-.089	.040	.469
jade bead	.061	.053	**.949**	.161	-.053	-.070	.100	-.032
worked shell	.061	.053	**.949**	.161	-.053	-.070	.100	-.032
unworked shell	**-.807**	.101	-.130	.168	-.130	-.083	.197	.065
obsidian	.046	.047	-.040	.088	-.066	**.991**	.069	.028
residential	-.100	-.150	.065	**.922**	.160	.102	-.090	-.001
plaza	**1.082**	-.215	-.059	.070	-.394	-.015	.180	.268
patio	.100	.150	-.065	**-.922**	-.160	-.102	.090	.001

Heavy loadings are indicated in bold. Together, the factors account for 95.1% of the variance.

subordinate burial dimensions. The small grouped factors that account for the bulk of the matrices document associations between variables that define dimensions of subordinate status. Among these there may be further vertical distinctions, but these are more subtle and are not easily ranked in social terms. In contrast to the superordinate dimension, the composition of these factors is sample specific; variables load differently at each site and over time. Differing covariation of variables in contemporaneous sites may illustrate the breadth of community participation in funerals. Elite interaction on a regional scale requires regionally recognized symbols of authority, while symbolic distinctions employed in lower-status funerals vary on a local level.

Chronological trends in attribute popularity are apparent. For instance, stingray spines load heavily on the Altar Early Classic PF1 but load on PF4 of Late Classic Dos Pilas, a pattern that could indicate either proliferation and diversification of elites at this time or emulation of elite ritual practices by lower-status groups. For Terminal Classic Seibal, exotic items are generally absent from the assemblage, and few of them load on PF1. While this pattern might reflect changes in trade systems

Table 4.12. Varimax rotated factor matrix for Late Classic Tamarindito burials

Variable	PF1	PF2	PF3	PF4	PF5	PF6	PF7
articulated	.105	**.868**	.041	-.044	-.286	.342	-.130
single	.085	**.901**	-.005	.060	.118	-.328	-.002
extended	.359	.322	-.028	-.410	**.694**	.223	.048
flexed on left	-.144	.208	.467	**.852**	-.103	-.067	-.084
flexed on right	-.139	-.165	-.122	-.236	**-.876**	.225	.139
head to north	.165	.295	.227	-.437	.026	**-.812**	.011
head to south	-.116	-.313	-.065	-.177	-.042	**.891**	.053
head to east	-.088	.034	-.175	**.911**	.068	.072	.095
simple	-.099	**-.822**	-.156	-.066	-.203	.228	-.303
simple crypt	-.472	**.749**	.149	.090	.156	-.132	.229
elaborate	**.989**	.004	-.013	-.020	.024	-.029	.087
jar	**.989**	.004	-.013	-.020	.024	-.029	.087
plate	.249	.346	-.283	.186	.065	.177	**.792**
vase	.359	.347	-.249	-.275	**.513**	.130	.368
bowl	.509	.228	.328	**.586**	.208	-.063	-.118
six vessels	**.989**	.004	-.013	-.020	.024	-.029	.087
stingray	**.989**	.004	-.013	-.020	.024	-.029	.087
jade bead	**.989**	.004	-.013	-.020	.024	-.029	.087
other jade	**.989**	.004	-.013	-.020	.024	-.029	.087
Spondylus valve	**.989**	.004	-.013	-.020	.024	-.029	.087
hematite	-.045	.096	**.872**	.207	-.042	-.057	-.100
chert	**.744**	.160	-.117	-.079	.245	-.118	-.171
obsidian	**.989**	.004	-.013	-.020	.024	-.029	.087
residential	-.262	.430	**-.550**	.261	.344	.127	-.440
patio	-.113	.111	**.907**	-.089	.128	-.074	-.112
ceremonial	.492	.156	-.100	-.178	-.426	-.261	**.639**
plaza	-.085	**-.901**	.005	-.060	-.118	.328	.002
axial	.262	**.485**	.072	.404	-.334	-.444	.085

Heavy loadings are indicated in bold. Together, the factors account for 85.1% of the variance.

generally, both univariate and principal factoring analyses reveal that skeletal positions and orientations also differ, indicating a change in the structure of symbolic status recognition.

Complete-linkage cluster analyses produced groupings of burials that reflect many of the patterns of variable association indicated by the principal factoring. The Preclassic samples from Altar and Seibal each contain four clusters (Figures 4.2 and 4.3). In each case, there are no obvious parallels between a specific cluster and the PFs, but instead the variables in a given cluster contribute to several PFs. Altar Cluster A is defined largely by PF1, containing multiple subadult burials. PF2 to PF6 contribute to Cluster B, which contains axial graves in ceremonial architecture accompanied by bowls, jade, and shell. Clusters C and D contrast graves in public space with few offerings against those with offerings in domestic space. At Seibal, the few Preclassic burials are divided among residential versus public contexts, by the presence of bowls, and by skeletal position.

In the Early Classic sample from Altar (Figure 4.4), the grouped PF1 contributes primarily

Table 4.13. Varimax rotated factor matrix for Terminal Classic Seibal burials

Variable	PF1	PF2	PF3	PF4	PF5	PF6	PF7	PF8	PF9
articulated	.136	**.871**	.136	.147	.137	.119	.133	.103	.099
single	.180	**.579**	.185	.240	.217	.430	.329	.324	.109
extended	-.168	**.628**	-.106	.316	-.266	-.304	.293	.276	.021
flexed on left	-.044	.118	-.133	-.093	-.021	**.811**	-.187	-.192	.026
flexed on right	-.062	.122	.515	-.127	**.738**	-.007	-.041	-.012	.119
seated	**.997**	.015	.019	-.005	-.019	-.035	.013	-.033	-.001
head to north	-.071	.128	**.732**	-.016	.466	-.02	-.096	.218	-.184
head to east	-.166	**.696**	-.268	-.223	-.145	.229	.181	-.217	.271
head to west	.569	.064	-.057	**.607**	-.038	-.004	-.124	.310	-.051
simple	-.062	.225	.061	-.116	-.005	-.051	-.045	**.870**	.146
pit	-.200	-.714	-.153	-.073	-.235	-.144	.087	-.291	-.132
slab	-.027	.044	-.037	**.912**	.028	-.044	-.132	-.051	.107
cap	-.075	**.623**	-.202	-.184	-.172	.149	-.495	-.322	.059
capped pit	**.737**	-.105	-.025	.000	.031	.205	.046	.112	-.064
cist	-.026	.022	-.009	.034	**.903**	-.030	-.019	.024	-.065
head cist	-.067	.239	-.091	-.082	.001	-.043	**.701**	-.098	-.120
simple crypt	-.051	.020	**.925**	-.028	.034	.059	-.022	-.166	.179
jar	**.997**	.006	.020	-.001	-.017	-.031	.018	-.027	.002
plate	.362	.294	-.055	.017	-.179	.010	**.609**	.031	.239
vase	.542	.119	**.749**	-.037	-.086	-.021	-.074	.187	-.144
bowl	.192	**.764**	.262	-.172	-.130	-.013	.250	-.196	-.176
≥ 6 vessels	**.997**	.006	.020	-.001	-.017	-.031	.018	-.027	.002
figurine	-.065	.115	-.002	**.850**	-.086	.018	.173	-.136	-.008
worked bone	**.997**	.006	.020	-.001	-.017	-.031	.018	-.027	.002
unworked bone	-.062	.067	.621	-.084	-.018	-.019	.083	.168	.700
jade bead	**.997**	.006	.020	-.001	-.017	-.031	.018	-.027	.002
worked shell	**.997**	.006	.020	-.001	-.017	-.031	.018	-.027	.002
polished stone	**.997**	.006	.020	-.001	-.017	-.031	.018	-.027	.002
residential	-.105	.260	.347	.026	-.194	**.729**	.220	.239	-.258
ceremonial	.210	**-.826**	-.123	-.153	-.189	-.301	-.130	-.192	-.046
plaza	-.059	.247	-.115	.504	-.094	-.122	-.138	.165	.684
axial	.157	**-.747**	.101	-.299	-.081	.294	.015	-.240	.022
patio	-.095	**.530**	-.157	-.220	**.531**	-.380	.013	-.163	-.159

Heavy loadings are indicated in bold. Together, the components account for 87.3% of the variance.

Table 4.14. Varimax rotated factor matrix for Terminal Classic Altar de Sacrificios burials

Variable	PF1	PF2	PF3	PF4	PF5	PF6	PF7	PF8
articulated	-.083	.046	.066	-.059	**.908**	.065	.029	-.005
cranium only	.132	.013	-.03	.065	**-.848**	-.062	-.039	.077
single	.069	-.026	-.195	**.920**	-.029	.053	.013	-.008
extended	.017	-.205	-.076	.077	.119	-.179	**.823**	.283
flexed on back	-.038	-.003	**.841**	-.278	.027	.029	-.002	-.019
flexed on left	-.054	-.133	-.121	.108	.148	-.158	-.145	**-.848**
flexed on right	-.203	-.111	-.385	.117	.227	.121	**-.558**	.542
seated	.208	**.763**	-.152	-.048	-.008	.176	.139	-.153
head to north	-.087	**.794**	.222	-.124	.016	.223	-.135	.123
head to south	.092	.090	.261	.236	.246	**-.693**	-.081	-.082
head to east	.093	**-.728**	-.353	-.103	.138	.412	.095	-.095
simple	.143	-.189	-.162	-.198	-.163	**-.827**	.008	-.059
pit	-.126	.030	.183	.218	.161	**.762**	-.133	.137
jar	.237	.027	**.757**	.159	.099	.031	-.065	.071
plate	.277	**.633**	-.275	.124	.204	-.036	.115	.220
vase	-.083	.375	-.122	.049	.036	.314	**.621**	-.111
bowl	**.485**	.271	-.186	.217	.326	.376	-.058	.231
worked bone	.302	.261	-.255	.015	.115	**.372**	.137	-.123
residential	**.922**	.091	.117	.099	-.095	-.192	.066	.082
ceremonial	**-.845**	-.090	-.071	.363	.041	.234	-.050	-.101
plaza	.063	-.009	-.080	**-.844**	.088	-.097	-.051	.049
axial	**.876**	-.039	.086	.088	-.234	.046	-.089	-.193

Heavy loadings are indicated in bold. Together, the factors account for 78.0% of the variance.

Table 4.15. Varimax rotated factor matrix for Terminal Classic Dos Pilas burials

Variable	PF1	PF2	PF3	PF4
cranium	-.389	**-.494**	-.630	-.433
single	.110	.178	.185	.111
flexed on back	-.056	-.065	.017	.987
flexed on left	-.083	-.071	**.800**	-.070
flexed on right	-.056	**.828**	.309	-.036
seated	**.999**	-.013	.023	.003
head to north	-.065	.657	-.061	.737
head to south	**.999**	-.013	.023	.003
head to east	-.091	.072	**.963**	-.108
simple	.035	**-.972**	.102	-.030
cap	-.035	**.972**	-.102	.030
worked shell	**.999**	-.013	.023	.003
residential	.356	-.086	**.656**	.422
axial	**.999**	-.013	.023	.003

Heavy loadings are indicated in bold. Together, the factors account for 88.9% of the variance.

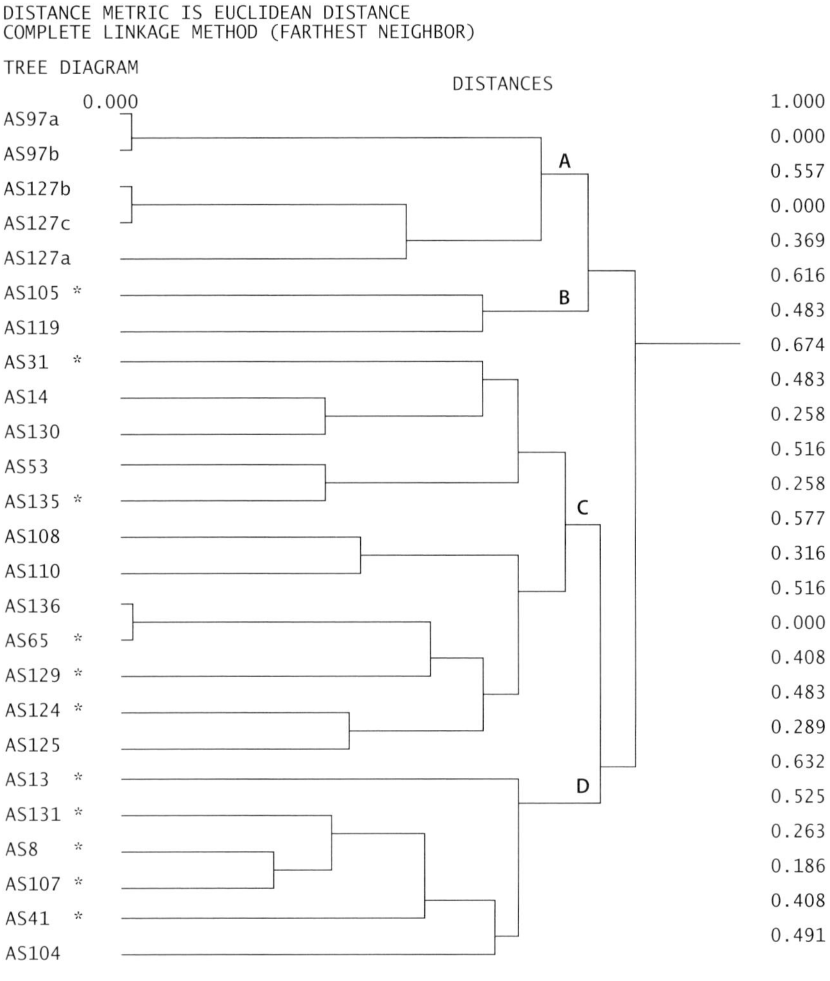

Figure 4.2. Tree diagram for Preclassic Altar de Sacrificios burial clusters

Skeletons sampled for chemical analyses are indicated by asterisks (*).

to Cluster D, but is also evident in Cluster A. In Clusters D and C, skeletal position and distinctions in artifacts reinforce the contrast between graves in ceremonial architecture and those in residential architecture. Clusters B and A group burials from diverse locations, grave forms, and grave goods that do not readily align with the remaining burials.

The Late Classic samples from Altar, Dos Pilas, and Tamarindito each illustrate one cluster (D, E, and A respectively) with very few burials, in contrast to most other clusters, which are large (Figures 4.5, 4.6, and 4.7). In each case, this small cluster is the last joined to the tree diagram and is characterized by variables that load on the preeminent PF1. Two of the skeletons in Dos Pilas Cluster E (DP30 and DP20) and the only Tamarindito burial in Cluster A (TA6) have been identified as probable members of royal dynasties. This supports the interpretation that the superordinate dimension corresponds to symbols of authority restricted to members of ruling dynasties. At Altar de Sacrificios, this superordinate dimension corresponds to Late Classic burials AS88 and AS128. The latter has been interpreted as the grave of a woman of the "ruling class" on the grounds of

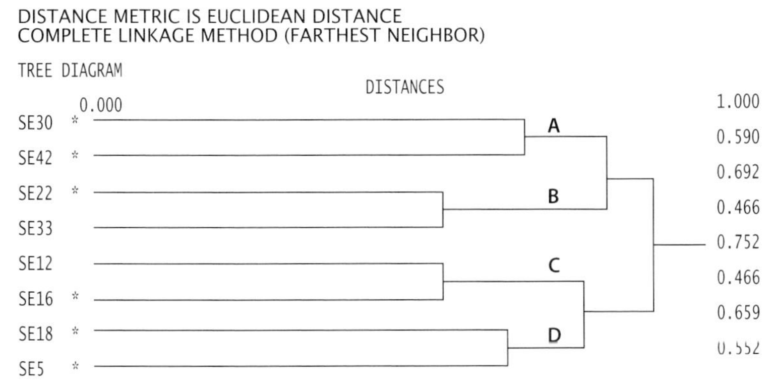

Figure 4.3. Tree diagram for Preclassic Seibal burial clusters

Skeletons sampled for chemical analyses are indicated by asterisks (*).

iconographic scenes on the Altar Vase, recovered from an associated burial (AS96) (Adams 1971:76–8), but there is no direct evidence for the identity of either burial.

The three subordinate clusters of Late Classic Altar represent divisions on the basis of location, grave type, and artifacts (Figure 4.5). A variety of skeletal positions are represented in each cluster. Cluster A contains axial residential burials in simple or cap graves with few artifacts, perhaps a single jar, plate, or bowl. Disarticulated burials also cluster here. In contrast, Cluster B contains articulated and cranial burials in simple graves, cists, and headcists; located in ceremonial architecture; and accompanied by plates, vases, or bowls. A third subordinate cluster, Cluster C, contains two graves that share eastern orientation; a plate, vase, jade bead, and chert as accompaniments; and burial in ceremonial location, variables that are grouped on PF6. One of these burials (AS96) has been interpreted as an elite sacrificial victim (Adams 1971), and this group may represent a high subordinate or intermediate status.

At Dos Pilas, Cluster C is distinguished from Clusters A, B, and D by burial in simple and cap graves rather than crypts, and by fewer ceramics and trade goods (Figure 4.6). The small Cluster B contains three burials that consisted only of a cranium. Cluster D (Plate 4.2) graves contain more ceramics, especially vases and bowls, than Cluster A burials, but the latter contain more jade and shell ornaments. Graves in both Cluster A and Cluster D are predominately simple crypts, with north being the dominant orientation for Cluster D, while east predominates for Cluster A. Cluster E contains three graves, including the likely tombs of Ruler 2 (DP30) and the "Woman from Cancuen" (DP20), which suggests a high elite or "royal" status for the third burial in the cluster, DP54. This burial was only partially excavated in 1994 from Str. N5-71, a small temple in the Murcielagos palace group.

In the small sample from Tamarindito (Figure 4.7), Cluster A contains the grave hypothesized to be that of the ruler "Chanal Balam" (TA6) (Valdés 1997) because of inscriptions on the stela in front of the structure. Cluster B contains flexed skeletons that were accompanied by tripod plates, while Cluster C contains extended skeletons with head to the north found in domestic contexts. Cluster D contains two skeletons that were buried together in a simple grave in an architectural terrace in the site center.

The Late Classic sample from Seibal contains three clusters that divide the sample according to location (Figure 4.8). Cluster A largely contains

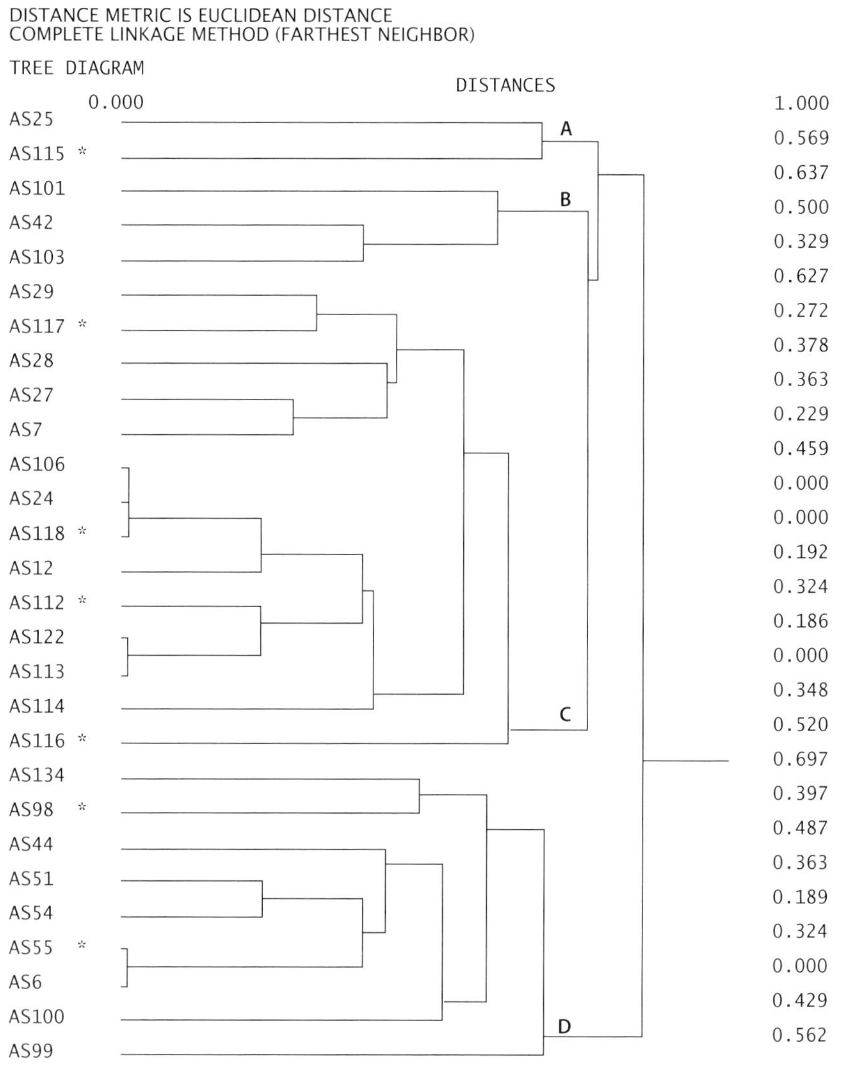

Figure 4.4. Tree diagram for Early Classic Altar de Sacrificios burial clusters

Skeletons sampled for chemical analyses are indicated by asterisks (*).

simple graves in patios, flexed on the back, with bowls, corresponding to the emphases of PF1 and PF4. Cluster B contains axial, simple graves, beneath plazas, flexed on the right side, with plates and bowls (PF2 and PF3). The final cluster, C, corresponds to axial cap graves in residential architecture, often flexed on the left, head to the east, with plates and vases. Cluster C might be considered the terminal cluster, but it contains a significant proportion of the sample, in contrast to the terminal clusters of Late Classic Altar and Dos Pilas.

Aguateca burials are divided into five clusters (Figure 4.9). Clusters B and D are the largest: Cluster B groups extended burials oriented to the north, in simple crypts, with plates and bowls; Cluster D groups flexed burials, also oriented to the north, in various grave types, and with few or

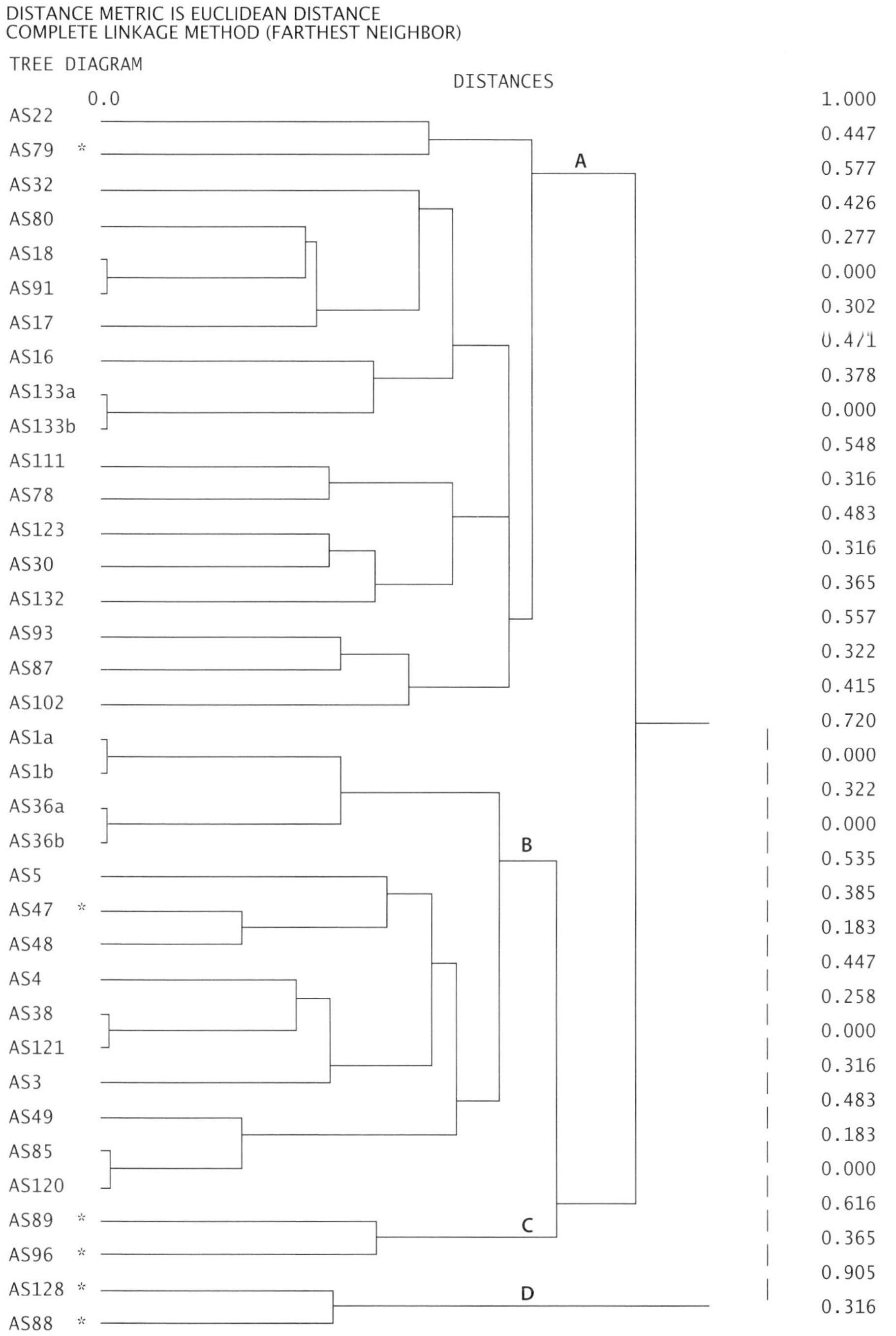

Figure 4.5. Tree diagram for Late Classic Altar de Sacrificios burial clusters

Skeletons sampled for chemical analyses are indicated by asterisks (*).

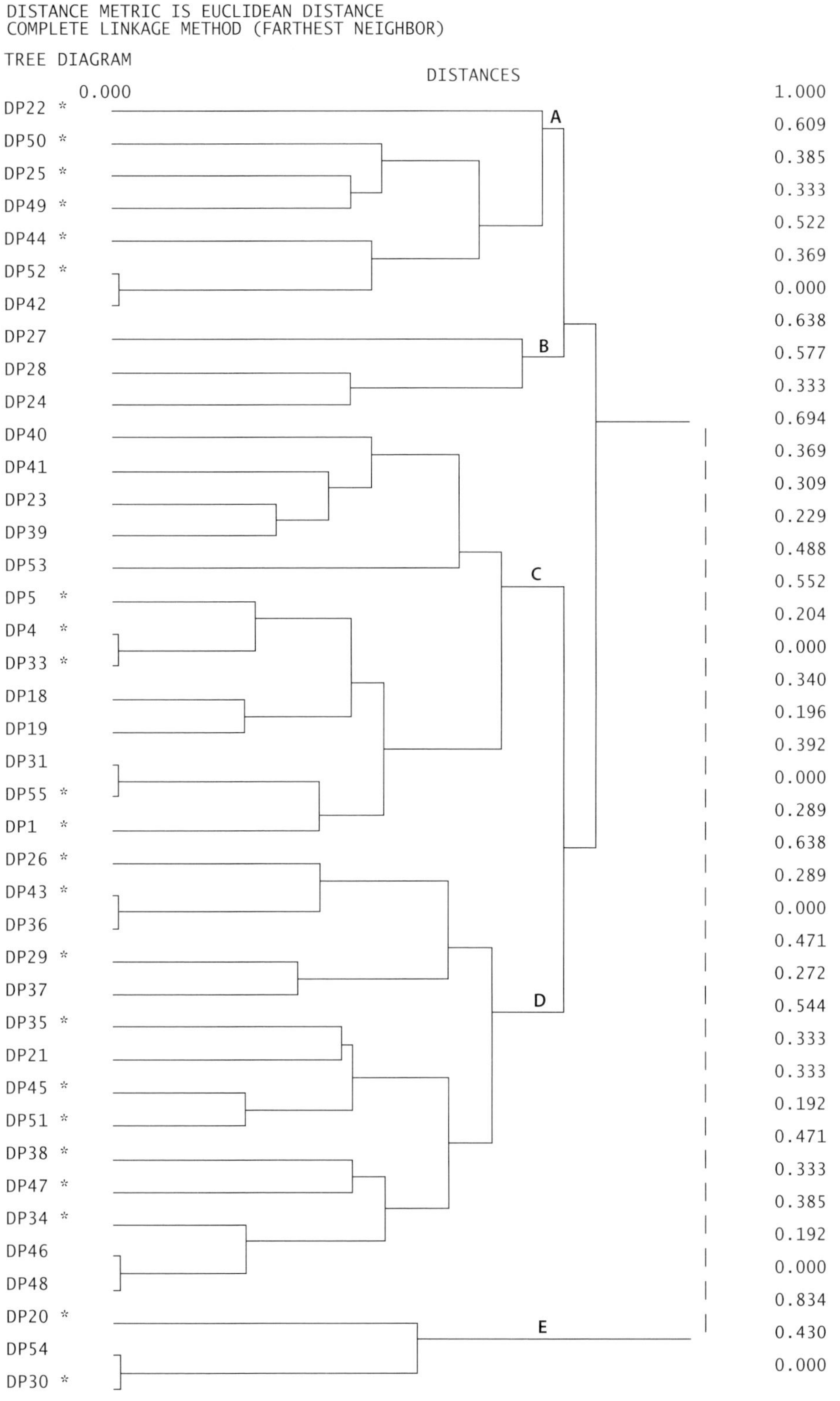

Figure 4.6. Tree diagram for Late Classic Dos Pilas burial clusters

Skeletons sampled for chemical analyses are indicated by asterisks (*).

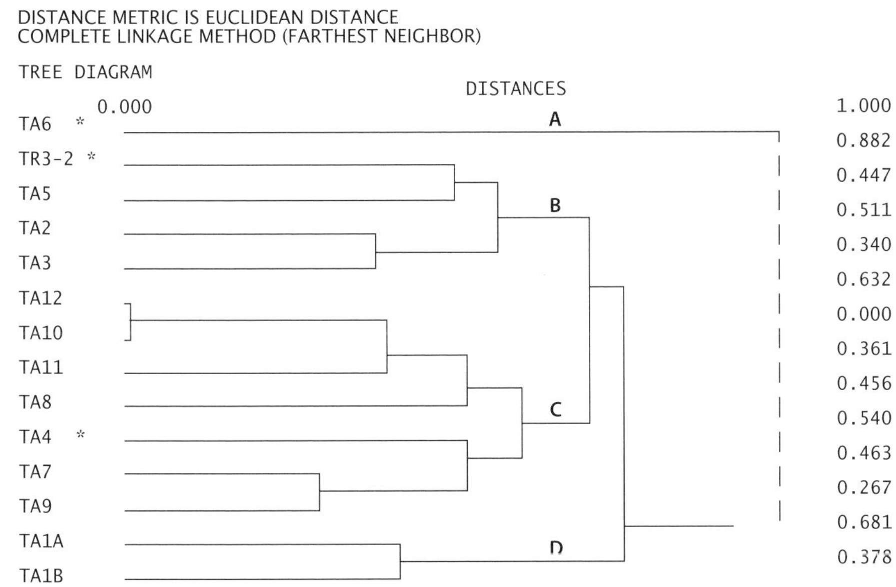

Figure 4.7. Tree diagram for Late Classic Tamarindito burial clusters

Skeletons sampled for chemical analyses are indicated by asterisks (*).

no goods. Two skeletons from a looted cap grave at Quim Chi Hilan were isolated in Cluster C, perhaps due to missing data on position and accompaniments. Two other burials form separate clusters, Clusters A and E, due to unique grave form or artifacts that might not have been singled out in a larger sample.

The Itzan sample is composed of four clusters (Figure 4.10). Cluster A contains capped pit graves in residential architecture; Cluster B contains cap graves below patios; Cluster C contains simple crypts, and cranial-only burials in residential architecture; while Cluster D contains the simple burial in the causeway. With a larger, more diverse sample, several of these clusters would likely have been joined below the 0.60 level.

The Terminal Classic sample from Seibal shows a pattern common to the Late Classic series from Dos Pilas and Altar (Figure 4.11). The terminal cluster contains a single burial characterized by the variables that compose PF1. Burial SE1 contains the characteristic attributes of the superordinate dimension but has been interpreted as a sacrificial victim on the basis of its female skeleton, seated position, and "domestic" vessels (Tourtellot 1990:87). None of these traits is sufficient to confirm sacrifice as cause of death. For instance, nondomestic vessels also accompany the bones (e.g., a Pabellon Modelled–carved vase). Females are found in Late Classic superordinate burials (e.g., AS128, DP20) and are known to have occasionally held important political offices. The remaining clusters in the Terminal Classic Seibal sample differentiate single burials in domestic contexts buried flexed on the right side (Cluster C) from those in varied domestic and public contexts (Cluster B).

There is little evidence in the Terminal Classic Seibal burials to support the idea of foreign invasion. Tourtellot (1990:139) had suggested that shifts to more consistent extended posture, eastern orientation, and burial in structures indicated immigration to the site. In addition, he cited the cessation of dental mutilation, the emergence of cranial deformation, and a change in stature. On reexamining the remains, however, I observed that

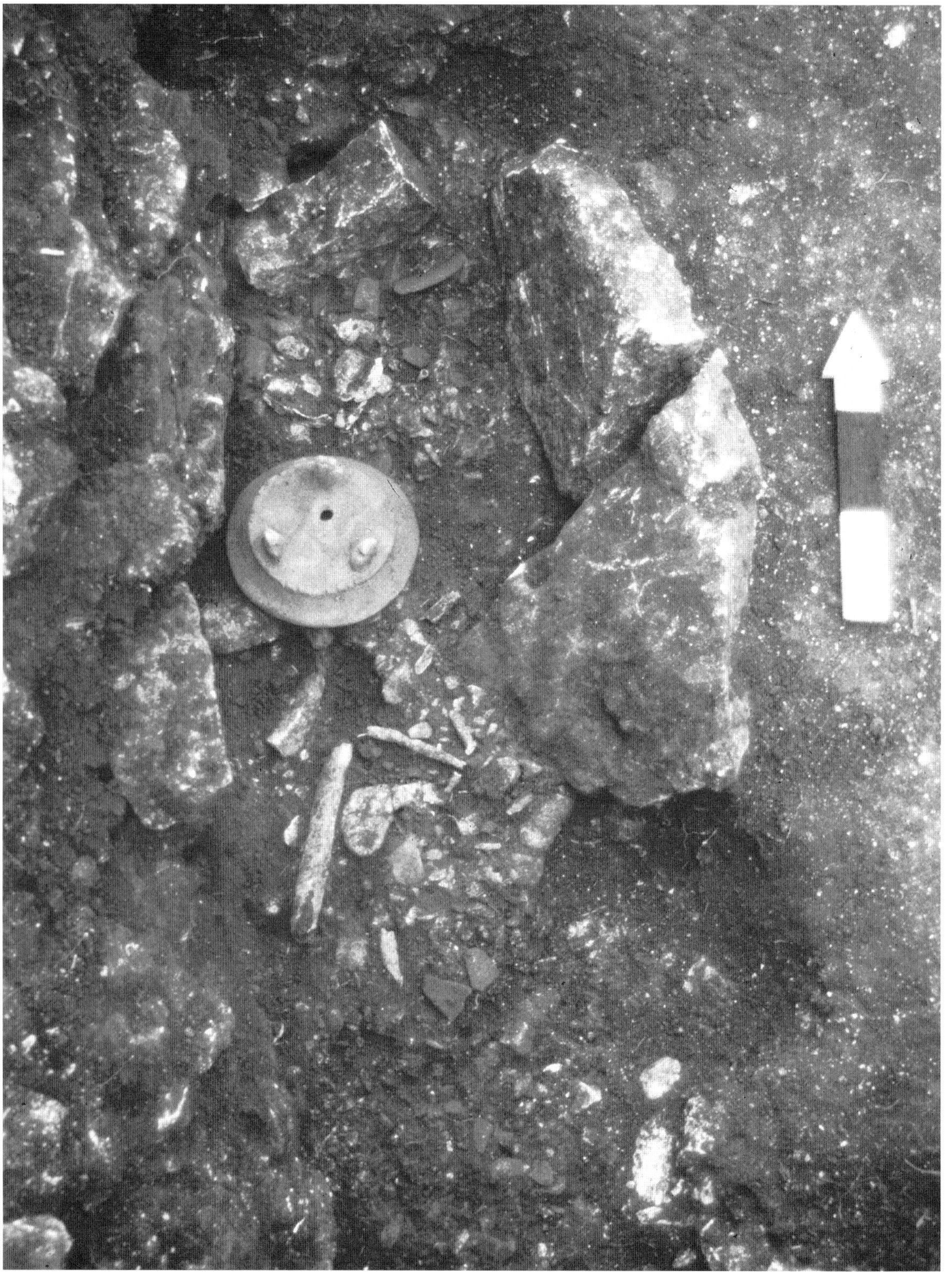

Plate 4.2. Burial DP48, a Cluster D simple crypt grave, after removal of the capstones.
The flexed skeleton is oriented with its head to the north, and the head is covered by a tripod plate.

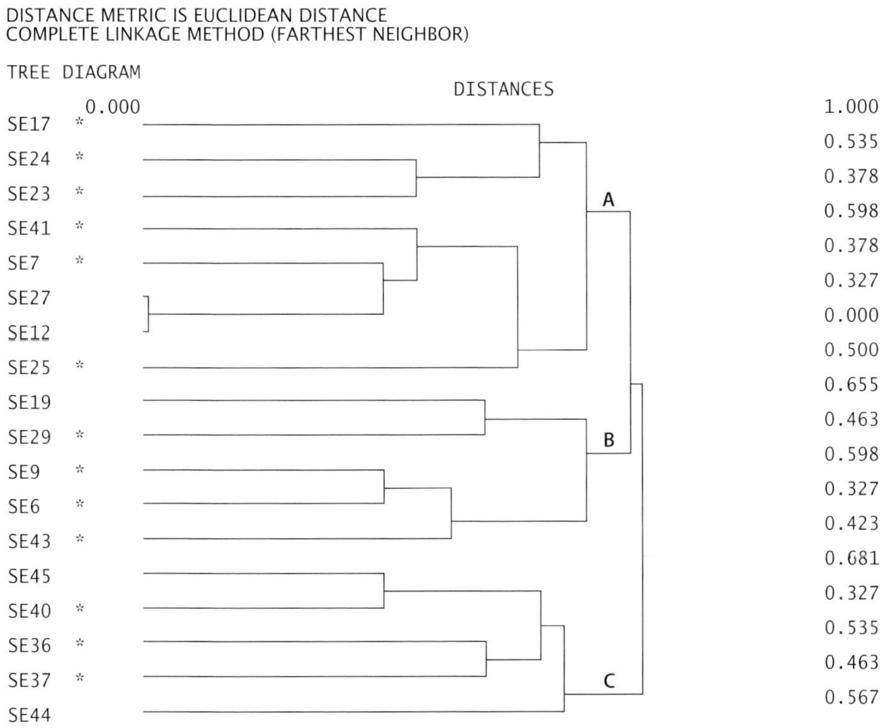

Figure 4.8. Tree diagram for Late Classic Seibal burial clusters

Skeletons sampled for chemical analyses are indicated by asterisks (*).

dental mutilation does indeed occur in several Bayal burials, and cranial deformation is present in earlier burials. Although the mean stature of males appears shorter, it is not statistically significant (Tepejilote 153cm±14.3, $n = 9$; Bayal 159cm±10.9, $n = 6$; $t = 0.78$, $p = 0.45$, d.f. = 13) (Wright 1994:158–61). Moreover, of the traits cited by Tourtellot, most have longstanding precedents in the Maya area and locally in the Pasión. Although the burial remains do not constitute evidence of foreign non-Maya intrusions into Terminal Classic Seibal, it is possible that changes in orientation and skeletal position might be related to an influx of local Pasión Maya peoples from sites that were abandoned at this time (Demarest and Escobedo 1998; Demarest 2006). This would account for the rapid increase in settlement density in central Seibal at this time (Tourtellot III 1988) and has implications for the mortuary and dietary trends that are the focus of this study.

In contrast to the pattern shown at Seibal, the Terminal Classic sample from Altar contains five clusters of burials (Figure 4.12). The clusters divide the sample on the basis of burial location, grave type, and orientation. Skeletal position is not patterned across clusters. Clusters A to D contain graves in ceremonial architecture that are distinguished by grave type (A and B in pits, C and D in simple graves) and orientation (A to north, B and C to east, D to south). No clusters identify "wealthy" burials, but Cluster D contains graves that are artifact poor. Cluster E groups axial residential burials in simple graves that show a range of orientations, positions, and accompaniments. In contrast to other samples where clusters are defined by several interacting variables, this diagram is more treelike than paradigmatic; the variables are not redundant and combine in an unstructured manner.

Finally, the small Terminal Classic sample

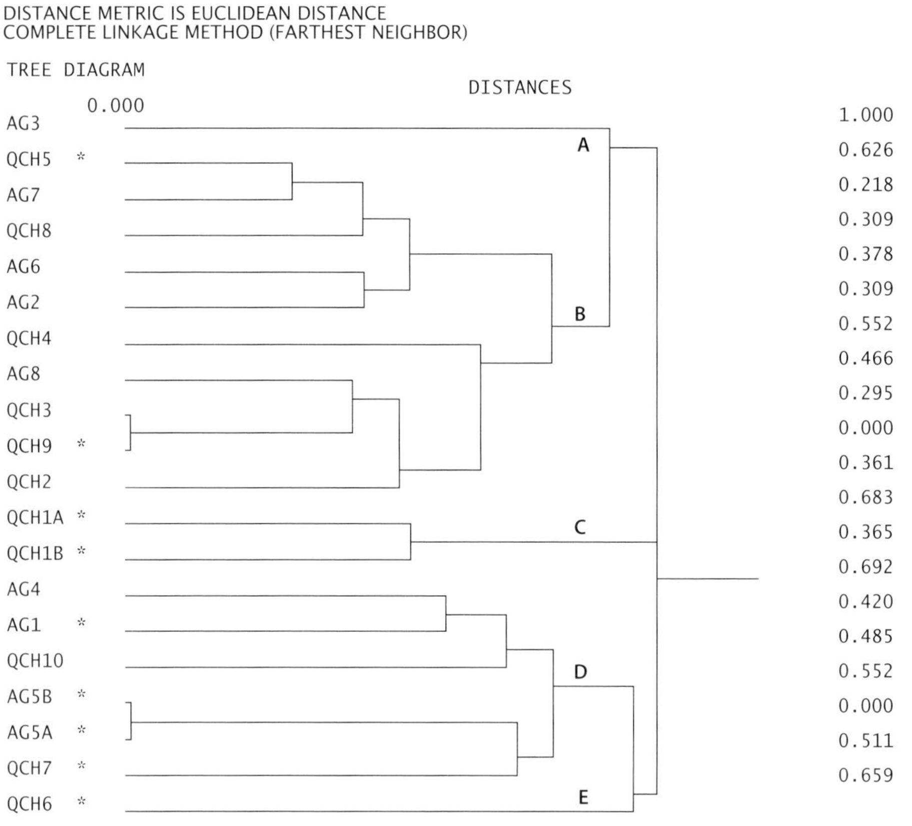

Figure 4.9. Tree diagram for Late Classic Aguateca burial clusters

Skeletons sampled for chemical analyses are indicated by asterisks (*).

from Dos Pilas is dominated by the decapitated crania of Cluster C, all sharing essentially identical attributes (Figure 4.13). The single subadult burial accompanied by a shell is isolated in its own Cluster A, as is the flexed cap grave in exterior space (Cluster D). Cluster C unites flexed burials without offerings below a low platform (Plate 4.3).

Some parallels can be seen in the definition of clusters between samples. As noted above, clusters are often distinguished by burial context and grave form. Excavation biases between sites and differential selection of grave types at the sites account for some differences in clustering between sites. It is likely that the general location of a burial had similar connotations across the region. Grave form shows significant site-specific patterning, however, making it difficult to identify equivalent clusters.

Apart from the superordinate dimension of variables that characterize the terminal cluster of some samples, it is difficult to rank the remaining clusters in terms of social strata; differences could represent either horizontal or vertical distinctions. The lack of common variable patterning between samples and site-specific variable use would necessitate different ranking criteria for each sample. Accordingly, no attempt will be made to identify equivalent clusters between samples. Instead, I will consider variability in dietary composition between clusters for each sample.

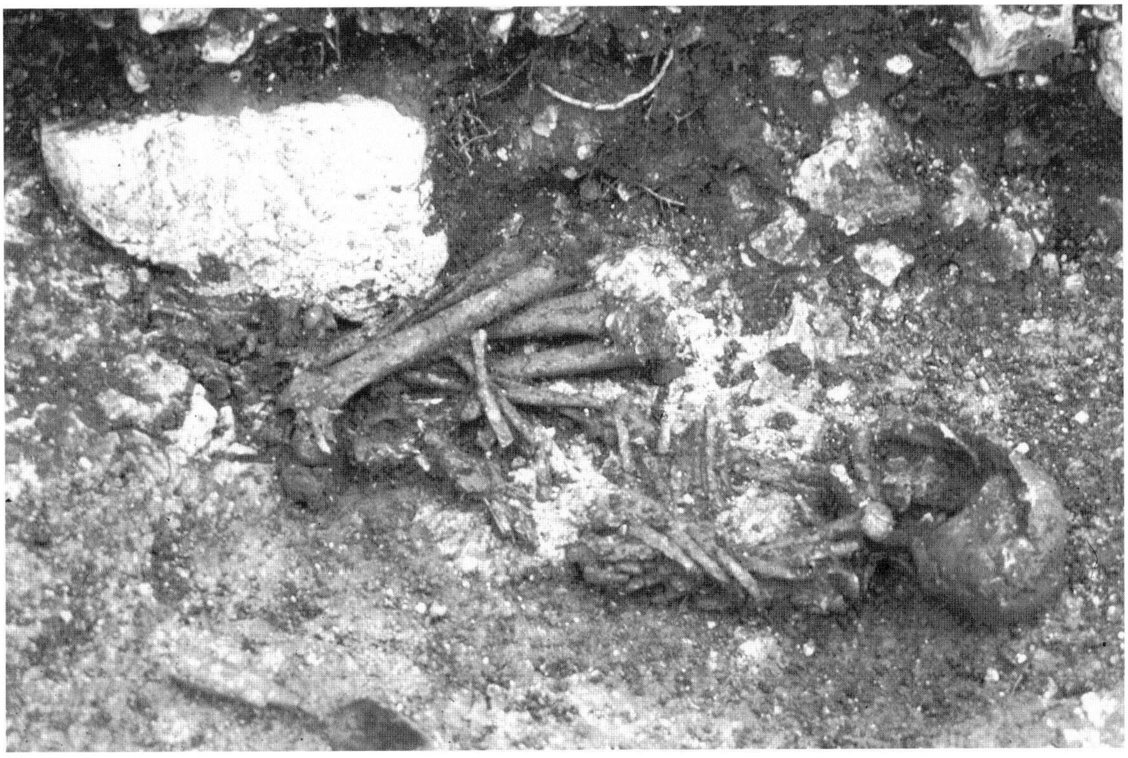

Plate 4.3. Burial DP13, a Terminal Classic cap grave, after removal of most of the cap stones. The skeleton is not accompanied by any grave goods.

teractions alone and perhaps emphasize kinship patterns and wealth distribution more than social office (*sensu* McAnany 1993).

Despite these difficulties, changes in the structure of Pasión society are illustrated in the organization of the mortuary domain over time and space. Emergence of the Late Classic elite is most apparent. Furthermore, patterns of variable covariation indicate changes in the formality of mortuary program organization. Over the Classic period, mortuary roles became increasingly formal and the superordinate stratum was emphasized by greater symbolic redundancy. Changes in attribute distributions illustrate changing rules governing trait expression. Most dramatic is the loss of this formal structure among Terminal Classic burials. Mortuary data from this final occupation indicate a loss of the superordinate dimension, except at Seibal where it was heralded by a very different set of symbols than in Late Classic times. Subordinate dimensions are less structured and show renewed emphasis on personal characteristics (age and sex), suggesting greater fluidity of social roles or perhaps rapid change in the definition of roles and mortuary symbols.

CHAPTER 5

Theoretical Foundations of Dietary Chemistry

As a major component in the articulation of prehistoric peoples with ancient landscapes, subsistence systems are a key focus of archaeological investigation. Archaeologists have pursued prehistoric foodways by examining food residues—botanical and faunal remains—recovered from archaeological sites and by considering technical aspects of culinary practices through material culture. Innovations in the chemical analysis of human bones over the last two decades provide a complementary avenue that allows comparison of actual diets consumed by individuals in extinct populations. These approaches are based on the principle that the chemical signature of foods consumed is recorded in the tissues of the consumer. Together, stable isotopic analysis and elemental analysis provide complementary approaches to examine the diet of past peoples.

Stable Isotopes

Most chemical elements exist in several different forms, known as isotopes. Atoms of different isotopes are identified by their nuclear weight; they contain the same number of protons but different numbers of neutrons. Isotopes are denoted by the number of protons plus neutrons in the nucleus, written as a superscript before the element symbol. Some isotopes are unstable or radioactive, as in the case of ^{14}C (carbon-14), which is used to date archaeological materials. Stable isotopes are not radioactive; their relative abundance in nature is determined by differences in the rate at which they react with other chemicals. The stable isotopic properties of a number of elements make them useful for examining ecological relationships in biology and anthropology. In this study, I consider only two elements: carbon and nitrogen. Their abundance in a natural ecosystem is determined by metabolic incorporation and fractionation in the food web.

Isotopic composition is measured as a ratio between two isotopes relative to a standard of known composition. By convention, the isotopic ratio (δ), expressed in permil (‰), is calculated as follows:

$$\delta = \{(R_{sample}/R_{standard}) - 1\} \times 1000$$

where R is the ratio of the heavier to the lighter isotope, for example, $^{13}C/^{12}C$. For carbon isotopes, the recognized standard is PeeDee Belemnite (PDB), a fossil limestone from South Carolina composed of *Belemnitella americana*. For nitrogen, the isotopic ratio of atmospheric N_2 (AIR) is used as a standard (Ambrose 1993; Schwarcz and Schoeninger 1991).

Relative to another data point, the isotopic composition of a tissue is said to be "heavy," or "isotopically enriched," when it contains proportionately more of the heavy isotope (that with an extra neutron). "Heavy" data have relatively larger values on the $\delta^{15}N_{AIR}$ scale and more positive values on the $\delta^{13}C_{PDB}$ scale. Conversely, measurements with relatively less of the heavy isotope are referred to as "light."

The natural distribution of the two stable isotopes of carbon, ^{13}C and ^{12}C, is largely a consequence of photosynthetic mechanisms employed by plants. During photosynthesis, less ^{13}C is incorporated into plants than is available in the air because this heavier isotope forms stronger chemical bonds in CO_2 and diffuses more slowly than the lighter ^{12}C. Two major photosynthetic pathways,

C3 and C4, incorporate the two isotopes differentially, producing distinct ratios in plant tissues. Photosynthesis metabolizes either a 3- or 4-carbon product during CO_2 fixation, for which the pathways are named (Edwards and Walker 1983; O'Leary 1988).

In plants using the C3 or Reductive Pentose Phosphate (RPP) Pathway (once called the Benson-Calvin cycle), CO_2 is carboxylated to ribulose 1,5-pentaphosphate (RBP) by the enzyme RBP carboxylase and then reduced to triose phosphate (C3). The tissues of C3 plants contain much less ^{13}C than is available in atmospheric CO_2. Kinetic isotope effects in carboxylation by the RBP enzyme produce a fractionation of 34‰ relative to that of air (−7‰$_{PDB}$) so that C3 plants have tissue $\delta^{13}C$ near −27.1±2.0‰ (Edwards and Walker, 1983:107–9, 467–70; O'Leary, 1988:334).

In contrast, plants using the C4 of Hatch-Slack pathway have much heavier isotopic values averaging −13.1±1.2‰. In the C4 pathway, bicarbonate (HCO_3^-) is fixed in mesophyll cells with phosphoenolpyruvate (PEP) to C3 precursor molecules producing the C4 acids malate, aspartate, and oxaloacetate. These C4 acids are shunted to the bundle sheath where decarboxylation takes place by PEP carboxykinase, and then follow through the RPP cycle. Isotopic fractionation by PEP carboxykinase (−2‰) is much less marked than by RBP. C4 tissue $\delta^{13}C$ is determined by the rate of diffusion of CO_2 in plant tissues and fractionation in the equilibrium of CO_2 to HCO_3^- (in which the heavier isotope is concentrated or enriched by 8‰). Thus, C4 plants are more enriched in ^{13}C than C3 plants are (Edwards and Walker 1983:299–307, 467–70; O'Leary 1988:334).

Plants that use a third pathway, Crassulacean Acid Metabolism (CAM), tend to have heavy $\delta^{13}C$ values like C4 plants but are more variable, occasionally resembling C3 isotopic signatures. Unlike either C3 or C4 daylight photosynthesis, CAM photosynthesis occurs at night, in the dark. The pathway is an adaptation to water stress as it allows these plants to keep their stomata closed during the day, minimizing water loss. CAM plants conduct dark acidification in which bicarbonate is fixed to produce the C4 acid malate, which is stored in vacuoles and then decarboxylated by PEP carboxykinase during the following day, and this CO_2 is shunted to the RPP pathway. As in C4 plants, bicarbonate ^{13}C enrichment and PEP carboxylation determine tissue $\delta^{13}C$. Many CAM species are obligate and always use this mechanism of photosynthesis, thus they have heavy $\delta^{13}C$ signatures like those of C4 plants. Others are facultative and also utilize a daylight mode of photosynthesis in which CO_2 is fixed by RBP carboxylase in a manner analogous to C3 photosynthesis, which lowers the net $\delta^{13}C$ of their tissues, producing intermediate values to either C3 or C4 plants (Edwards and Walker 1983:449, 465–70).

Smaller variations in the $\delta^{13}C$ of plants can be caused by several other environmental and biochemical mechanisms independent of photosynthetic pathway. The biochemical composition of various plant foods may explain some of the differences between species. For instance, plant lipids are slightly depleted relative to the whole plant (DeNiro and Epstein 1978), but cellulose is slightly enriched (Tieszen 1991). Variation in the lipid and fiber content of plant foods thereby produce variation in the overall isotopic signal. Moreover, genetic differences between strains within a species may produce differences in $\delta^{13}C$ on the order of 2–3‰ (Tieszen 1991). Comparisons of modern and prehistoric maize specimens find little difference in carbon isotopic composition when corrected for an anthropogenic decline in atmospheric CO_2 isotopic composition since industrialization (Tieszen and Fagre 1993a:44).

In dense forests, the reassimilation of respired CO_2 can have a significant effect on the $\delta^{13}C$ of plants. Carbon dioxide released in plant respiration is depleted in $\delta^{13}C$, so its use in subsequent soil respiration further lowers the $\delta^{13}C$ of plant tissues. This "canopy effect" produces lower $\delta^{13}C$ near the forest floor than at the canopy, so forest plants may have $\delta^{13}C$ as low as −35‰ (van der Merwe and Medina 1991).

Aquatic plants may differ significantly from terrestrial plants. In marine systems, dissolved ^{13}C is enriched relative to atmospheric levels. Most marine plants use the C3 pathway and have $\delta^{13}C$ close to −19‰ (Ambrose 1993). In coral reef ecosystems $\delta^{13}C$ is more positive still (Keegan and DeNiro 1988). Freshwater carbon isotopic signals are largely dependent upon the relative contribution of terrestrial C3 and C4 plants to detritus from which dissolved carbon originates (Fry et al. 1983).

The isotopic composition of plants is preserved in the tissues of animals that consume them. The isotopic signal is transferred to animals with some fractionation between trophic levels. For carbon isotopes the trophic level effect is generally stated to be small, but a broad range of values have been reported from laboratory experiments, from shifts of +1‰ in small mammals to values up to 6.0‰ for large animals (summarized in Ambrose 1993:Table 5). A diet-collagen fractionation of 3–5‰ is often cited (DeNiro 1987; Krueger and Sullivan 1984; Schwarcz et al. 1985; van der Merwe and Vogel 1978) and is supported by recent data on a variety of wild fauna (Lee-Thorp et al. 1989; Schoeninger 1985).

Recent work has begun to use bone mineral $\delta^{13}C$ for dietary reconstruction, but this has not been free of debate. Initial reservations focused on the susceptibility of bone apatite to carbonate diagenesis (Schoeninger and DeNiro 1982, 1983; Sullivan and Krueger 1981, 1983), a difficulty that continues to limit the interpretive power of apatite data in many environments (Wright and Schwarcz 1996). However, experimental work has demonstrated that apatite $\delta^{13}C$ actually tracks the bulk dietary $\delta^{13}C$ more faithfully than does collagen $\delta^{13}C$ (Ambrose and Norr 1993; Tieszen and Fagre 1993b). The contributions of dietary proteins, lipids, and carbohydrates to collagen syntheses were the source of speculation for many years (Chisholm 1989; Chisholm et al. 1982; Klepinger 1984; Krueger and Sullivan 1984; Lee-Thorp et al. 1989; Schwarcz 1991; Sillen et al. 1989) and are not completely understood at present. It now seems likely that dietary protein is at least partially routed to collagen synthesis and that lipids may not contribute to it (Ambrose and Norr 1993; Schwarcz 1994; Tieszen and Fagre 1993b). By comparing collagen and apatite $\delta^{13}C$, we may be able to learn more about complex diets that contain many foods of different isotopic compositions.

In addition to differences in dietary fractionation and routing, analysis of different tissues can also provide a means to examine diet over different periods of time due to the different turnover rates among tissues. Body tissues that are more metabolically active have faster turnover rates than less active tissues and can record more narrow fluctuations in diet over time (Tieszen et al. 1983). Bone collagen has a very long turnover rate, probably recording an average diet over the last 10 to 30 years of life (Ambrose 1993). Apatite $\delta^{13}C$ values may turn over more rapidly but have not received detailed study as yet (Ambrose 1993:111).

Nitrogen isotopes document similar biological processes in ecosystems, but unlike carbon isotopes, nitrogen isotopes are not differentially affected by photosynthesis. In plants, the relative proportions of ^{15}N and ^{14}N, designated as $\delta^{15}N$, are dependent upon the source of the nitrogen that is incorporated into plant tissues. Most nitrogen taken up by plants comes from the soil, where it occurs as nitrates and ammonium. Soil nitrogen is fixed by bacteria and undergoes complex nitrification processes before it can be taken up by plants in inorganic form. As a result of kinetic isotopic effects in nitrification, soil $\delta^{15}N$ is heavier than atmospheric N_2. Plants that rely on soil nitrogen sources have $\delta^{15}N$ between −2 and +8‰. Some plants have nitrogen-fixing symbiotic bacteria and obtain N_2 directly from the air, so have much lighter $\delta^{15}N$ values. Legumes obtain most of their nitrogen from this bacterial fixation and typically have values near 0‰ (DeNiro 1987; Shearer and Kohl 1988).

Since soil nitrogen characteristics are highly variable, nitrogen isotopic ratios also differ between ecosystems (Ambrose 1993). The balance between soil nitrogen fixation and denitrification contributes to heterogeneity of soil $\delta^{15}N$ and is affected by climatic variables. Hot, arid climates and high soil salinity inhibit soil N_2 fixation, thereby raising the $\delta^{15}N$ of soils and the plants that grow upon them (Ambrose 1991; Heaton 1987). Cool, damp climates promote N_2 fixation in soils, lowering ^{15}N abundance. Damp forest soils are typically low in $\delta^{15}N$, in part because of the decomposition of litter, particularly in tropical rain forests that contain many leguminous trees (Shearer and Kohl 1988; Virginia et al. 1988).

Unlike carbon, the fractionation of nitrogen isotopes between trophic levels appears to be fairly consistent, with a factor of +3–4‰ recorded for a broad range of trophic distinctions (DeNiro and Epstein 1981; Schoeninger 1985; Schoeninger and DeNiro 1984). This enrichment appears to occur in transamination of dietary protein for use in structural growth (Macko et al. 1986), so proteins from different animal tissues tend to have similar $\delta^{15}N$ (DeNiro and Epstein 1981). Because nitrogen is obtained only from dietary protein, the contributions of different macronutrients need not be considered. As with carbon, nitrogen isotopes in collagen reflect a mean diet over the last 10 or more years of life. Environmental discrepancies in soil $\delta^{15}N$ dictate that trophic relationships be evaluated within narrow ecological parameters (Heaton et al. 1986).

Nitrogen isotopes are characteristically about 4‰ higher in marine plants than in terrestrial plants because dissolved nitrate in water is isotopically heavy. Zooplankton that provide the basis of carnivorous food chains also utilize nitrate, producing heavy $\delta^{15}N$ in the tissues of consumers after fractionation through several trophic levels. Where nitrogen-fixing blue-green algae contribute significantly to water nitrogen, however, as in tropical coral reef and mangrove habitats, marine $\delta^{15}N$ values may be similar to those of terrestrial ecosystems (Ambrose 1993; Keegan and DeNiro 1988; Schoeninger et al. 1983; Schwarcz and Schoeninger 1991). Freshwater ecosystems also show analogous enrichment of $\delta^{15}N$ (Katzenberg 1989; Schwarcz et al. 1985). However, in some tropical lakes, nitrogen fixation by blue-green algae may lower $\delta^{15}N$, resulting in signatures similar to those of terrestrial environments (Schwarcz and Schoeninger 1991).

Together, the stable isotopic ratios of carbon and nitrogen in archaeological human bone provide considerable information about the composition of the prehistoric diet. Carbon isotopic methods were first used to document the introduction of maize—a C4 cultigen—into North America (van der Merwe and Vogel 1978; Vogel and van der Merwe 1977) and then to identify its early development in Formative Mexico (DeNiro and Epstein 1981; Farnsworth et al. 1985). Subsequent studies have fine-tuned regional patterns in the evolution of horticultural economies in North America (Boutton et al. 1984; Buikstra 1992; Buikstra et al. 1988; Buikstra and Milner 1991; Schwarcz et al. 1985; Spielmann et al. 1990) and South America (Ericson et al. 1989; Hastorf and Johannessen 1993). On the Pacific coast of Guatemala, isotopic data indicates that maize agriculture was well underway by 800 B.C. (Blake et al. 1992).

Nitrogen isotope ratios provide a means to evaluate the relative contributions of marine and terrestrial foods to the diets of coastal populations in temperate regions (Chisholm et al. 1982; Schoeninger and DeNiro 1984; Schoeninger et al. 1983). Although maize consumption provides a potential confound with marine reef species in tropical areas, isotope ratios still provide insight into the nature of subsistence adaptations (Keegan and DeNiro 1988; Norr 1991).

African food webs incorporate foods of diverse isotopic signatures that are further affected by regional variation in nitrogen isotopes with water stress. Research has focused on discriminating between agriculturalists and pastorists and separating marine and terrestrial foods, both of which have proven complex (Ambrose and DeNiro 1986; Sealy and van der Merwe 1986; Sealy et al. 1987; Sillen et al. 1989). In prehistoric Nubia, White (1990; White and Schwarcz 1994) employed isotopic analyses to document changing patterns of the consumption of C4 grains (millet and sorghum) relative to the C3 grains (wheat and barley).

As research progresses, it has become clear that accurate paleodietary reconstruction with isotopes depends on two issues. First, a complete understanding of the isotopic composition of food items available on the prehistoric menu is necessary. Therefore, most studies include analyses of potential food items, especially in areas where previous work has not sampled flora and fauna. Second, the mechanism of collagen synthesis remains incompletely understood. Therefore, isotopic data is best suited for identifying trends in the relative proportions of food classes, rather than for estimating precise dietary percentages.

Alkaline Earth Elements

The inorganic phase of bone is composed of a poorly crystalline form of hydroxyapatite, $Ca_{10}(PO_4)_6(OH)_2$. In addition to calcium (Ca), other alkaline earth elements, notably strontium (Sr) and barium (Ba), occur in bone in low levels reflecting their relative abundance in the diet. Both Sr and Ba may occur directly in the structure of the hydroxyapatite crystal where they replace Ca by ionic substitution since they have the same valence as Ca (Burton et al. 1999; Elias et al. 1982; Schroeder et al. 1972). This structural incorporation also means that Sr and Ba may be subject to relatively little diagenesis, unlike elements that bond to the surface of crystals. Recent research in elemental analysis of bone has focused on these two elements because neither is known to have a biological function, so the abundance observed in bone should reflect diet faithfully, without bias from metabolic factors regulating uptake or storage of the elements (Ezzo 1992b; Price and Kavanaugh 1982).

Levels of both Ba and Sr in bone reflect the concentration of these elements in the soils on which dietary plants are grown, and, in turn, on which animals feed. Plants draw up minerals from soil moisture for use in growth. Recently it has been shown that plants discriminate against Ba and Sr in favor of Ca in this uptake, so that plant tissues show lower Ba/Ca and Sr/Ca than do soils. The extent of this discrimination differs between plant species and is easily masked by geographic differences among plants of a single species (Burton et al. 1999; Elias et al. 1982; Runia 1987).

Similarly, animals discriminate against the heavier alkaline earth elements, so that Sr/Ca and Ba/Ca ratios in animal tissues are lower than in the foods they consume. This discrimination occurs mainly at the level of intestinal absorption, where Ca is taken up preferentially over other heavier alkaline earth (Comar 1963; Comar et al. 1957; Marcus and Wasserman 1965). Moreover, Sr and Ba are excreted preferentially from the kidneys, further reducing the net incorporation of these elements relative to Ca (Liniecki 1971). Further discrimination occurs in the mammary gland in lactating females (Sillen and Smith 1984).

Elias et al. (1982) documented stepwise decreases in Sr/Ca and Ba/Ca between species of different trophic levels in an alpine ecosystem. Decreases in these elements occurred between soil and sedge, sedge and vole, and vole and marten, illustrating discrimination against Ba and Sr at each step in the food web. Similar results for a large number of species from a Wisconsin ecosystem have recently confirmed this principle (Burton et al. 1999). This pattern appears to hold between species in direct predator-prey relationships but may be obscured if only broad classes of dietary behavior (e.g., herbivores vs. carnivores) are considered (Sealy and Sillen 1988). The degree of discrimination appears to be greater for Ba than for Sr, perhaps because of the larger ionic radius and heavier mass of Ba (Burton et al. 1999; Elias et al. 1982; Marcus and Wasserman 1965).

In aquatic systems alkaline earth elements are taken up in a slightly different manner than in terrestrial systems. In general, aquatic fauna absorb Ca directly from the water, and the contribution of dietary mineral is less important. For instance, mollusks absorb water Ca through the exposed surface of the mantle (van der Borght and van Puymbroeck 1966), and fish absorb Ca via the gills. Although the larger alkaline earths undergo some biopurification in this absorption, this discrimination is generally less than that of terrestrial vertebrate digestive systems but can reveal some interesting ecosystem characteristics. For instance, in the Ca-deficient Amazon watershed, fish bone contains very high levels of Ba (Geisler and Schneider 1976). Mollusks show a strong linear relationship between water and shell Sr/Ca ratios (Buchardt and Fritz 1978), indicating a constant discrimination factor. Discrimination against Sr is greater for fish and mollusks than for crustacea (Rosenthal et al. 1970).

This process seems to be equivalent in marine and freshwater animals of the same taxa. However, marine and freshwater systems differ significantly in alkaline earth content. Freshwater mineral levels are derived from precipitation and the solubility of soil minerals that enter the watershed in runoff. Ca and Sr are much more abundant in marine (salt)water than in freshwater, and the Sr/Ca ratio is also higher. Thus, in coastal areas where marine protein is consumed it can be expected to contribute high Sr/Ca to the diet, which might be confused for herbivory in a strictly terrestrial subsistence economy. This stands in contrast to the low Ba/Ca of saltwater, which contributes to a very low Ba/Sr ratio of marine biota in comparison to freshwater or terrestrial foods, providing a means to identify marine food (Burton and Price 1990b).

Early research in trace element anthropology also attempted to employ magnesium (Mg) and zinc (Zn) to estimate dietary components (e.g., Blakely and Beck 1981; Gilbert 1975). Both elements occur in disparate proportions in a number of food groups and are stored in bone mineral, though they are not incorporated into the crystal lattice. In addition, Mg and Zn are regulated metabolically. Bone Mg has recently been shown to reflect dietary levels only minimally (Klepinger 1990), and it also appears to be fairly susceptible to postmortem diagenetic alteration (Klepinger et al. 1986; Lambert et al. 1985). Zinc is an important component of some enzymes and helps to regulate cell replication (Hambidge et al. 1986). Documented differences in Zn concentration in bone of different trophic levels cannot be discounted (Morgan and Schoeninger 1989), but the argument (Ezzo 1994; Price et al. 1992) that elements which serve a metabolic function and are not incorporated into the crystal structure of hydroxyapatite should not be dietarily useful is compelling. For these reasons, I focus on Sr and Ba.

Because of the principle of biopurification, differences in the abundance of the heavier alkaline earth elements in prehistoric bone were initially interpreted as trophic level indicators and used to estimate meat consumption. Skeletons containing low Sr/Ca or Ba/Ca are interpreted as having consumed more meat than those with higher ratios. Although this pattern does hold for individual trophic relationships within a single ecosystem, interpreting elemental ratios for omnivores like humans is now known to be much more complicated.

Recent modeling has shown that heavy reliance on maize decreases the consumption of other plant foods that are high in Ca, so that the contribution of Ca (and thereby Sr or Ba) from meat is proportionately increased (Burton and Wright 1995; Wright 1994:180–83). Because plant foods typically contain a lot of Ca, they contribute proportionately more to the total pool of alkaline earths consumed (Ca + Sr + Ba) than do low-Ca foods like meat. Hence, small variations in the amount of meat consumed do not have a significant effect on total dietary alkaline earth ratios because the contribution from meat is typically small. Thus, alkaline earth ratios shed light on the relative sources of dietary calcium. Since there are significant differences in Sr/Ca ratios among plant species, and because plants and animal foods vary widely in Ca content, accurate elemental characterization of food sources is critical to interpreting elemental ratios of prehistoric bone.

By reorienting the focus to sources of Ca in prehistoric bones, the anomalously low Sr/Ca ratios documented in a population of maize agriculturalists (Katzenberg 1984) can be more easily explained. Katzenberg interpreted her data from Ontario to be the result of the low Sr content of maize. Maize does contain little Sr relative to meat. However, the critical issue is the relative contribution of the Ca of a food to the total Ca (Burton and Wright 1995). Maize does not have anomalous Sr/Ca in comparison with other plants, but it is exceptionally low in Ca. Thus, the low Sr/Ca of maize agriculturalists actually reflects the low elemental ratio signal of meat consumed, which is not masked by the higher Sr/Ca of plants due to consumption of this low-Ca staple.

Although maize itself is low in Ca, it is often prepared in ways that dramatically increase its calcium content. Nearly all maize-reliant cultures in the Americas soak maize in a lime solution to dissolve the tough outer skin (pericarp) of the kernels and to soften them prior to grinding (Katz et al. 1974). This also has the advantage of improving the amino acid balance of the grain and diminishes the likelihood of niacin deficiency (pellagra) (Bressani and Scrimshaw 1958). Such alkaline processing leads to dramatic increases in the Ca content of maize foods (Bressani et al. 1958; Calloway et al. 1974; Kuhnlein 1981; Serna-Saldivar et al. 1991; Serna-Saldivar et al. 1992). Accordingly, where alkaline processing is practiced, high maize consumption should be indicated by high Ba/Ca and Sr/Ca in bone mineral because the Ca content of maize is augmented by traditional maize preparation techniques (Burton and Wright 1995; Ezzo 1992a; Wright 1999). The exact ratio expected would depend on the source of lime used. Similarly, the elemental ratios of many food sources would be swamped by consumption of other high-Ca food items, such as fishmeal or perhaps dairy foods (Burton and Wright 1995).

It has been suggested that mollusk consumption produces high levels of Sr in consumer skeletons (Schoeninger and Peebles 1981) in view of the high total Sr content of molluskan tissue. Although the ratio of Sr to Ca should reflect the geological source of water since mollusks are similar to fish and other aquatic fauna, feasting on mollusks could influence the total signature of a consumer significantly because mollusks store significant Ca in the foot as reserves for shell regeneration (Sminia et al. 1977, Watabe 1976:#1006).

These sorts of interpretive issues are important for evaluating the possible dietary factors influencing the elemental composition of prehistoric bone mineral. Although some researchers concerned about diagenesis have advocated comparison of absolute Sr ratios in archaeological bone, instead of Sr/Ca (Lambert et al. 1982; Pate and Brown 1985), normalizing elemental abundances to Ca permits comparison of elemental composition between foods of differing Ca content. Emphasis on alkaline earths that substitute directly for Ca in bone mineral highlights this difference and underscores the importance of the Sr/Ca or Ba/Ca ratio as the unit of analysis in both bone mineral and food menu items.

Like analyses of stable isotopes, elemental studies have attempted to evaluate subsistence changes over time and space, with a focus on the emergence of horticulture in North America (Blakely and Beck 1981; Katzenberg 1984; Lambert et al. 1982; Szpunar 1977). However, elemental analysis has principally been employed to examine status-specific meat consumption within prehistoric populations. Such status differences have been sought in the northeast of North America (Brown 1973; Hatch and Geidel 1985), the American Southwest (Ezzo 1992a), Mexico (Blitz 1995; Schoeninger 1979a; Schoeninger 1979b), coastal Guatemala (Chinchilla Mazariegos 1990; Chinchilla et al. 1992), and the Harappan civilization of Pakistan (Radosevich 1993).

The high Sr content of marine waters prompted the application of elemental analyses for evaluating the contribution of marine fauna to Alaskan populations (Connor and Slaughter 1984; Harritt and Radosevich 1992), coastal Peruvians (Baraybar 1999), and Iron Age Spanish populations (Subira and Malgosa 1991). Results of these attempts are somewhat ambiguous, probably because the Sr/Ca compositions of all food items in the prehistoric menu are incompletely documented. Consideration of the Ba content of bones in conjunction with Sr provides a more successful approach for detecting marine food consumption (Burton and Price 1990a, 1990b).

Bone Preservation and Diagenesis

The biochemical and geochemical processes outlined above form the basis of powerful tools for the study of both ecological systems and human subsistence strategies (Grupe and Herrmann 1988; Lambert and Grupe 1993; Price 1989b; Rundel et al. 1988; Sandford 1993). However, before either stable isotopic or alkaline earth elemental data from prehistoric bone can be interpreted in dietary terms, care must be taken to ensure that biogenic chemical signatures can be demonstrated.

After interment, bone is subjected to a variety of processes that can alter both the organic and inorganic phases, rendering them less useful for dietary analysis. Soft tissue decomposition, groundwater action, and microbial activity lead to gradual decay of bone tissue in most environments. The organic matrix of bone may be damaged by the enzymatic activity of bacteria, fungi, and yeasts that erode tunnels or pockets in bone tissue. This damage, in turn, weakens the structure of the bone and promotes chemical weathering of the mineral fraction, which occurs more rapidly in acidic conditions (Hackett 1981; Hagihara et al. 1988; Hanson and Buikstra 1987). This decomposition may weaken the collagen structure without change to the amino acid composition of the protein (Beeley and Lunt 1980) or may produce radically different amino acid profiles (Schoeninger et al. 1989). Organic degradation may have profound effects on the nitrogen isotope ratio of gelatin extracted from bone, due to kinetic effects in the hydrolysis of peptide bonds between amino acids (Bada et al. 1989).

Evaluation of collagen integrity in prehistoric bone samples is necessary to verify that isotopic signals obtained are biogenic. Atomic ratios of carbon to nitrogen (C/N) are most commonly employed to evaluate collagen integrity. Modern bone collagen has a C/N ratio of about 3.2. Bones with C/N ratios between 2.9 and 3.6 appear to have reliable isotopic compositions (DeNiro 1985). Prehistoric samples with ratios beyond this range may have suffered some selective loss of amino acids or the incorporation of other organic materials that would affect isotope ratios. The yield of collagen obtained from archaeological bones is also a sensitive indicator of preservation. Archaeological bones with less than 5% collagen have been regarded as suspect, but reliable collagen isotopic signatures have been obtained from bone with as little as 1% collagen (Ambrose 1990). Poorly preserved collagen may show low elemental concentrations of C and N as well as anomalous ratios between the two elements. Amino acid profiles provide a further means to evaluate collagen integrity (Hare 1980; Schoeninger et al. 1989).

Collagen degradation initiates weathering of the inorganic phase of bone by the substitution of hydrogen ions for Ca ions in hydroxyapatite, breaking down the crystal lattice. Calcium and other trace elements are then leached away in soils (White and Hannus 1983). Bone may suffer from contamination by extraneous minerals through a variety of mechanisms. For instance, soil minerals may crystallize in bone pores such as osteocyte lacunae and canaliculi (Parker and Toots 1980). Bacteria and fungi may also draw a number of soil elements into the bone matrix and deposit oxides containing heavy metals (Grupe and Piepenbrink 1988; Parker and Toots 1972). More insidious alteration, referred to as diagenesis, involves the structural incorporation of extraneous mineral. This may occur through the adsorption of soil carbonates onto the surface of hydroxyapatite crystals. Under certain conditions, soil minerals may crystallize as geological hydroxyapatite, a form that is indistinguishable from biogenic apatite (Pate and Brown 1985).

Although some have expressed skepticism about the feasibility of recovering biogenic signals of alkaline earth elements and stable carbon isotopes from interred bone mineral (Hancock et al. 1989; Schoeninger and DeNiro 1982; Tuross et al. 1989), a number of methods provide fruitful approaches to the problem. Initial studies examined correlations in bone and soil, attempting to evaluate chemical gradients (Lambert et al. 1983, 1984). This technique is useful in cases of extreme differences, but gradients may often be too small for detection. Diagenetic apatite can be distinguished by X-ray diffraction peaks, fluorine content, and infrared peaks (Lee-Thorp and van der Merwe 1991; Schoeninger et al. 1989; Sponheimer and Lee-Thorp 1999; Wright and Schwarcz 1996). Mechanical surface removal and acid washing appear to minimize the effects of contamination and diagenesis, thus providing biologically acceptable mineral compositions (Lambert et al. 1990; Price et al. 1992; Sillen and LeGeros 1991). Statistical techniques examining the cooccurrence of a broad array of elements in addition to dietary discriminators provides a means to evaluate the nature of soil contamination (Buikstra et al. 1989; Price 1989a).

Materials and Methods of Chemical Analysis

I use stable isotopic analysis of carbon and nitrogen in bone collagen and ratios of alkaline earth elements in bone mineral to examine Pasión Maya diet. Chapter 6 presents an examination of the chemical signatures of ancient menu items from the Pasión ecosystem. Chapter 7 contains an evaluation of archaeological bone preservation and paleodietary reconstruction through Pasión prehistory. Sampling and analytic methods common to both chapters are discussed here.

Sampling

To gain an understanding of the nature of dietary distinctions that might be revealed by isotopic and elemental analysis, I collected modern floral and faunal samples during the spring of 1992. Floral sampling was targeted at indigenous species available or known to have been exploited prehispanically, including both cultivated and wild species. Most floral samples are from the Parque Arqueológico Dos Pilas or from the nearby Kekchi villages, Nacimiento and Sepens. A few samples were also obtained at Aguateca and Altar de Sacrificios. All floral samples were cleaned so that only the edible portion was sampled. Samples were sun-dried, packed in coin envelopes, and then placed in plastic bags with silica gel.

Most of the faunal remains were obtained in the nearby Kekchi villages and are the remains of meals consumed within the previous year or two, but were bones kept around the house (mandibles, crania) and not removed from kitchen middens. Snake bones were cleaned by placing them over anthills for a few days. Fish were caught in the lagoon at Aguateca and their vertebrae cleaned, sun-dried, and packed in silica gel. I collected molluskan shells at Aguateca and Dos Pilas and along the Pasión and Usumacinta Rivers near Altar de Sacrificios. I also collected flesh samples of fish and snails that I salted, sun-dried, and packed in silica gel. I sampled archaeological faunal bone recovered by Petexbatun project excavations at Dos Pilas, Aguateca, and Punta de Chimino. In addition to comparing prehistoric fauna with modern controls to examine diagenesis, the archaeological fauna further expand the dietary baseline data for the region.

I selected bone samples from all Pasión human skeletal remains that appeared to be well preserved. Skeletons sampled were limited to those interred in surface architecture (not caves). Most samples were selected from the midshaft of the femur, but other long bones were sampled for a few burials from which no femur was available. In each case, I attempted to sample dense, thick cortical bone rather than trabecular bone or elements with thin cortices, as these may be subject to greater diagenesis (Lambert et al. 1982) and different rates of bone turnover (Chisholm 1989; Grupe 1988). I attempted to select only elements that did not show surface erosion and did not have a soft, chalky cortex, as these likely contain little collagen.

Soil samples were collected for as many burials as possible in order to examine patterns of elemental transport between bone and soil. Beginning in 1991, Petexbatun project excavations aimed to collect three soil samples from each burial excavated. These samples were selected adjacent to the best preserved femur and at 10 and 20 cm from the femur in the horizontal plane; however, fewer samples could be selected in some burial features due to space restrictions. I collected marrow cavity samples for a few Petexbatun burials excavated before the implementation of this procedure. During excavation, soil pH was determined for many Petexbatun project burials using a commercial soil pH indicator kit. For the previously excavated series from Altar de Sacrificios, Seibal, and Itzan, I extracted soil samples from the marrow cavities of the bone sampled or an antimere. I obtained a total of 17 samples from Altar skeletons and 5 samples from Itzan burials, but soil had been more fully cleaned from the Seibal skeletal collection, so only 2 samples could be obtained in this manner. Two samples each were subsequently collected from the site center and riverbank at Seibal.

Stable Isotopes

I cleaned archaeological bone specimens of adhering soil in the field, and cancellous and surface bone was removed in the laboratory. Collagen was extracted and mass spectrometry conducted in the laboratory of Dr. M. J. Schoeninger in the Department of Anthropology at the University of Wisconsin, Madison. Bone samples were cleaned mechanically and ultrasonicated in doubly purified water. Cleaned samples were dried to a constant weight at 35°C, and bone chunks (approximately 1 mm diameter) were placed in stoppered tubes with 0.5 M EDTA that had been titrated to pH 7.2 with HCl, and stored at 4°C with continuous agitation. The solution was changed daily until demineralization was complete. "Collagen" pseudomorphs were rinsed at least 15 times with doubly purified water to completely remove EDTA, then soaked in 0.125 M NaOH overnight to remove humic acid contaminants, and again rinsed to neutrality with purified water. "Collagen" obtained by this process was freeze-dried in preparation for mass spectrometry.

Approximately 5 mg of this freeze-dried residue was loaded into quartz tubes with excess silver, elemental copper, and cupric oxide; the tubes were then evacuated and sealed. The tubes were heated to 800°C for six hours and slowly cooled to room temperature. CO_2 and N_2 were purified, cryogenically separated, and collected in Pyrex tubes under vacuum. Atomic C/N ratios were determined by measuring CO_2 volume manometrically and N_2 volume with a Baratron pressure gauge. Stable carbon isotope ratios in CO_2 were measured on a Finnegan MAT Delta E isotope ratio mass spectrometer and are reported in δ notation relative to PDB limestone. Stable isotopes of N_2 were analyzed on a Finnegan MAT 251 isotope ratio mass spectrometer, with results reported in δ notation relative to AIR. Precision of the results is +/−0.2‰ for $\delta^{13}C$ and +/−0.2‰ for $\delta^{15}N$, as measured on an internal laboratory glycine standard.

Collagen extracts from modern faunal specimens were prepared in the laboratory of Dr. L. Tieszen in the Department of Biology at Augustana College, Sioux Falls, South Dakota. Bone pieces were cleaned and dried overnight. Lipids were removed by soaking the bones for 24 hours in a solution of methanol, chloroform, and water (2:1:0.8), and then rinsing the samples with deionized water. The samples were demineralized with 0.3 N HCl at 4°C with continuous agitation. The solution was changed daily for one week or until the sample became translucent, indicating that it was decalcified. After rinsing in distilled water, this "collagen" extract was soaked in 0.125 M NaOH at 4°C for 24 hours to remove humic contaminants, and again rinsed in distilled water. To remove residual lipids, the pseudomorph was soaked for 30 minutes in the methanol/chloroform/water solution and rinsed. Collagen was solubilized by placing the pseudomorphs in pH 3.0 water at 90°C for 12 hours, then filtered and freeze-dried.

The samples were then loaded into a Carlo Erba NA1500 carbon/nitrogen analyzer, where the sample is combusted at 1030°C and reduced to N_2 and CO_2 at 650°C. The elemental analyzer also measured the C/N ratios of the samples. The gases were separated on a chromatographic column, and isotope ratios were measured on a VG SIRA mass spectrometer.

Isotope ratios of modern plant specimens were also obtained at Augustana College. Plant tissues were dried at 75°C in a drying oven and ground in a Wiley mill through 40-mesh sieve. The powdered samples were analyzed directly without further preparation. Snail flesh samples were rinsed to remove salt, soaked in chloroform/methanol/water solution (2:1:0.8) for 12 hours, dried, macerated, and analyzed isotopically at Augustana College. Fish flesh was analyzed likewise at the University of Wisconsin, Madison.

After the first phase of research, a few more human and archaeological faunal samples were prepared at McMaster University, Hamilton, Ontario, Canada. These samples pertain to human material from Tamarindito, Arroyo de Piedra, Punta de Chimino, Dos Pilas burials above DP51, and the decapitated crania from Operation DP1. The human collagen was prepared according to the EDTA protocol described above, and collagen samples were combusted at 550°C and isotope measurements obtained on a VG SIRA mass spectrometer. The new faunal material consisted of a number of canid and felid samples also identified toward the end of the Petexbatun Project. These were prepared at McMaster according to the same protocols as at Augustana College, but C/N ratios were measured manometrically. Due to financial constraints, elemental analyses were not carried out on these additional remains.

Alkaline Earth Elements

All elemental analyses were conducted at the Laboratory for Archaeological Chemistry at the University of Wisconsin, Madison, according to standard procedures developed in that laboratory and under the supervision of Dr. James H. Burton. Discolored surface bone was removed by mechanical abrasion with a Dremel "moto-tool" in order to minimize surface contaminating elements (Lambert et al. 1990). Samples were then rinsed with deionized water in a sonic water bath and soaked overnight in 1 M acetic acid to dissolve diagenetic carbonates (Price et al. 1992, Sillen

1989:#503; Sillen 1990; Sillen and LeGeros 1991). Samples were ashed at 725°C for eight hours. For each sample, 50 mg of bone ash was weighed into test tubes and dissolved in 1 ml of concentrated nitric acid at 120°C for one hour, then diluted to a total volume of 17 ml (1/340 dilution) and analyzed by Inductively Coupled Plasma Emission spectroscopy (ICP-AES) for Al, Ba, Ca, Fe, K, Mg, Mn, Na, P, Sr, and Zn. Detection limits for the ICP are very low and, when multiplied by the bone dilution factor, are well below the concentrations measured in bone for the elements studied. The N.I.S.T. bone standard, H5, and two internal laboratory standards, B5407 and B0126, were analyzed with each sample run to monitor accuracy and precision.

Modern bone specimens were prepared similarly, but surface bone was not removed. Modern shell samples were rinsed with deionized water and sampled without chemical cleaning. Fifty milligrams of each shell sample was dissolved in hot, concentrated nitric acid, diluted (1/340), and analyzed like the bone samples. Plant samples were oven-dried, macerated, digested in hot, concentrated nitric acid (0.050 g/2 ml nitric acid), diluted (1/340), and analyzed for the same elements as the bone samples. In 1995 some plants were reanalyzed using a new protocol that allows detection of elements down to about 1 ppm. After digestion in nitric acid at room temperature (as above), the plant samples were heated to 115°C for one hour to complete the digestion. Then they were diluted with deionized water to a total volume of 17 ml, filtered, and analyzed for Ba, Ca, and Sr. Background intensities were measured on both sides of the peaks for all elements and were subtracted from the signal intensity.

Soil samples were oven-dried and 200 mg samples of each weighed into polypropylene vials. Twenty ml of 1 M hydrochloric acid was added to each vial, and the samples were kept at 26°C for two weeks with intermittent agitation. This solution was decanted and analyzed by ICP for the same set of elements. Derived from methods for soil-phosphate analysis (Burton and Simon 1993), this procedure measures only the ions that are soluble and thus available for interchange with bone mineral.

I examined the possibility of diagenetic contamination of archaeological bone samples from four avenues. Calcium/phosphorus ratios (Ca/P) were scrutinized to evaluate the overall integrity of archaeological bone hydroxyapatite (Sillen 1989; White and Hannus 1983). Elemental relationships were examined in human bones for each site by correlation and principal components analysis (Buikstra et al. 1989). Elemental discrimination of trophic level relationships in archaeological fauna was compared with modern faunal data (Ezzo 1992b; Sillen 1981). I also studied the correlation of soil element concentrations with bone values (Nelson and Sauer 1984) and the distribution of soil elements in soil surrounding bone (Francalacci and Borgognini Tarli 1988; Lambert et al. 1984).

Because most elemental concentrations are not normally distributed and sample sizes are small, I use nonparametric tests in most aspects of the diagenetic and dietary comparisons. Parametric tests are not appropriate for isotopic and elemental comparisons because social differentiation within samples can produce deviation from normality. Specific details and justification of the statistical analyses are presented with the results as they are best explained in the context of each comparison. In most tests I rejected the null hypothesis when $p < 0.05$.

CHAPTER 6

Defining the Parameters of Pasión Diets

The reconstruction of past subsistence behavior from bone chemistry requires detailed consideration of potential menu items and their chemical signatures. A substantial body of research has focused on ancient Maya food choices, identifying various cultigens, wild flora, and fauna that were consumed. To date, investigations of chemical dynamics in the Neotropical rain forest ecosystem are limited. Through isotopic and elemental analysis of local flora and fauna, I examine chemical parameters of foods that may have been exploited by the ancient inhabitants of the Pasión region. These data provide a baseline for interpreting human data in Chapter 7. Chemical effects of food-processing techniques may further complicate the interpretation of bone chemical data. I consider the impact of alkaline processing of maize on the isotopic and elemental composition of the diet and its implications for paleodietary reconstruction.

Maya Menus: Ethnohistoric and Archaeological Inference

By analogy with modern Maya peoples, prehispanic Maya subsistence is generally considered to have been based on maize agriculture, supplemented by cultivation of beans and squash. Modern diets in the Maya area rely heavily on maize as a staple cereal. Maize may provide up to 70% of caloric intake, as in rural modern Guatemala (Flores et al. 1964). Most protein is supplied by beans rather than meat. Continuity of dietary practices can be assumed to a considerable extent, but major changes in agriculture were brought about by the Spanish conquest. In addition to new crops that were introduced, including rice, plantains, and citrus fruits, culinary practices changed to suit Spanish tastes. With political reorganization of New Spain, indigenous foods, along with indigenous peoples, were redefined as a subordinate class. Despite the biases imposed by this transition, a variety of approaches can help to reconstruct prehispanic foodways.

Ethnohistoric, iconographic, paleobotanical, and chemical data indicate that maize was an important cultigen in prehispanic times. The name "maize" is derived from an Arawak term brought to Central America by the Spanish (Marcus 1982). To both the Yucatec and Kekchi Maya, the tropical grass *Zea mays* is called *"ixim"* (Marcus 1982; Secaira 1992), but it is known as *"näl"* to the Lacandon Maya (Marcus 1982; Nations and Nigh 1980; Secaira 1992). As well as being a dietary staple, maize played a pivotal role in prehispanic religion (e.g., Tedlock 1985) and continues to function as a symbol of national identity today (Rojas Lima 1988).

In the Maya Lowlands, the earliest evidence for maize domestication comes from pollen that dates to 3500 B.P. or perhaps slightly older (Pohl et al. 1996; Spross Hansen 1990). Pollen profiles show a decrease in primary forest pollen during the Preclassic period that presumably reflects agricultural expansion at this time (Pohl et al. 1996; Vaughan et al. 1985; Wiseman 1983).

Maize was prepared in a variety of dishes. Today, the bulk of maize is consumed as tortillas; however, it is likely that tortillas were not as important to the Maya during the Classic period. Ceramic *comales* on which tortillas are cooked are quite rare in Classic Maya ceramic inventories, in contrast to ceramic inventories from central Mexico. Comales recovered from Early

Classic deposits at Kaminaljuyu may reflect central Mexican influence at this site (Taube 1989). A few comales were found in Bayal deposits at Seibal (Sabloff 1975:154) and are rare forms in the Late Classic Petexbatun ceramic inventory (Foias, personal communication 1993). The Maya "maize bread" described in colonial documents (e.g., Tozzer 1941:90) is probably the tamale, a steamed cake of maize dough filled with beans or meat and wrapped in a corn husk. Iconography of maize plants and the maize god on ceramic plates suggests that these vessels may have been made to hold maize foods. Ceramic plates holding maize balls that resemble tamales are depicted on Classic period vessels. Taube (1989) argues that the term *"wah,"* now used to denote "tortilla," originally described tamales. Iconographic and epigraphic references to *wah* abound, indicating that the tamale held ceremonial significance as well as providing a staple food (Love 1989; Taube 1989).

Like tamales and tortillas, most maize foods are produced from ground maize, or *masa;* rarely, corn is roasted on the cob or eaten as fresh young cobs (*elotes*). Maize was traditionally ground with a metate and mano after it had been soaked in a lime solution made with either burned limestone or slaked snail shells (Nations 1979b). This alkaline processing dissolves the pericarp of the maize kernels, improves the isoleucine/leucine ratio of maize, and raises the availability of niacin, thereby reducing the risk of pellagra (Katz et al. 1974). Interestingly, Redfield and Villa Rojas (1934:39) noted that ritual maize foods (*zaca*) are not treated with lime in Yucatan. Similarly, maize *bokix*, a ritual food eaten by Tzotzil men on the first day of planting, is also unprocessed (Guiteras-Holmes 1961:30).

Ground maize is added along with honey to boiling water to form a gruel called *atole,* a common beverage and breakfast food. Prepared with a variety of different spices and condiments, *atole* is also used as a medicament for a variety of illnesses (Benedict and Steggerda 1937). Hieroglyphic inscriptions on Classic period deep bowls indicate that these contained *ul* or *sakha,* providing evidence that *atole* was consumed prehispanically (Houston et al. 1989). This *sakha* could also have been *pozole*, another gruel that is produced in Yucatan and Chiapas from *masa* that is partially fermented and contains nitrogen-fixing bacteria and fungi, which make it storable for several weeks (Ulloa and Herrera 1986). This dough is taken to the fields by laborers, where it is mixed with water and consumed (Benedict and Steggerda 1937). Interestingly, in Yucatan *pozole* is prepared with a distinct alkaline treatment (Redfield and Villa Rojas 1934:38–39), and Tozzer (1907:52) indicated that the Lacandon do not treat *pozole* maize with any lime.

Two other grains were used by the Maya but were probably very minor dietary components. Goosefoot, or epazote (*Chenopodium ambrosoides*), is used mainly as a flavoring for cooking beans (Benedict and Steggerda 1937; Redfield and Villa Rojas 1934; Shattuck 1933). Although amaranth, a C4 plant that is isotopically similar to maize (DeNiro and Epstein 1981), was an Aztec crop (Ortiz de Montellano 1990), amaranth pollen found in Maya raised fields cannot be securely distinguished from wild secondary successional species, so its use by the Maya is unclear (Miksicek 1983).

Beans, *Phaseolus vulgaris,* provide an important protein supplement to the maize of modern Maya diets, providing as much as 30% of the protein consumed (Flores and Garcia 1966). Beans are usually eaten boiled with epazote or mashed to a thick paste, and they are a common filling for tamales. Squashes, particularly the chayote, *Sechium edule*, are eaten as vegetables. Pumpkin seeds, *Cucurbita pepo*, are roasted, ground, and mixed with masa for preparation of tamales and other maize foods (Love 1989).

The fruits of the breadnut, or ramon tree (*Brosimum alicastrum*), are often described as starvation foods in both modern communities and ethnohistoric accounts (Marcus 1982). Yet, modern Itza Maya in the Petén consume ramon as both tortillas and *pozole* (Atran 1993). Puleston argued that ramon could have provided an alternate staple crop to maize because the nuts are easily collected, can be stored over long periods, and have high nutritional value (Puleston 1968, 1971, 1982). Commonly found growing at archaeological sites, ramon groves were thought to be descendants of orchards planted by the Classic Maya near their homes (Folan et al. 1979; Puleston 1968). However, this pattern appears to be a result of the reproductive strategy and habitat preferences of the tree (Lambert and Arnason 1982; Peters 1983). No carbonized remains of ramon have been recovered from archaeological excavations (Lentz 1991:279). Moreover, ramon pollen is lowest during the Classic period, a finding which hints that ramon trees were not selectively spared in agricultural forest clearing (John Jones, personal communication 1999).

Bronson (1966) first proposed that root crops may have been an important staple to the Maya. During the 16th century, the Yucatec Maya cultivated the sweet potato, or *camote* (*Ipomoea batatas*); manioc (*Manihot escuelenta*); and jícama (*Pachyrrhizus erosus* and *Calopogonium coeruleum*). The Old World yam (*Dioscorea alata*) was also grown and given a Maya name, *macal*, that may have been transferred from a Prehispanic root crop, *Xanthosoma violacium* (Marcus 1982). It has been suggested that root crops may have been the focus of early agriculture in the Maya Lowlands that were later supplanted by maize cultivation (Harris 1972). Manioc pollen dating to 3400 B.C. has been recovered at Cob Swamp (Pohl et al. 1996), and pollen dating to 2500 B.C. has been reported from Cobweb Swamp (Jones 1994) in Northern Belize. It is possible that manioc pollen is underrepresented at Maya sites because the crop was propagated from cuttings, so its flowering and subsequent dispersal of pollen was at a minimum (John Jones, personal communication 1999).

Although given little attention until recently, wild palm fruits may have been a significant component of prehistoric diet. Fruits, influorescences, and the "heart" of a number of native palms are consumed today (Lundell 1939). Carbonized endocarps of *coyol* nuts, *Acrocomia mexicana*, were common in archaeological deposits at Copan (Lentz 1991), prompting Lentz to suggest that *coyol* was widely consumed during the Late Classic period. *Coyol* nuts are eaten raw or used to make wine by a number of modern Maya groups (Lentz 1990).

A variety of domesticated fruits were consumed, including avocados (*Persea americana*), guavas (*Psidium guajava*), and papaya (*Carica papaya*). Fruit-bearing trees were probably planted around Maya houses as they are today. These include the mamey (*Calocarpum mammosum*), soursop (*Anona muricata*), custard apple (*Anona reticulata*), cherimoya (*Anona chirimola*), nance (*Byrsonima crassifolia*), star-apple (*Chrysophyllum cainito*), ciruela (*Spondias mombin*), frijolillo (*Cassia occidentale*), and wild grape (*Vitis spp.*). In addition to its edible fruit, the seed of the zapote, *Pouteria zapota*, is ground to make *atole* (personal observation, Chichicastenango, 1992).

Succulents are rare in the humid southern part of the Maya Lowlands, so consumption of plants using the Crassulacean Acid Metabolism (CAM) photosynthetic pathway are unlikely to affect dietary $\delta^{13}C$ values dramatically. The prickly pear cactus, or nopal (*Opuntia spp.*), produces fruits called *tuna* in addition to its edible fleshy leaves. *Opuntia* were cultivated in the dry northern lowlands at the time of conquest (Marcus 1982). The cactus is much rarer in the southern lowlands but occurs in some well-drained soils, as at Aguateca. The bromeliad *piñuela* (*Bromelia karatas*) produces edible fruits used to make *atole* and is abundant in the southern lowlands in both wild and cultivated forms (Lundell 1939). Although it is now a ubiquitous crop, the pineapple (*Ananas comosus*) may not have been grown by the prehistoric Maya as it is not mentioned in ethnohistoric texts (Lundell 1939).

Cacao beans held a special role in prehistoric Mesoamerican economies. Cacao was roasted and ground for use in the preparation of chocolate drinks, *kakaw*, that may have been sumptuary foods, restricted to elite consumption. The Aztecs used cacao in beverages and to produce *mole* sauces for meat dishes, which were consumed only by the upper social strata (Alcocer 1938). Dilute chocolate drinks are consumed by the Maya (Benedict and Steggerda 1937; Shattuck 1933) and were important ritual and elite drinks in 16th century Yucatan (Tozzer 1941:90). Cacao residues have been identified in a ceramic vessel from an Early Classic tomb at Río Azul, which also bears a hieroglyphic inscription about cacao (Stuart 1988b). Iconographic scenes often depict principal lords together with tall, cylindrical vessels that are hieroglyphically identified as cacao containers (Houston et al. 1989), hinting that cacao consumption was status linked. In addition to its culinary uses, cacao beans served as currency at the time of contact (Coe 1994).

Prehispanic meals were undoubtedly seasoned by a number of spices mentioned in the ethnohistoric literature; most prominent among them are chili peppers (*Capsicum spp.*). Chaya (*Jatropha aconitifolia*), allspice (*Pimienta officinalis*), and vanilla (*Vanilla fragrans*—a C4 plant) are other indigenous plants that were used to flavor prehispanic foods (Benedict and Steggerda 1937; Miksicek et al. 1981). Achiote (*Bixa orrellana*) was used to color Maya sauces a brilliant red.

At Ceren in El Salvador, several houses and adjacent *milpas* were preserved by a thick deposit of volcanic ash. Excavations there have documented prehistoric cultivation of maize, tomatoes, chiles, cacao, beans, achiote, guava, piñuela, yuca, conacaste (*Enterolobium cyclocarpum*), and jocotes (*Spondias spp.*) (Sheets 1992:37).

In addition to wild and cultivated plant foods, Maya diet included a variety of animal protein sources. Archaeological faunal analyses document prehistoric exploitation of deer (*Odocoileus virginianus* and *Mazama americana*), peccary (*Tayassu pecari* and *tajacu*), agouti (*Dasyprocta punctata*), paca (*Agouti paca*), tapir (*Tapirus bairdii*), armadillo (*Dasypus novemcinctus*), rabbit (*Sylvilagus sp.*), spider monkey (*Ateles goeffroyi*), and howler monkey (*Alouatta villosa*). There has been some speculation that deer were semi-domesticated, at least during the Postclassic period (Pohl 1985). Both turkeys (*Meleagris gallopavo*) and dogs (*Canis familiaris*) are confirmed domesticates that were raised as livestock. Wild forest birds, including the currassow (*Crax rubra*), guan, and parrots (*Amazona spp.*), were undoubtedly hunted (Emery 1997; Pohl 1985).

At coastal sites, skeletal remains of marine fauna are very common (Hamblin 1984). Marine fish and mammals were heavily exploited in Postclassic times and may have been salted and dried for trade inland (Lange 1971). The rivers and lakes of the southern Maya Lowlands provided protein from both aquatic fauna and terrestrial species that are easily captured in the area (Nations and Nigh 1980). At Seibal, freshwater faunal consumption is indicated by bones of catfish (Siluriformes) and ciclids (Ciclidae), turtles (*Pseudemys, Dermatemys,* etc.), and crocodiles (*Crocodylus moreleti*) (Pohl 1985). Freshwater molluskan exploitation is indicated by shells of the apple snail (*Pomacea flagellata*) (Moholy-Nagy 1978) and the river snail *jute* (*Pachychilus spp.*) (Healy et al. 1990).

Although archaeological data document this broad diversity of foods that were exploited, it is difficult to evaluate from these data the relative importance of each food to the diet of individual members of Maya society. Chemical analysis provides one means to approach chronological, spatial, and social variation in dietary behavior. Unlike paleobotanical and archaeozoological research, however, dietary chemistry cannot identify specific foods consumed. The above review serves to identify a baseline menu of foods that might account for the dietary signatures observed in bone chemistry.

Chemical Dynamics in the Pasión Ecosystem

Stable Isotopes

The isotopic composition of modern Pasión plant samples along with summary elemental data is given in Table 6.1. Most of the plants analyzed conform to a C3 photosynthetic pathway, as indicated by the low values of $\delta^{13}C$. These C3 plants show values well within the typical range, having a mean $\delta^{13}C$ of $-27.88 \pm 1.64‰$ ($n = 30$, excluding cacao as per below). Due to the humid climate and canopy effect that lower the $\delta^{13}C$ of plants in this forested environment, this value is slightly lower than the C3 mean ($-27.1 \pm 2.0‰$) given by O'Leary (1988). There is a slight, but not significant, difference in $\delta^{13}C$ between plants grown in open *milpas* ($-26.3 \pm 4.4‰$, $n = 14$) and those collected from the forest ($-28.2 \pm 2.0‰$, $n = 16$, excluding cacao; 2-tailed $t = 1.53$, $p = 0.14$, d.f. $= 28$). For the most part, no systematic differences occur in $\delta^{13}C$ between plant types. Some of the nuts show slightly lighter $\delta^{13}C$ (chapay, corozo, zapote), but the difference is not great, and these are also forest species so it is not possible to separate the relative influence of the canopy effect and interspecific metabolic variations on the total $\delta^{13}C$.

The cacao seed is markedly light in $\delta^{13}C$, at −34.14‰. Since this fruit was from a small understory tree, its low value might be due to the canopy effect (van der Merwe and Medina 1991), but the high lipid content of cacao is probably more significant. Lipids account for almost half (46.3%) of the mass of dried cacao seeds (I.N.C.A.P. 1961:92), a value much higher than that in other plant tissues sampled. Typically, lipids are isotopically light in comparison to other plant biochemicals (Tieszen and Boutton 1988), so the low value for the cacao seed may simply reflect this bias. Since lipids probably are not used to synthesize collagen, however, it can be assumed for the purposes of this analysis that the $\delta^{13}C$ composition of cacao is similar to that of other C3 plants.

The two maize samples and the nopal cactus (*Opuntia*) show distinct C4 signatures (mean = −10.74±0.64‰, $n = 3$). In fact, the nopal signature is even heavier than the maize, indicating that this CAM plant is primarily using dark acidification. The piñuela leaf shows a more typical CAM value, −16.7‰, due to the combined effects of daylight photosynthesis and dark acidification. Given the similarity of these C4 values, it is obvious that isotopic analysis will not be able to distinguish between maize and nopal consumption in this region. It is possible that cacti were planted near prehispanic Pasión homes as is done today in the northern Yucatan peninsula; however, nopal are currently extremely rare in the region, probably because of the high humidity. Piñuela consumption is more likely to contribute to heavy human $\delta^{13}C$ and would be impossible to isolate against the background of a maize-based diet.

It was not possible to measure the nitrogen isotopic composition of most Pasión plant samples because of the low nitrogen content (%N) of the tissues. Most plants fell between 0.5 and 5.5‰. The zapote nut is the lightest at 0.56‰, and beans are somewhat heavier at 3.94‰. Two squash samples are anomalously high (7.53, 8.78‰), raising the possibility that they are diagenetically enriched or had been fertilized artificially. Excluding the squash, these values are somewhat higher than those observed by Norr (1991) in lower Central America (nonlegumes: 1.4–2.4‰), but fit into the ranges observed for nonsaline sites in Africa (−1.0±6.0‰; Heaton 1987).

The isotopic composition of plants and animal foods is illustrated in Figure 6.1 in relation to Pasión human collagen. In the top graph, actual values obtained are shown for each animal bone sampled and for a few key cultigens; the ranges measured for plant tissues are indicated by boxes. The boxes incorporate the $\delta^{13}C$ of all plants sampled, but $\delta^{15}N$ could only be measured for a few samples, so the range shown here is based on the limited sample and excludes the problematic squash. Individual data for a few key plants are also given. Both modern and archaeological fauna are illustrated, as the archaeological fauna amplify the ecological breadth of the modern samples. Criteria for including archaeological samples are discussed more fully below with respect to sample preservation. In the second graph, an idealized model of human food values is presented. Shaded boxes depict the meat values expected for fish, mollusks, dogs, and herbivores. For fish, meat values are estimated to be offset from bone collagen by −3.0‰ in $\delta^{13}C$ and +1‰ in $\delta^{15}N$, values which represent a compromise between the offset published by Keegan and DeNiro (1988) for reef fish ($\delta^{13}C$: −3.4‰; $\delta^{15}N$: +1.7‰) and the bone collagen–flesh differences measured for two *Petenia splendida* fish from the Laguna Petexbatun. Herbivore meat values were calculated from the observed ranges of deer, peccary, agouti, and turtles with a collagen-flesh offset of −2.4‰ in $\delta^{13}C$ (DeNiro and Epstein 1978; van der Merwe 1982) and +0.6‰ in $\delta^{15}N$ (DeNiro and Epstein 1981). The mollusk box represents the values obtained for two *Pachychilus* meat samples. Since *Pomacea* and *Amblema* have shell carbonate $\delta^{13}C$ equivalent to *Pachychilus*, I assume a similar meat value. Carbon isotopic ranges for modern plants and meat estimates are shifted by +1.5‰ to account for the anthropogenic decline in $\delta^{13}C$ (Tieszen and Fagre 1993a). The isotopic composition of modern and archaeological fauna is given in Table 6.2 for each sample analyzed, along with measures of sample quality.

Table 6.1. Isotopic and elemental data for modern Pasión plant samples

N	Species (Common name)	Location	$\delta^{13}C$	$\delta^{15}N$	%N	%C	Ba/Ca	Sr/Ca	Ba/Sr	Ca(ppm)
115	*Opuntia sp.* (nopal cactus)	Aguateca	-10.01		0.3	26.7	.221	.213	1.04	152939
116	*Capsicum sp.* (chili pepper)	Aguateca	-30.10		2.2	48.7	.320	.323	.99	4185
121	*Brosimum alicastrum* (ramon)	Aguateca	-27.70		1.8	42.2	.552	.335	1.65	2209
122	*Brosimum alicastrum* (ramon)	Aguateca					.394	.320	1.23	1753
127	*B. alicastrum* (ramon tortilla)	Aguateca	-25.17		1.2	36.3	.526	3.684	.14	1938
128	*Phaseolus vulgaris* (beans)	Paso de Caribe	-27.12		3.8	43.3	.829	.449	1.85	869
130	*Astrocaryum mexicanum* (chapay nut)	Dos Pilas	-31.44		0.9	51.6	1.388	.945	1.47	519
131	*Astrocaryum mexicanum* (chapay nut)	Dos Pilas	-31.62		0.9	52.9	.963	1.280	.75	664
133	*Orbignya cohune* (corozo nut)	Dos Pilas	-29.65		0.0	58.0	.521	.397	1.31	1210
134	*Orbignya cohune* (corozo nut)	Dos Pilas	-28.30		0.0	58.2	.422	.342	1.23	1374
136	*Pouteria mamosa* (zapote fruit)	Dos Pilas	-27.10		0.8	44.1	.438	1.310	.33	2627
137	*Pouteria mamosa* (zapote seed)	Dos Pilas	-27.82	0.56	2.8	55.5	.464	.344	1.35	4444
138	*Bixa orellana* (achiote seeds)	Sepens	-29.71		2.0	43.4	.207	.384	.54	1640
145	*Ipomoea batatas* (camote/potato)	Sepens	-26.44		0.7	41.9	.635	.611	1.04	2505
146	*Capsicum sp.* (chili pepper)	Nacimiento	-27.75		2.4	0.8	1.117	.635	1.76	788
147	*Annona sp.* (anona fruit)	Sepens	-28.98		1.8	46.8	.316	.545	.58	2534
148	*Annona muricata* (soursop)	Sepens	-27.72	5.21	2.5	43.9	.374	.533	.70	2891
149	*Carica sp.* (wild papaya)	Sepens	-26.37	5.49	4.0	42.2	.096	.298	.32	23565

150	*Theobroma cacao* (cacao)	Sepens	-34.14	3.69	2.6	59.4	.631	.855	.74	2013
153	*Pouteria mamosa* (zapote fruit)	Dos Pilas	-28.13		0.6	43.8	1.127	.635	1.77	1464
154	*Pouteria mamosa* (zapote seed)	Dos Pilas	-30.04		2.9	62.6	1.406	.609	2.31	854
155	*Dialium guianense* (wild tamarind)	Dos Pilas	-26.11		1.3	43.2	.857	.917	.93	665
156	*Zea mays* (maize)	Nacimiento	-11.20	6.07	1.9	44.3	1.371	1.029	1.33	146
157	*Brosimum alicastrum* (ramon)	Dos Pilas	-27.03		1.4	42.0	.968	.654	1.48	795
158	*Dioscorea alata* (macal/yam)	Dos Pilas	-25.06		2.2	34.9	2.897	4.602	.63	3038
159	lingua de vaca (epiphyte)	Dos Pilas	-26.81		-0.5	40.9	.602	.839	.72	3671
160	*Psidium guajava* (guava)	Dos Pilas	-27.27		1.5	46.6	.765	.344	2.23	640
161	*Persea americana* (avocado)	Dos Pilas					.463	.799	.58	1252
162	*Licania platypus* (sunzapote)	Dos Pilas	-29.28		0.9	50.1	.612	.365	1.68	1095
163	(junco palm leaf)	Dos Pilas	-26.66	4.01	3.8	41.9	.864	1.860	.46	6284
176	*Cucurbita sp.* (pepitoria squash)	Nacimiento	-27.35	8.78	6.0	55.4	1.256	.802	1.56	573
177	*Phaseolus vulgaris* (beans)	Sepens	-27.75	3.94	3.9	40.9	1.187	.731	1.62	657
183	*Byrsonima crassifolia* (nance)	Nacimiento	-27.10		0.8	47.4	.205	.413	.49	3652
190	*Zea mays* (maize)	Altar	-11.02	3.50	1.4	43.4	4.888	3.016	1.62	96
191	*Zea mays* (maize cob)	Altar					2.202	1.276	1.73	886
196	*Cucurbita sp.* (pepitoria squash)	Altar	-27.12	7.53	4.8	39.1	2.024	1.418	1.43	7609
242	*Bromelia karatas* (piñuela)	Dos Pilas	-16.72		2.2	42.4	-	-	1.00	6525
243	water lily	Laguna Petexbatun	-24.55		4.0	38.2	1.274	4.531	.28	14124

The terrestrial fauna fall intermediate to C3 and C4 plant signals in terms of $\delta^{13}C$ composition. Herbivore (deer, peccary) bone collagen is about 5‰ more positive than C3 plants for most samples, paralleling the diet-collagen spacing noted for other large herbivores. However, two archaeological deer samples (#24 and #28) are sufficiently more positive to suggest some consumption of C4 plants. This likely reflects the tendency of deer to browse in *milpas*, where maize leaves would contribute isotopically heavier carbon to the total collagen signal. Intentional feeding of maize to deer would also produce this effect, if deer were domesticated. Semi-domestication of deer is suggested by Landa's description of tame herds of deer and by the rearing of young deer by Maya women in their homes (Pohl 1985; Tozzer 1941). Among the remains examined here, the most secure evidence for domestication comes from a cache of subadult deer limbs excavated from Str. N5-21 at Dos Pilas (Chinchilla Mazariegos 1991). One femur shows a healed midshaft complete fracture, an injury that would predispose a juvenile animal to rapid death in the wild. The animal survived after the injury for several months, which is an unlikely outcome unless it had been protected from predation (Emery 1991). A sample from this animal (#25) does not show anomalously heavy $\delta^{13}C$ (−21.6‰), indicating that it was not fed significant quantities of maize. While heavy maize consumption by deer would support the hypothesis of domestication, the converse is not true. Domesticated deer could also have been fed C3 plant foods.

A larger series of Petexbatun *Odocoileus* remains were analyzed by Emery and colleagues (2000) after the work described here had been completed. They found a mean $\delta^{13}C$ of −20.55±1.0‰, which falls well within the range shown here. The $\delta^{13}C$ of Petexbatun deer collagen does not vary systematically by site or chronological period, which suggests that agricultural pressures did not dramatically affect deer feeding behavior (Emery et al. 2000). Stability in deer $\delta^{13}C$ has also been reported at Colha in northern Belize (White et al. 2001).

Several other "wild" fauna show evidence of maize consumption in both the past and present. Although modern white-lipped peccary (*Tayassu pecari*) values are similar to deer in $\delta^{13}C$, with values perhaps slightly lighter, near −24‰, modern collared peccary (*Tayassu tajacu*) differ substantially, with much more positive $\delta^{13}C$, at −17.6 and −12.9‰. The latter value approaches the range measured for prehistoric Pasión humans! Although there are difficulties with linear modeling of complex diets like that of omnivorous peccary, the high $\delta^{13}C$ of this modern animal implies a 50% contribution of carbon from C4 sources, assuming a fully herbivorous diet. Like deer, collared peccary often graze in *milpas*, where corn stalks and cobs may be a significant component of their diet. White-lipped peccary do not do this, which likely accounts for the difference (Emmons 1990). The prehistoric specimens do not show such a difference between the two peccary species, with most falling around −20‰. Indeed, one white-lipped peccary is the most enriched at −18‰.

Discrepancies in $\delta^{13}C$ between modern and archaeological fauna are also seen for *Agouti* samples. The two modern *Agouti*s show C3 signals (average −22.7‰), while the two Late Classic specimens average −9.2‰, indicating significant maize consumption in the past. The $\delta^{13}C$ of one prehistoric *Dasyprocta* also indicates significant maize consumption at −14‰, but a second indicates a pure C3 diet. Although the sample sizes are small, these discrepancies indicate that for both peccary and agoutis, modern faunal comparisons cannot adequately constrain the dietary signal of prehistoric food items.

Presumably, intentional feeding explains the ^{13}C enriched collagen of prehistoric Petexbatun dogs. Most of the dogs sampled were clearly dependent on maize for most of their food, having average $\delta^{13}C$ of −9.1±0.6‰ (n = 5), but one canid had very light collagen (−19.19‰), which might indicate a nondomesticate or a misidentification. This average is significantly more enriched than Preclassic dogs from either Cuello or Colha (Tykot et al. 1996; White et al. 2001), indicating proportionately greater maize consumption by Pasión dogs than Belizean ones.

One sample of domestic turkey that was raised in the modern village of Nacimiento shows

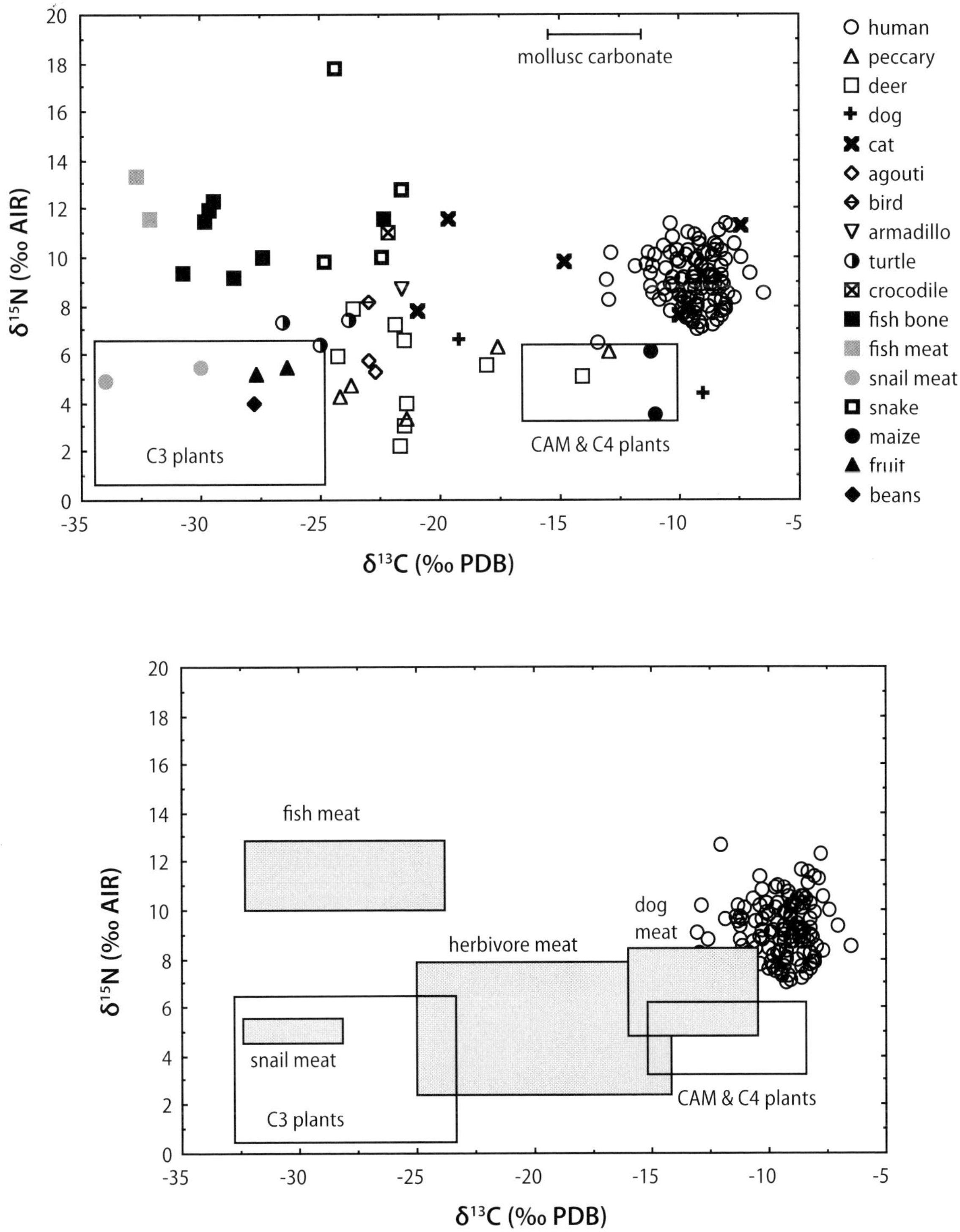

Figure 6.1. Isotopic composition of Pasión flora and fauna, relative to human data

Table 6.2. Isotopic and elemental composition of animal tissues

(a) Archaeological bone samples

N	Site	Species	Tissue	δ13C	δ15N	C/N	%C	%N	Ca/P	Ba/Ca	Sr/Ca	Ba/Sr
25	Dos Pilas	Cervidae	femur	-21.64	2.23	3.13	45.27	16.85	2.08	.40	.93	.43
24	Aguateca	*O. virginianus*	femur	-18.13	5.60	3.23	45.60	16.46				
233	Dos Pilas	*O. virginianus*	astragalus	-21.40	4.00	3.00		.	2.23	.44	.34	1.28
234	Dos Pilas	*O. virginianus*	tarsal IV centrale					2.27	.36	.47	.77	
27	Punto de Chimino	*O. virginianus*	femur	-21.48	6.60	3.19	45.99	16.81	2.13	.52	.84	.61
26	Punto de Chimino	*Mazama americana*	humerus	-21.50	3.10	3.30		.	2.18	.50	.47	1.05
28	Aguateca	*M. americana*	humerus	-14.04	5.08	3.23	43.51	15.71				
379	Tamarindito	*M. americana*	radius	-22.47		3.28						
232	Punto de Chimino	Tayassuidae	mandible					.	2.26	.47	.52	.90
231	Punto de Chimino	*Tayassu cf. pecari*	metatarsal	-21.40	3.30	3.04	45.97	17.65	2.26	.45	.89	.51
383	Arroyo de Piedra	*T. pecari*	innominate	-18.505		3.31						
318	Arroyo de Piedra	*T. tajacu*	radius	-19.62		3.26						
319	Arroyo de Piedra	*T. tajacu*	humerus	-20.77		3.14						.
382	Tamarindito	*T. tajacu*	tibia	-20.74		3.34						
316	Dos Pilas	*Agouti paca*	humerus	-9.29		3.24						
381	Dos Pilas	*Agouti paca*	femur	-9.25		3.04						
230	Punto de Chimino	*cf. Dasyprocta*	humerus					.	2.27	.23	.24	.96
317	Dos Pilas	*Dasyprocta punctata*	femur	-14.45		3.33						
380	Tamarindito	*D. punctata*	humerus	-20.91		3.44						

215	Dos Pilas	turtle	carapace					.	2.16	.41	1.02	.40
225	Punto de Chimino	turtle	carapace					.	2.23	.49	1.32	.37
226	Punto de Chimino	turtle	carapace						2.16	.40	1.10	.37
227	Punto de Chimino	turtle	carapace	-23.80	7.40	2.80			2.26	.41	1.60	.26
228	Punto de Chimino	turtle	carapace	-25.00	6.40	2.90			2.26	.48	6.77	.07
216	Dos Pilas	large felid	phalange	-14.80	9.80	3.15	44.87	16.63				
217	Dos Pilas	large felid	metapodial					.	2.17	.25	.57	.45
218	Dos Pilas	small felid	metapodial					.	2.08	.01	.37	.02
322	Arroyo de Piedra	large felid	calcaneus	-10.01	7.57	3.67						
323	Dos Pilas	*Felis sp.*	ulna	-7.45	11.26	3.02						
324	Tamarindito	*Felis sp.*	humerus	-20.91	7.77	3.09						
320	Arroyo de Piedra	*Felis sp.*	talus	-19.76		3.27						
321	Aguateca	*Felis sp.*	phalanx	-16.53		2.94						
325	Arroyo de Piedra	*Felis sp.*	phalanx	-18.49		3.17						
327	Arroyo de Piedra	*Canis sp.*	ulna	-19.19	6.57	2.92						
328	Dos Pilas	*Canis sp.*	ulna	-8.96	4.37	3.33						
329	Dos Pilas	*Canis sp.*	longbone	-9.57	7.91	2.91						
330	Aguateca	*Canis sp.*	radius	-9.90		3.27						
326	Arroyo de Piedra	*Canis sp.*	ilium	-8.78		3.14						
331	Arroyo de Piedra	*Canis sp.*	radius	-8.32		3.28						
378	Aguateca	*Meleagris gallopavo*	not noted	-8.11		3.37						
229	Punto de Chimino	*Crocodylus moreleti*	dermal scute	-22.10	11.00	2.90			2.28	.27	.60	.46

continued on next page

(b) Modern faunal samples

N	Site	Species	Tissue	$\delta^{13}C$	$\delta^{15}N$	C/N	%C	%N	Ca/P	Ba/Ca	Sr/Ca	Ba/Sr
171	Sepens	*O. virginianus*	antler	-21.86	7.20	3.27	30.07	10.72	2.10	2.67	.06	41.46
180	Flores	*O. virginianus*	femur	-23.63	7.86	3.35	20.20	7.03	2.13	.59	1.54	.38
184	Dos Pilas	*M. americana*	ribs	-24.26	5.92	3.24	23.58	8.50	2.16	.20	.28	.71
151	Maravillas	*Tayassu tajacu*	femur	-12.99	6.07	3.27			2.13	.05	.07	.65
170	Dos Pilas	*Tayassu tajacu*	mandible	-17.60	6.32	3.21	26.86	9.75	2.22	.00	.07	.07
168	Dos Pilas	*Tayassu pecari*	mandible	-23.66	4.73	3.24	31.32	11.28	2.27	.01	.33	.03
167	Dos Pilas	*Tayassu pecari*	zygomatic	-24.17	4.29	2.90	26.47	10.65	2.19	.02	.47	.05
164	Sepens	*Agouti paca*	femur						2.11	.29	.15	1.95
165	Sepens	*Agouti paca*	rib	-22.97	5.78	2.97	17.88	7.03				
166	Dos Pilas	*Agouti paca*	zygomatic	-22.64	5.28	3.29	20.72	7.35	2.16	.92	1.39	.66
237	Flores	*Agouti paca*	ribs						1.96	.07	.24	.28
152	Sepens	*Dasypus novemcinctus*	carapace	-21.75		2.60	21.78	9.77	2.20	.22	.66	.33
181	Sepens	*Dasypus novemcinctus*	carapace	-21.62	8.66	3.26	28.42	10.18	2.21	.17	2.68	.06
172	Dos Pilas	*Felis cf. pardalis*	canine root	-19.64	11.58	3.27	21.32	7.60	1.96	.05	.22	.25
235	Punto de Chimino	*Chrysemys cf. scripta*	carapace	-26.57	7.29	3.34	29.57	10.32	2.56	.18	1.16	.16
185	Dos Pilas	*Meleagris gallopavo*	ribs	-9.93	8.29	3.37	15.73	5.45	2.12	.04	.15	.26
238	Dos Pilas	*Tinamus major*	egg membrane	-22.94	8.11	3.38	46.62	16.07				
238	Dos Pilas	*Tinamus major*	egg shell	-11.40	(carbonate)				114	.02	.08	.25
173	Dos Pilas	rat snake	vertebra	-24.84	9.81	10.46	4.39	0.49	1.99	.04	.09	.44
174	Dos Pilas	rat snake	vertebra						2.10	.03	.13	.22
175	Dos Pilas	*Micrurus sp.*	vertebra	-21.62	12.74	3.84	5.53	1.68	2.09	.15	.15	1.02
186	Dos Pilas	*Porphidium nummifer*	vertebra	-24.35	17.76	2.90	14.6	5.87	2.15	.09	.07	1.29

187	Dos Pilas	*P. nummifer*	vertebra						2.16	.09	.07	1.32
188	Aguateca	*Bothrops asper*	vertebra	-22.37	10.01	3.09	20.72	7.81	2.09	.14	.25	.58
31	Aguateca	colorada fish	vertebra	-28.60	9.20				1.94	.28	1.30	.21
239	Aguateca	colorada fish	vertebra	-27.39	10.00	3.88	20.01	6.01	2.11	.20	1.12	.18
32	Aguateca	guapote fish	vertebra	-30.80	9.30				1.92	.09	.69	.13
240	Aguateca	guapote fish	vertebra	-29.86	11.51	3.53	14.68	4.85				
33	Aguateca	*Petenia splendida*	vertebra	-29.50	12.30				1.95	.07	.63	.12
36	Aguateca	*Petenia splendida*	meat of #33	-32.70	13.30							
34	Aguateca	*P. splendida*	vertebra	-29.60	11.90				1.94	.05	.65	.08
35	Aguateca	*P. splendida*	meat of #34	-32.10	11.60							
241	Aguateca	*P. splendida*	vertebra						2.17	.05	.81	.06
179	R. Salinas	*Ictalurus*	cranium	-22.28	11.59	3.33	14.31	5.02	2.08	.02	2.04	.01
194	Altar	*Pomacea flagellata*	shell	-13.20					9668	.24	.99	.24
30	Aguateca	*P. flagellata*	shell						4422	.09	.43	.21
195	Dos Pilas	*P. flagellata*	shell	-15.50					6313	.11	.40	.28
29	Aguateca	*P. flagellata*	shell						29454	.12	.87	.14
141	Dos Pilas	*Pachychilus glaphyrus*	shell	-13.80					3561	.04	.49	.09
141	Dos Pilas	*Pachychilus glaphyrus*	meat	-33.59	4.87							
142	Dos Pilas	*P. glaphyrus*	shell	-13.80					6182	.03	.44	.07
142	Dos Pilas	*P. glaphyrus*	meat	-30.00	5.49							
197	Altar	*Amblema sp.*	shell	-11.40					4239	.06	1.36	.05
236	Altar	*Amblema sp.*	shell	-12.40					4579	.16	1.53	.10
182	Dos Pilas	freshwater crab	chitin	-21.22	3.21				84	.92	1.77	.52

a distinct C4 signature at −9.9‰ (hidden below the human data points in Figure 6.1) because spoiled maize is fed to domestic animals (Secaira 1992). A prehistoric specimen from Aguateca is even more ^{13}C-enriched, indicating that this practice is of great antiquity. The wild bird eggshell has light membrane $\delta^{13}C$, indicating that the bird which laid the egg consumed mostly C3 plants in the forest. Somewhat high $\delta^{15}N$ in egg membrane protein may indicate a more omnivorous diet, although a secondary trophic effect is also possible.

Herbivore bone collagen is characterized by a broad range of $\delta^{15}N$, showing variable trophic enrichment from the plant signatures. Several of the deer and peccary are only 1 to 2‰ heavier than the C3 plants, suggesting that leguminous plants might contribute to their diet. This is not surprising as many leguminous species occur in the primary forest and in secondary regrowth. The presence of nitrogen-fixing bacteria that live on the surface of many tropical forest leaves might also contribute to the low $\delta^{15}N$ of deer. For peccary, soil organisms ingested while foraging for palm nuts might also be implicated in low values. The agouti have $\delta^{15}N$ values comparable to deer and white-lipped peccary, reflecting herbivory.

Carnivores show further enrichment of $\delta^{13}C$ over the majority of herbivore data, with an average $\delta^{13}C$ of −15.4±5.0‰, but are quite variable, ranging from −20.9‰ to −7.4‰. The value obtained from canine dentine of a modern small cat (probably ocelot, *F. pardalis*) falls at the light end of this range, at −19.6‰. Since cats are essentially carnivorous, this value must reflect some fractionation of meat $\delta^{13}C$, but for some may also be due to preying on other maize-eaters, such as agouti. Although these cats also consume snakes and fish (Emmons 1990), the $\delta^{15}N$ levels are in line with single trophic-level enrichment from consumption of terrestrial herbivores alone. Thus, high $\delta^{13}C$ in cat collagen presumably reflects trophic enrichment in ^{13}C, further elevated by the heavy $\delta^{13}C$ of C4-eating prey.

Snake collagen is more negative than the cat values and resembles herbivore $\delta^{13}C$, perhaps due to the consumption of frogs that might have lighter values like other aquatic fauna. Although we cannot assume identical isotopic fractionation and metabolic processes among mammals and reptiles, snake $\delta^{15}N$ values are comparable to the mammalian carnivores, suggesting an analogous trophic effect in nitrogen metabolism. One pit viper (*Porphidium nummifer*) shows exceptionally high $\delta^{15}N$ (17.8‰), perhaps due to consumption of some carnivorous prey.

Freshwater fauna contrasts the terrestrial trend with highly variable $\delta^{13}C$ and generally high $\delta^{15}N$. Freshwater turtle collagen $\delta^{13}C$ and $\delta^{15}N$ is comparable to that of terrestrial herbivores, perhaps because turtles consume both aquatic and terrestrial foods. Crocodile collagen is similar in $\delta^{15}N$ to that of terrestrial carnivores. The $\delta^{13}C$ level is somewhat low, −22.1‰, and implies consumption of very light prey, such as fish.

Collagen carbon in modern fish (blanco, guapote, colorada) from the Laguna Petexbatun is exceptionally light, with $\delta^{13}C$ of vertebrae averaging −29.75‰. Dried and salted meat samples from two "blanco" bass (*Petenia splendida*) indicate that meat is further depleted by about −2.8‰ (−32.05, −32.74‰). This low value could reflect the decomposition of very light terrestrial plant detritus in streams and rivers that contributes to dissolved inorganic carbon in water, which is further depleted by −5 to −30‰ (depending on rate of water flow) during photosynthesis by aquatic plants (Fry and Sherr 1988). A catfish cranium sample (*Ictalurus sp.*) from the Salinas River is less distinctive, −22.3‰, perhaps owing to dietary peculiarities of this species or the swifter current in this river. Unfortunately, the only aquatic plant sampled, a water lily from Laguna Petexbatun, has a typical C3 signature, −24.6‰, probably because it photosynthizes atmospheric CO_2. Fish are particularly enriched in $\delta^{15}N$ owing to stepwise trophic-level fractionation. Indeed, fish $\delta^{15}N$ is comparable to that produced by carnivory in felids, snakes, and crocodiles.

Yet, other aquatic species show much heavier $\delta^{13}C$. Carbonate in molluscan shells (*Pomacea, Pachychilus,* and *Amblema*) resembles a C4 signal (−11.4 to −15.5‰), a result that may suggest heavy dissolved carbonate, contradicting the previous hypothesis. However, the flesh of two *Pachychilus* from Dos Pilas is very light in carbon, at −30.0 and −33.6‰, resembling the flesh of Petexbatun fish. Because snails are detritivores, the $\delta^{15}N$ of snail flesh is lower than most aquatic fauna, resembling terrestrial herbivores.

Chitin from a freshwater Dos Pilas crab is characterized by values akin to herbivore collagen, but crab meat would have been much more enriched in ^{15}N, approximately 13.2‰, because the chitin-flesh offset is particularly large (flesh $\delta^{13}C$ = chitin − 2.4‰; $\delta^{15}N$ = chitin + 10.0‰; Schimmelman 1985).

Human bone collagen falls clearly into the range of maize dependency, being slightly heavier in $\delta^{13}C$ than maize. However, were maize the sole component of the diet, human collagen $\delta^{13}C$ should be heavier still, near −6 to −5‰, because of the offset between diet and collagen $\delta^{13}C$ of +5‰. C3 plant or animal consumption must be keeping this value down. The $\delta^{15}N$ values are also heavy and lie above the values of terrestrial herbivores. In fact, human $\delta^{15}N$ is comparable to felid and crocodylid $\delta^{15}N$, indicating a significant contribution of nitrogen from animal protein. Human consumption of domestic dogs, and agoutis that live in maize fields, presumably also contributes to the heavy $\delta^{13}C$ and $\delta^{15}N$.

Alkaline Earth Elements

Because elemental distributions throughout the food web ultimately are dependent upon the geological distribution of elements in soils (Burton et al. 1999), my investigation of elemental patterns in the Pasión ecosystem begins with consideration of soil data. Table 6.3 contains descriptive statistics for soil samples from each site. Raw data for each sample can be found in Wright (1994). The limestone parent material that underlies the region leads to very high soluble Ca in Pasión soils. Barium and Sr levels are low at all sites and, relative to Ca, approximately an order of magnitude lower than in soils from the American Midwest (Burton et al. 1999). The high kurtosis and skewness in soil element data at each site indicate that soil element distributions are not normally distributed in these small samples and that nonparametric tests are generally appropriate for analysis of these data.

Intersite differences in the concentration of a number of elements indicate that soils from Altar de Sacrificios are most distinctive. Altar soils show lower concentrations of soluble Ca and Mg, but higher Fe, K, Ti, Zn, and Ba. Elemental differences are to be anticipated between Altar and the remaining sites because of its unique location on the floodplain of the Pasión River. Soils at Altar are composed largely of alluvial deposits of highland origin. These highland sediments occur in the Pasión and Salinas valleys but are rare in the smaller Petexbatun drainage, which receives only slight sedimentation from rainy-season backup of the Pasión (N. Dunning, personal communication 1993). Moreover, underlying parent material at Altar is composed of Paleocene-Eocene marine sediments, in contrast to the Cretaceous Neocomian-Campanian carbonate horst below the other sites (Dunning et al. 1997). Soil characteristics also differ between sites inasmuch as that the floodplain soils are poorly drained hydromorphic calciaquolls, while the better-drained karstic upland soils are lithic rendolls and rendic entisols (Dunning et al. 1991).

Because dietary incorporation of Sr and Ba occurs by substitution for Ca, the abundance of these elements is examined here in relation to the Ca content of soils (Figure 6.2). Strontium concentration shows a high positive linear correlation with Ca content (Spearman's Rho = 0.891, $p = 0.0001$). In contrast, Ba is negatively correlated with Ca (Rho = −0.755, $p = 0.0001$). Together, these patterns contribute to the higher Ba/Sr ratio in the Ca-poor soils at Altar than in the Ca-rich soils of the other sites (Table 6.3). The low Sr levels in the Ca-poor soils simply reflect the low Ca concentration, given the highly linear relationship between these two elements. The two samples from the riverbank at Seibal show particularly low Ca in comparison to the site center and marrow samples, but have equivalent Sr, and fall above the line with anomalously high Sr/Ca. Samples from two burials at Tamarindito broadly cluster with soils from Itzan but lie below the line, perhaps due to greater leaching of Sr from these better-drained upland areas.

The relationship appears to be more complex

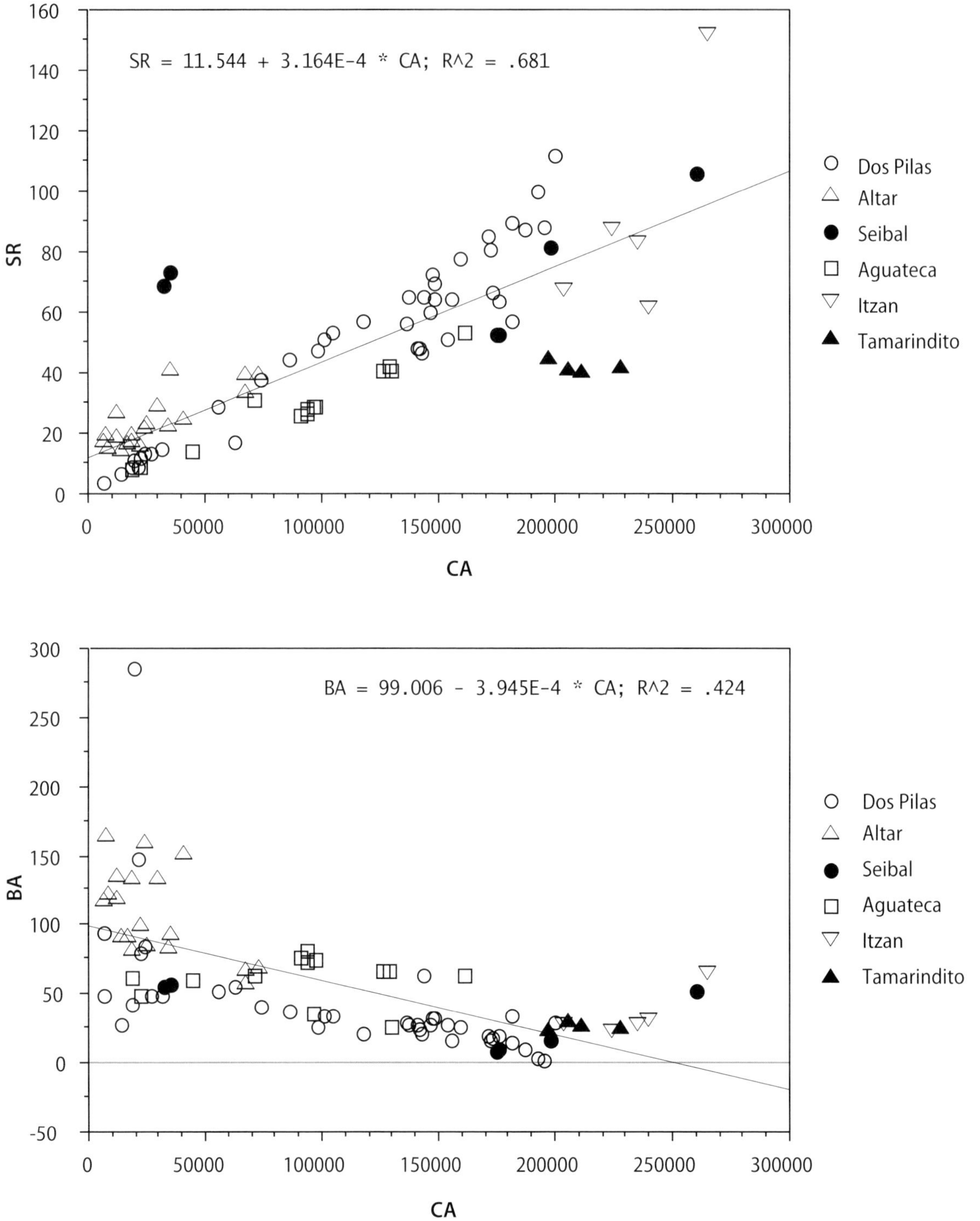

Figure 6.2. Alkaline earth concentrations (ppm) in Pasión soils by site

Sr and Ca show a strong positive linear correlation, while Ba and Ca show a strong negative correlation.

Table 6.3. Descriptive statistics for elemental concentrations in soils by site

Element	mean	s.d.	Kurtosis	Skew	Element	mean	s.d.	Kurtosis	Skew
(a) Altar de Sacrificios (n=19)					**(b) Dos Pilas (n=41)**				
Al	10779	1464	-.753	-.533	Al	9525	3555	-.058	-.278
Ba	107	32	-1.090	.205	Ba	43	47	15.978	3.743
Ca	28002	20733	.092	1.129	Ca	112750	63683	-1.260	-.445
Fe	15785	2496	-1.023	-.493	Fe	5316	3140	.264	.955
K	1271	455	5.554	2.246	K	347	153	.523	.046
Mg	18013	11507	.505	1.351	Mg	52034	33152	-.874	.014
Mn	531	117	-.484	-.218	Mn	774	860	7.765	2.593
Na	212	54	5.578	2.361	Na	196	56	.348	-.091
P	3056	2634	6.288	2.455	P	1320	1868	11.426	3.097
Sr	24	9	-.587	.843	Sr	50	29	-.897	-.057
Ti	114	31	-.419	-.462	Ti	16	10	1.324	1.348
Zn	68	12	.080	-.338	Zn	18	7	1.177	.773
Ba/Sr	5.186	2.262	-1.129	-.245	Ba/Sr	3.043	5.991	6.807	2.749
Sr/Ca	.001	.001	.138	1.177	Sr/Ca	.00046	.00005	.016	-.342
Ba/Ca	.007	.006	1.107	1.352	Ba/Ca	.002	.003	7.901	2.929
(c) Itzan (n=5)					**(d) Aguateca (n=13)**				
Al	5081	896	-1.638	.006	Al	15937	4215	-1.430	-.500
Ba	34	17	.118	1.400	Ba	61	16	.181	-1.002
Ca	233732	22521	-.796	.086	Ca	90350	42419	-.673	-.294
Fe	2750	520	-1.284	.255	Fe	8582	3366	-1.006	-.208
K	636	397	-.815	.766	K	495	289	-1.451	.629
Mg	50538	34092	-1.789	-.391	Mg	38357	19588	-.492	-.103
Mn	202	64	-1.480	.383	Mn	726	164	.557	-.293
Na	281	58	-1.551	.373	Na	285	247	1.757	1.869
P	5889	2038	-.809	-.105	P	2778	2924	1.307	1.332
Sr	90	36	-.159	1.182	Sr	29	13	-.654	-.062
Ti	16	4	-1.415	-.196	Ti	19	7	-1.334	-.163
Zn	29	22	.094	1.392	Zn	39	18	-1.626	.386
Ba/Sr	.375	.093	-1.210	-.096	Ba/Sr	3.033	4.499	11.144	3.040
Sr/Ca	.00038	.00012	-.407	.858	Sr/Ca	.001	.001	6.419	2.607
Ba/Ca	.00014	.00005	.050	1.339	Ba/Ca	.002	.004	7.325	2.663

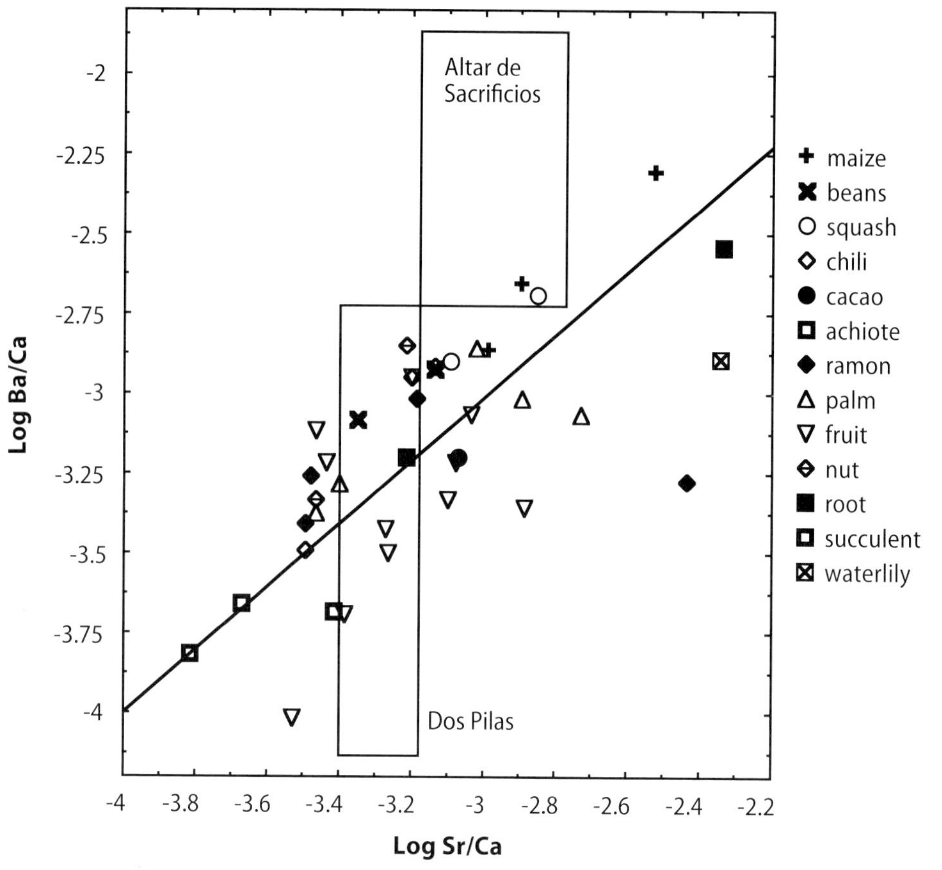

Figure 6.3. Log Ba/Ca and Log Sr/Ca in Pasión plants

Boxes delineate the mean soil values for Altar de Sacrificios and Dos Pilas, ± 1 s.d. The diagonal line indicates Ba/Sr = 1.

for Ba (Figure 6.2). Ba is less strongly correlated with Ca in soils with greater than 80,000 ppm Ca (Rho = −0.489, $p = 0.001$) than in the series overall, but it is much more abundant in soils of lower Ca concentration at Altar de Sacrificios, probably reflecting the different geochemical origin of these soils. A few samples from Dos Pilas are also low in Ca and cluster with the Altar soils. These samples are from the north edge of the site where there is a transition to denser limestone that causes an upwelling of subsurface streams. The two riverbank samples from Seibal do not show high Ba like the Altar samples, so highland sediments may not be so significant in floodplain soils at that site as at Altar. The very high Ca in Itzan and Tamarindito soil samples might be due to weathered bone mineral, in part, given the almost total disintegration of skeletal remains at both these well-drained sites.

Given these patterns, the Ba/Sr composition of groundwater available for uptake into plants is expected to differ across the region. The majority of plant samples were collected near Dos Pilas or in nearby villages that are located on rendzina soils. Ba and Sr content of the plants sampled, relative to Ca, is illustrated in Figure 6.3. The raw data are in Wright (1994). The boxes indicate the Ba/Ca and Sr/Ca content of soils within one standard deviation of the mean for Altar and Dos Pilas. Although the soil values obtained by acid extraction are probably not precisely the concentrations available to plants and so cannot be used to confirm biopurification in plant uptake, they serve to illustrate the relative availability of Ba and Ca in the two soil types.

Most plant tissues contain Ba and Sr in approximately similar proportions to the soils at Dos Pilas. The broad spread of floral Sr/Ca ratios undoubtedly reflects the larger regional origin of the samples than of soils at Dos Pilas. The effect of intersite soil heterogeneity is apparent in the maize values. The two maize samples from Altar are higher in both Sr/Ca and Ba/Ca than the sample from Nacimiento, near Dos Pilas, paralleling the direction of soil differences between the sites. Overall, Ba and Sr content of the plants is highly correlated (Rho = 0.810, $p = 0.0001$), indicating fairly consistent discrimination between species in root uptake. However, some patterns are worth noting. The typical Maya cultigens—maize, beans, and squash—show higher Ba/Ca values than many other foods, in part because one squash and two maize samples were obtained from Altar. Nonetheless, Dos Pilas domesticates are also relatively high. The two succulents, nopal and piñuela, are at the opposite extreme, low in both elements. Most plants contain slightly more Ba than Sr, lying slightly above the Ba/Sr = 1.0 line, but many fruits are low in Ba, falling below this line. Cacao is similar to the fruits. The two species of palm differ in both Sr and Ba content, with corozo nuts lower in both elements than chapaya. Ramon nuts are similar in composition to most nonfruit samples. Gaspar Riqueña, an institute guard at Aguateca, prepared ramon tortillas that I sampled. After removing the flesh, he boiled the nuts for one hour, removed the pericarp, and ground the endocarp into masa. Tortillas formed from this masa were wrapped in plantain leaves to facilitate turning and cooked on the comal. This tortilla preparation caused an increase in Sr/Ca as compared to unprepared ramon but did not affect Ba/Ca, indicating either Sr enrichment from the water in which the nuts were boiled or contamination from the aluminum pot. The water lily is similarly high in Sr, foreshadowing an aquatic distinction.

The effect of plant foods on the bone mineral content of a consumer depends on the Ca content of the food. The *Opuntia* leaf contains much more Ca than other plants sampled and could affect bone chemistry if eaten in sufficient quantities. In contrast, maize kernels contain much less Ca than other plants and would contribute few dietary minerals unless treated with lime.

Ba and Sr composition of the modern faunal specimens is illustrated in Figure 6.4. The Ba/Ca and Sr/Ca composition of plants is indicated by the two boxes. The higher position of the cultivated triad reflects both interspecies differences as well as site soil differences as discussed above. Trophic-level fractionation between flora and terrestrial fauna is readily apparent in the lower concentrations of both Ba and Sr in faunal bone. Overall, the terrestrial fauna are aligned with the plants close to the Ba/Sr = 1.0 line. The fauna lie slightly below the line, due to greater discrimination against Ba than Sr in mineral metabolism (Burton and Price 1990a; Elias et al. 1982). The more strictly herbivorous species (deer, agouti) show high Ba/Ca and Sr/Ca, close to the plant values, reflecting the high Ca content of their largely folivorous diet. Interestingly, an agouti from Sepens that was trapped near its burrow in a *milpa* falls on the edge of the staple triad box. The peccaries, domestic turkey, and mangolol eggshell are low in Ba/Ca due to their omnivorous diet. The snake bones and ocelot tooth contain lower ratios of both elements than the herbivorous mammals, but higher ratios than the peccaries. As both cats and snakes consume their prey whole, the high Ca contribution of partially digested bone may underlie the intermediate location of both carnivores relative to other species.

Few geographic differences are apparent in herbivore values. One deer from Sepens that shows very high Ba/Ca in addition to high Mg and K may be contaminated or may not have been hunted locally. A second deer purchased in Flores is high in Sr that may also be an environmental distinction. Otherwise, samples from the Pasión region proper are homogeneous, indicating that elemental heterogeneity across the region is averaged out by large and shifting herbivore ranges.

A useful distinction among the faunal data is the clear separation of freshwater from terrestrial species. The Sr/Ca ratio in fish bones and snail shells is much higher than in the bones of terrestrial vertebrates. Freshwater turtle and crab also

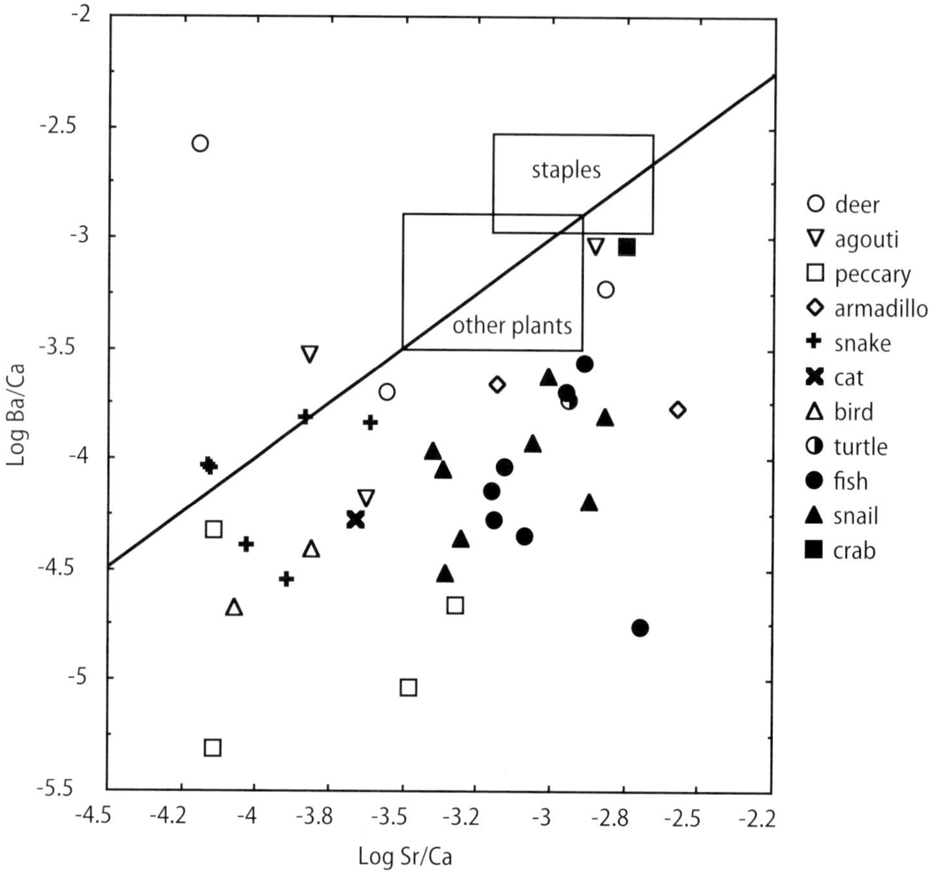

Figure 6.4. Log Ba/Ca and Log Sr/Ca in modern faunal samples. Boxes delineate the mean values for the staple foods (maize, beans, squash) and other wild or cultivated plants, ± 1 s.d.

The diagonal line indicates Ba/Sr = 1.

show high Sr/Ca values. As Ba/Ca ratios do not differ, the Ba/Sr of freshwater fauna (0.19) is lower than terrestrial fauna (1.91), paralleling the marine/terrestrial distinction noted elsewhere (Burton and Price 1990b). Mean Ba/Sr for Pasión aquatic fauna is also somewhat lower than values for freshwater fauna (0.63; log Ba/Sr = −0.2) reported by Burton and Price (1990b) but are not nearly as low as in marine systems (0.0004; log Ba/Sr = −2.4). Recall that the water lily also showed higher Sr/Ca than terrestrial plants. Given the low Sr of Pasión soils and the lack of Sr differences between soils of different geological origin in the region, the high freshwater Sr values must be a consequence of Sr leaching from soil into the watershed. In contrast to temperate ecosystems in which the bulk of minerals are stored in the soil, in tropical ecosystems minerals are bound up in forest biomass, leaving soils relatively nutrient deficient. Heavy rainfall leaches minerals from soil and carries them away in runoff (Golley et al. 1975; Jordan et al. 1972). Highly soluble Sr may be more prone to leaching and more concentrated in runoff than Ba, which is bound up in barite and soil sulfates. Differential leaching of Sr relative to Ba was also documented in the Bajo de Santa Fe at Tikal (Cowgill and Hutchinson 1963). Moreover, Elias and others found higher Sr/Ca ratios in stream water than in soil moisture but no difference for Ba/Ca in a temperate subalpine ecosystem (Elias et al. 1982). Given higher tropical leaching, this pattern might be magnified in tropical ecosystems.

Paleodiet and Alkaline Processing of Maize

Maize is a primary staple food for many New World cultures; however, several of its chemical characteristics can pose nutritional problems at high levels of consumption. The pericarp contains phytate, a chemical that inhibits the absorption of iron and zinc in the digestive tract (Layrisse et al. 1969). Secondly, maize protein contains very little niacin, lysine, and tryptophan and has a high leucine/isoleucine ratio. Tryptophan is a precursor necessary for endogenous synthesis of niacin. Niacin deficiency causes pellagra, a form of malnutrition that can also be induced by consumption of foods with excessive leucine. Many Amerindian cultures have adapted to high levels of maize consumption by developing techniques to process maize with alkali before consumption (Katz et al. 1974). Alkaline processing effectively combats the nutritional difficulties of maize-reliant diets by changing the chemical and physical composition of corn. By soaking or boiling maize in an alkaline solution, the pericarp is dissolved from the exterior of the kernel, then subsequently rinsed away, eliminating most of the phytate. Alkaline treatment also changes the protein composition of maize by liberating the glutelin fraction, which lowers the leucine/isoleucine ratio and increases available lysine, tryptophan, and niacin, improving the overall nutritional quality of the grain (Bressani et al. 1958; Bressani and Scrimshaw 1958; Katz et al. 1974).

Chemical changes induced in maize by alkaline processing could have implications for the reconstruction of prehistoric diets through an analysis of the isotopic and elemental composition of human bone. With respect to $\delta^{13}C$, changes in the relative solubility of proteins from different compartments of the maize kernel might affect the total isotopic composition because these compartments differ in $\delta^{13}C$ (Tieszen and Fagre 1993a). The main goal of alkaline processing is removal of the pericarp, which is generally more positive than the embryo. Selective loss of protein, fiber, and vitamins from the endosperm, which is more positive than either the embryo or pericarp, could also lower the effective $\delta^{13}C$ of maize. Moreover, individual amino acids within maize differ isotopically (Hare et al. 1991), so relative changes in amino acid content might affect the total $\delta^{13}C$. Alternately, loss of isotopically light lipids might raise the $\delta^{13}C$ of maize (White and Schwarcz 1989:466).

Alkaline processing also has a significant impact on the mineral content of maize. Untreated maize is very low in Ca and, consequently, in dietarily informative trace elements (Ba and Sr). Several studies have documented dramatic increases in Ca content with alkaline processing using plant ash (Calloway et al. 1974; Kuhnlein 1981) and burned limestone (Bressani et al. 1958; Bressani and Scrimshaw 1958). However, alkaline processing techniques may vary dramatically between cultures and for the preparation of different maize foods within cultures. In some cases the lime solution is not discarded, while in others the treated kernels are rinsed or reboiled in clean water. Among the Maya, lime may not be used for the preparation of some ritual foods (Redfield and Villa Rojas 1934:39; Guiteras-Holmes 1961:30). These differences could have a substantial effect on the final Ca content of maize and on the Ca contribution of maize to the total diet and skeletal mineral reservoir. Moreover, different sources of lime have been reported from the Maya area that could affect the chemical changes induced, including burned limestone, burned and slaked mollusk shells, and tree-bark ash.

There has been some speculation that alkaline processing might not have been practiced throughout Maya history (White and Schwarcz 1989), so changes in maize chemistry are of fundamental importance to diachronic reconstruction of Maya diets with bone chemistry. In order to examine the potential effect of alkaline processing on maize $\delta^{13}C$ and trace element content for dietary reconstruction in the Pasión region, this study examines the effect of two different alkaline processing methods on three maize varieties (Wright 1994, 1999).

Yellow, white, and black maize were prepared with lime purchased in Antigua, Guatemala. This lime is prepared for maize treatment by burning limestone in a slow wood fire. The lime contained approximately 34.9% Ca and 83 ppm Sr, hence had a Sr/Ca ratio of approximately 0.00027. Ba in the lime was below the detection limits of the ICP (1 ppm), indicating a very low Ba/Ca ratio.

I processed each maize sample according to two methods reported ethnographically in the Maya area. The first method is commonly used in preparation of *nixtamal* (softened, treated unground maize) for use in tortillas and tamales, and involves soaking the maize overnight in the lime solution. Specifics of the preparation used here follow the protocol of Bressani and Scrimshaw (1958; Bressani et al. 1958). According to Redfield and Villa Rojas (1934:38–39), another method, in which maize is boiled in fresh water after the initial alkaline soak, is used to prepare *nixtamal* for *pozole* gruel in the Yucatan. To control for possible changes in maize that occur from boiling in water alone or from contamination from the cooking vessel, I also analyzed maize that was boiled without lime treatment. Details of the treatment procedures are given in Wright (1994:222) and (1999:207).

Because the Lacandon prefer to treat their maize from slaked *Pachychilus* snail shells (Nations 1979b; Tozzer 1907), I also treated yellow maize with snail shell lime. But in lieu of *Pachychilus* from the Pasión region, *Pomacea* was used. Pomacea lime contains 69% Ca, 636 ppm Sr (Sr/Ca = 0.000922), and 79 ppm Ba (Ba/Ca = 0.000114) as measured by ICP-AES.

I selected three samples per maize variety from each treatment method for elemental and isotopic analysis. Unprocessed dried kernels were also analyzed from each variety. Isotopic and elemental analyses were conducted at Augustana College and the University of Wisconsin using techniques described above.

The method of treatment has little effect on the $\delta^{13}C$ of *nixtamal* (see Wright 1994:223–24). Tested with a 2-way ANOVA, $\delta^{13}C$ does not differ significantly among treatment methods ($F = 1.529$, $p = 0.23$). Instead, maize variety has a highly significant effect on $\delta^{13}C$ ($F = 22.14$, $p = 0.0001$). Black maize is heavier than either white or yellow maize, which do not differ substantially from each other. These differences probably result from both varietal genetic and altitudinal differences (Tieszen 1991; Tieszen and Fagre 1993a). The different varieties do not appear to be affected differently by the different methods of alkaline processing ($F = 0.946$, $p = 0.48$). These data confirm the lack of impact of alkaline processing on cellulose $\delta^{13}C$, which was previously reported (Marino and DeNiro 1987) for a single analysis each of treated (−10.6‰) and untreated maize (−10.9‰). Thus, reconstruction of prehistoric diet using $\delta^{13}C$ should not be unduly affected by alkaline processing with lime. Genetic differences between maize varieties in $\delta^{13}C$ are more substantial but are less than 1‰ among the types tested here, so are unlikely to have significant consequences within a population.

Treatment with alkaline solutions has a dramatic effect on the mineral content of maize. Because the maize varieties sampled are extremely low in Ca (below the 100 ppm analytical limits of the ICP), in order to calculate Ca increases the Ca content of unprocessed maize was arbitrarily set at 100 ppm, a high estimate. Maize grown in the Pasión region (see Table 6.1) contains more Ca than the maize analyzed here. The Ca content of untreated maize likely reflects the Ca content of soils on which it is grown. Ca is more abundant in the limestone-derived soils of Petén than in the volcanic highland and coastal soils on which the maize used here was grown.

Both white and yellow maize show increases in Ca on the order of 20 times when treated for *nixtamal* by lime soaking. Boiling the treated maize in water for *pozole* reduced this significantly but still produced an increase of 7 to 11 times over unprocessed maize. The difference between these two methods is highly significant ($F = 10.17$, $p = 0.008$, all varieties). However, some of this increase is due solely to the effects of boiling in Chicago water, since the boiled maize shows an increase in Ca near 6 times for all varieties. A similar effect might be found in the karstic Maya Lowlands. Recall that a large increase in Sr/Ca was caused by boiling ramon nuts for tortilla preparation at Aguateca. Thus, alkali processing of maize for *pozole* would raise the maize contribution to total alkaline earth element intake only slightly. The more common technique used for preparation of tamales and tortillas increases Ca content to a much greater extent.

This effect is most apparent for white and yellow corn. Ca was not exceptionally increased in the black corn with lime soaking (8 times) and indeed is higher for the samples that were subsequently boiled (9 times). However, it is difficult to ascertain whether this is a difference in the solubility of lime from processed black corn or simply reflects idiosyncratic variation. The ANOVA indicates that both the effect of maize variety ($F = 3.528$, $p = 0.0624$) and the interaction of variety with treatment method on Ca content are statistically significant ($F = 3.467$, $p = 0.064$). That maize varieties absorb Ca differentially is also supported by the data obtained by Bressani et al. (1958) on *nixtamal* prepared for tortillas by two Guatemalan women. A greater Ca increase was measured for each family in preparation of white maize (24 times) than yellow maize (13 times), paralleling the trends obtained here for white and yellow maize.

Despite its higher Ca content, *Pomacea* lime has slightly less effect on yellow maize Ca, using either the *nixtamal* (10 times unprocessed) or *pozole* (6 times) preparations. However, these differences may reflect idiosyncratic variation since only one sample each of Pomacea-treated lime was analyzed (Wright 1999:208). Larger increases of 20 to 70 times are recorded for preparation of Hopi maize products with *chamisa* ash that is not decanted or rinsed from the maize (Calloway et al. 1974; Kuhnlein 1981).

These results indicate that alkaline processing is unlikely to affect isotopic reconstructions of prehistoric diet but that it may have a substantial effect on elemental ratios and perhaps change the relative importance of maize as a Ca source in the diet. The magnitude of this effect may be dependent on local elemental distributions. Different techniques of alkaline processing could indeed have significant effect on dietary reconstruction. For instance, men consuming *pozole* in the field would receive less Ca from this maize than women consuming *atole* or tamales in the home would. Changes in the use of different processing methods could be mistakenly identified as dietary differences.

Implications for Pasión Diets

Given the nutritional shortcomings of maize, it is probable that the ancient Pasión Maya processed their maize with an alkaline solution. At Lamanai, the presence of lime-encrusted colanders has been used to argue that alkaline processing was practiced there (White and Schwarcz 1989). Given the heavy leaching in the Pasión environment, an absence of lime residue on Classic period ceramics does not indicate a lack of alkaline processing. Encrusted lime on Pacific-coast ceramics may be due to boiling mollusks (Pye 1995:233–5), which could also have been practiced at Lamanai. Because alkaline processing is ubiquitous in cultures that rely heavily on maize throughout the New World (Katz et al. 1974), it is likely that the technique is of considerable antiquity.

Modern Maya maize processing techniques produce an increase in Ca of 10- to 20-fold when burned limestone is used. A Ca increase of 20 times would bring Pasión maize to the mean Ca content of most other plants, but a 10-fold increase would place maize toward the low end of the floral range. Slaked snail shells have a slightly lesser effect. Regardless of the exact Ca increment, alkaline processing would raise the Ba/Ca or Sr/Ca of maize to the level in the lime used. If burned local limestone was used, the ratios could be slightly elevated, with the increment equivalent to that of fractionation between plants and the soil on which they grow (Runia 1987), since Pasión soils are derived from the weathered limestone bedrock.

Tozzer (1907:51) noted that the Lacandon produced lye from ashes of mahogany bark (*Swietenia macrophylla*) that was used to make a specific maize drink, *saqnum*. Katz et al. (1974:770) observe that wood-ash alkali takes the form of potassium hydroxide, so use of plant ash might not produce such dramatic Ca increases. The relative contribution of Ca to ash alkalinity will depend on the relative content of Ca versus K and Na, which are often more abundant in plant tissues than Ca. Although chamisa ash does elevate Ca levels substantially in Hopi maize (Calloway et al. 1974), Ca concentrations given by the I.N.C.A.P. tables (I.N.C.A.P. 1961:13–5) for ash-treated maize *arepa* from Ecuador, Columbia, and Venezuela, as well as ash-treated tortillas (Guatemalan?), are not substantially higher than those given for untreated corn and are markedly lower than those for lime-treated maize products. A measurement of the Ca, K, and Na content of mahogany bark would be necessary to evaluate the effect of this treatment. If the Ca content of the bark is low and the alkali produced is primarily potassium and/or sodium hydroxide, then processing with mahogany ash would not produce a significant change in the Ca content of treated maize, and the effect of maize consumption on bone chemistry would be equivalent to that of untreated maize.

Although limestone is the usual source of lime in Yucatan, the Lacandon claim that local Chiapas limestone does not produce good lime (Tozzer 1907:51) and therefore prefer slaked *Pachychilus* shells (Baer and Merrifield 1971; Nations 1979b). Moreover, *Pachychilus* is preferred over *Pomacea* as a source of lime (Nations 1979b). Given the proximity of the Lacandon to the Pasión research area (indeed, Lacandon settlements some 80 to 150 years old are documented near Dos Pilas [Palka 1998], from whence these groups moved to Chiapas), it is possible that ancient perceptions of the quality of Pasión limestone for alkali were analogous. The use of molluscan shells would produce quite different results on maize Ba/Ca and Sr/Ca levels than terrestrial sources of lime. The mollusks, like other aquatic fauna, show very low Ba/Sr, due to disproportionately high Sr that has leached into the watershed. Hence, alkaline processing with mollusk lime would be confounded with consumption of other aquatic foods in elemental ratios in bone.

Since maize was probably consumed daily (on the basis of modern analogy) and Classic populations were much larger than 20th century Lacandon numbers, we must consider whether local molluscan populations could withstand predation on the level necessary for widespread alkaline processing. In a study of modern *Pomacea* population dynamics and prehistoric harvest pressure at Lamanai, Emery (1986) concluded that *Pomacea* was very efficiently harvested but that it would not have provided a significant dietary source because the energy expended to recover the snails, which are buried deep in lagoon mud, outweighed the caloric yield. In contrast, *Pachychilus* lives in shallow, fast-flowing streams, it is more easily collected, and populations may be large enough to sustain substantial harvest pressure (Emery 1989). Baer and Merrifield (1971:153) observe that shells of *Pachychilus* eaten by the Lacandon throughout the year are stored for lime production in one annual batch, so the production of lime in itself may not put undue stress on snail populations.

Differences in local access to molluscan species and quality limestone might produce heterogeneity in lime sources exploited at different sites. For instance, limestone is not found in the immediate environs of Altar and was imported for the construction of Late Classic monuments. *Pomacea* snails and *Amblema* clams are the most abundant mollusks at Altar and might have been the focus of local lime production, unless limestone was imported from elsewhere. All other Pasión sites had ready access to all potential sources of lime. Presumably, mahogany-bark lye could have been produced at all sites.

CHAPTER 7

Paleodiet of the Pasión Region

Isotopic and elemental analysis of ancient human bone is a productive avenue from which to investigate dietary transitions in Pasión prehistory. Environmental models of collapse imply specific changes in diet that should be reflected in bone chemistry. In order to use this data to evaluate dietary changes in the context of the collapse models, however, it is necessary to confirm the biological integrity of the chemical signals. In this chapter, I examine the human chemical data to evaluate bone preservation and paleodietary trends in Pasión history.

Previous Chemical Analyses of Maya Diet

Mesoamerica, and especially the Maya area, has been a focus of chemical analyses of diet since their inception. The first archaeological application of elemental analyses to questions of dietary inequality was Schoeninger's study of strontium at Chalcatzingo, Morelos (Schoeninger 1979a, 1979b). Shortly thereafter, White (1986; White and Schwarcz 1989; White et al. 1994) used stable isotopes and trace elements to investigate Mayan subsistence at Lamanai in northern Belize. Isotopic analysis indicated a decline in maize consumption from the Preclassic through Terminal Classic periods, but a dramatic rise in the Postclassic and Historic occupations. These isotopic changes are accompanied by changes in Sr and Zn concentrations that support the isotopic interpretations. She linked this rise to the technological innovation of alkaline processing that allowed greater reliance on maize in the Postclassic and later times. In stark contrast to the pattern at Lamanai, $\delta^{13}C$ at Pacbitun, Belize, increased from Preclassic through Late Classic periods (White et al. 1993) and indicated very high maize consumption during the Late Classic.

Few other elemental studies of Maya material have been carried out. One exception is Bennett's (1985) analysis of trace elements at the colonial site of Tipu, Belize. Bennett (1985) found some evidence of variability in elemental ratios among Historic interments of the Franciscan mission church, though specific social correlates of diet are difficult to ascertain in this case.

Reed's isotopic analyses (1994, 1998, 1999) of Late Classic skeletons from Copan show similar values of $\delta^{13}C$ to those obtained at Pacbitun. The data also indicate greater variety of dietary signatures in high-status skeletons in comparison to low-status interments, suggesting that a greater diversity of foods were available to the Copan elite.

In a broad survey of skeletons from across the Maya Lowlands and from both Early and Late Classic periods, Gerry found that burials which clustered together in terms of mortuary characteristics did not show discrete dietary patterning (Gerry 1993, 1997). However, he did find significant regional differences in isotopic ratios, which suggest that dietary patterns were also governed by broad environmental distinctions (Gerry 1993; Gerry and Krueger 1997). In particular, maize consumption was much lower in northern Belize than in the Peten and at Copan. The distinctive Belizean diet is also observed in isotopic data from Preclassic Cuello (Tykot et al. 1996) and K'axob (Henderson 1998). Presumably, these geographic patterns confound status-related differentiation within Gerry's burial series. Moreover, funerary symbols also varied across Maya space and time (Ruz Lhuillier 1968; Welsh 1988) and may further obscure any social patterning in the isotope data.

These data suggest a broad range of dietary variability in Maya skeletons over temporal, spatial, and social variables. Most importantly, they illustrate the ability of chemical analyses to detect dietary trends in Maya subsistence that may be useful in evaluating factors that could have contributed to the collapse of this civilization, which is the focus of the present research.

Prehistoric Pasión Diets and Collapse Models

Changes in diet that lie at the core of environmental models of the Maya collapse should be apparent through chemical analysis. Models that emphasize overpopulation, agricultural stress, and ecological deterioration provide the most explicit dietary implications. Although the varied "environmental collapse" models emphasize slightly different aspects of the interaction of the Classic Maya with their environment, they ultimately rely on similar dietary mechanisms. Differences between models largely reflect the development of the field over the last two decades with respect to specific agronomic strategies employed by the Maya and the nature of political interactions between polities.

For the purpose of simplicity, the following dietary expectations rely heavily on the arguments of Santley, Killion, and Lycett (1986), who have provided the most explicit articulation of the dietary and health implications of environmental collapse models. The basic argument focuses on increasing reliance on maize agriculture to the exclusion of other crops and wild foods. Farmers intensified maize cultivation because of the high yields per unit of land that this crop can provide. Erosion of agricultural swidden plots, sedimentation of terraces, and flooding of raised fields led to the expansion of agricultural systems to all utilizable soils. This expansion was also motivated by the rising population of all Late Classic centers and consequent food demands. Agricultural expansion resulted in deforestation of an ever-increasing proportion of the lowlands. With less mature forest remaining, cropping cycles were shortened so that fields were left fallow for shorter periods, exacerbating soil exhaustion and further fueling the expansive cycle.

Reduction of natural forest habitats placed limits on the availability of collected foods not found in *milpas* or *acahuales*. In particular this would affect wild fruits, palms, and seasonings. Most critically, reduction of interconnecting forest belts restricted the habitats of fauna that provided most of the animal protein consumed. Habitat circumscription and elevated predation from rising populations stressed faunal populations, ultimately leading to decreases in animal protein consumed and greater reliance on maize and beans as the major sources of dietary protein.

These two trends—increasing maize reliance and decreasing animal protein consumption—lie at the root of hypothesized nutritional deficiencies that could have reversed demographic trends of the Late Classic period and led to population collapse. If environmental conditions were prime movers in the collapse, nutritional stresses would need to be maintained; otherwise, if environmental pressures were relaxed, a rebound in the population would occur.

Thus, dietary chemistry should demonstrate that maize was a primary nutritional staple for the Pasión Maya. It should also reveal increasing maize consumption over time in the skeletal remains. This would be reflected in progressively rising $\delta^{13}C$ from Preclassic through Terminal Classic periods at all sites. Nitrogen isotopic values should decrease over time as a result of the shift from animal to plant sources of protein. Trace element data should illustrate the same trend, with decreasing Ba/Ca and Sr/Ca over time.

Moreover, these trends should be apparent at all sites. Skeletons from earlier occupations might show dietary diversity according to local environmental distinctions. The hypothesized agricultural expansion and environmental stress would eliminate this heterogeneity, with all local resources under heavy pressure. Dietary signals should then converge toward a common Terminal Classic signature.

Dietary expectations are more difficult to develop for patterns among social strata since few authors deal with dietary distinctions in the social hierarchy when discussing the collapse. Santley et al. (1986) argue that taxation of producers might have declined on a per capita basis toward the end of the Classic period but that the increasing population density would have maintained the total support available for the aristocracy. Thus, chemical data should illustrate increasing differentiation between mortuary clusters over time. In the Terminal Classic, when protein resources were most severely stressed, this distinction should indicate clear channeling of meat resources toward the top of the socioeconomic pyramid.

Deviation from these expectations would indicate that factors other than environmental stress and population pressure played a significant role in determining dietary partitioning in Pasión prehistory. Broad distinctions between sites might suggest politically mediated collapse mechanisms. Social distinctions deviating from the model described above should provide an avenue for investigating the nature of social changes and shed light on social dynamics that might have been involved in the political failure and depopulation.

Preservation and Diagenesis

Although a number of steps were taken in the preparation of archaeological bone samples to minimize or remove diagenetic effects, before inferring dietary patterns it is necessary to examine the data carefully to ensure that diagenetic alteration of the isotopic and elemental values cannot be detected. For the purpose of diagenetic investigation, I examine the human material for each site without reference to chronological period. Although duration of interment might influence the magnitude of elemental change, heterogeneity in soil composition and hydrology is probably more significant, in view of the dramatic variability observed in macroscopic bone preservation within each time period. Division of the samples by chronological placement would reduce sample sizes, making statistically significant trends more difficult to identify.

Stable Isotopes

Intact "collagen" pseudomorphs were obtained from most human specimens following EDTA decalcification. Of 145 human samples prepared, only 14 human samples dissolved entirely, producing no organic residue. The remaining samples (91%) produced good white or yellow pseudomorphs. Only 1 of 32 archaeological faunal samples dissolved. All of the samples that were lost on decalcification had marked surface erosion and/or a chalky texture, indicating that significant decay had occurred. Isotopic ratios and measures of "collagen" integrity are listed in Table 7.1 for all human data, while faunal data is in Table 6.2.

Two human samples that gave very low $\delta^{13}C$ values (DP25 = −22.19; DP34 = − 25.12‰) are outliers and are likely affected by diagenesis. Certainly, the direction of deviation is consistent with contamination from external C3 organics that would be predicted in this forested environment. Unfortunately, C/N ratios were not obtained for these samples due to the low "collagen" yield. Since it is not possible to confirm that they are valid dietary signatures, the data for these two samples are excluded from the statistical analysis.

Carbon to nitrogen ratios provide a means to evaluate the integrity of "collagen" recovered. The majority of samples produced pseudomorphs with C/N ratios within the acceptable range of 2.9 to 3.6 (DeNiro 1985). Two samples with high C/N and one with low C/N may not be collagen and are excluded from statistical analysis (SE24 = 4.2; SE32 = 4.4; DP-PD1B = 1.86) although their isotopic values do not appear especially anomalous. Within the acceptable range, variation in C/N ratio has little effect on $\delta^{13}C$ (Figure 7.1). Samples from all sites are spread across the range of C/N measured. The correlation between C/N ratios and $\delta^{13}C$ is low whether all samples are included ($r = -0.13$, $n = 110$) or if only those with C/N of 2.9 to 3.6 are considered ($r = -0.16$, $n = 106$). Thirty-three archaeological faunal samples show C/N ratios between 2.8 and 3.7 (mean = 3.17), only two of which lie outside the acceptable range.

The concentration of carbon and nitrogen (%C and %N) in the pseudomorphs was measured in the Augustana College Carlo Erba elemental analyzer for 63 human samples. Ambrose (1990) argues that dietary isotopic signatures are retained in "collagen" if C accounts for > 3% by weight and N accounts for > 1%. Pasión pseudomorphs contain much higher levels of C and N than these

Table 7.1. Isotopic and summary elemental composition of human bone, with measures of sample quality

Burial	$\delta^{13}C$	$\delta^{15}N$	C/N	%C	%N	Ca/P	Sr/Ca	Ba/Ca	Ba/Sr
Altar de Sacrificios									
AS8	-9.85	7.70	3.07	18.41	48.37	2.22	.58	1.92	3.33
AS13	-9.61	8.23	3.15	16.02	43.23	2.21	.68	1.17	1.71
AS31	-9.61	7.57	3.2	.	.	2.14	.53	.78	1.49
AS39	-8.71	9.27	3.09	17.65	46.75	2.20	.28	.37	1.32
AS40	-8.19	7.90	3.19	16.06	43.85	2.23	.58	.72	1.24
AS41	-11.21	9.39	3.3	.	.	.	.	.	.
AS43	-9.36	8.73	3.09	17.55	46.44	2.23	1.08	.66	.61
AS47	-7.69	8.33	3.11	17.81	47.44	2.20	1.27	.42	.33
AS52	-8.25	7.62	3.14	17.25	46.49	2.25	.83	.93	1.12
AS55	-13.02	9.12	3.02	16.88	43.65	2.26	.43	1.05	2.45
AS57	-9.41	7.41	3.15	16.50	44.52	2.22	.44	.47	1.08
AS58	-8.15	8.86	3.13	16.99	45.61	2.22	.68	.30	.44
AS60	-9.78	9.21	3.17	16.17	43.95	2.15	.55	.47	.85
AS62	-10.38	11.41	3.13	16.33	43.80	2.19	.36	.66	1.84
AS63	-10.66	8.70	3.3	.	.	2.21	.39	.71	1.80
AS65	-11.14	8.50	3.11	17.48	46.52	2.17	.44	.97	2.19
AS66	-10.31	9.18	3.1	.	.	2.21	.62	.71	1.13
AS67	-8.48	10.32	3.2	.	.	2.18	.44	.54	1.24
AS70	-9.27	7.03	3.2	.	.	.	.	.	.
AS74	-8.35	8.71	3.14	17.10	46.05	2.24	.50	.81	1.63
AS75	-8.77	10.17	3.14	17.46	46.93	2.25	.38	.64	1.68
AS79	-9.78	8.19	3.11	16.32	43.46	2.17	.53	.65	1.23
AS86	-8.09	8.05	3.13	17.60	47.29	2.19	.55	.68	1.23
AS88	-8.54	10.54	3.11	17.67	47.12	2.20	.79	1.10	1.38
AS89	-6.52	8.53	3.3	.	.	2.11	.36	.20	.56
AS90	-8.28	9.02	3.18	15.34	41.83	2.21	.87	.62	.71
AS92	-8.50	8.20	3.2	.	.	.	.	.	.
AS96	-8.08	7.87	3.1	.	.	2.27	.50	1.13	2.26
AS98	d	.	.	.	.	2.24	.30	.24	.82
AS105	d	.	.	.	.	.	.	.	.
AS107	-10.55	9.56	3.14	15.96	42.98	2.29	.68	1.30	1.91
AS112	-9.12	8.74	3.3	.	.	2.12	.42	.54	1.29
AS115	-9.22	7.93	3.0	.	.	2.25	.54	.84	1.57
AS116	-9.33	7.73	3.2	.	.	2.13	.37	.51	1.38
AS117	-8.27	7.74	3.2	.	.	2.14	.70	.89	1.27
AS118	-9.54	8.77	3.1	.	.	2.31	.82	1.26	1.54
AS124	-10.36	7.81	3.1	.	.	2.19	.54	1.06	1.97
AS128	-8.94	10.22	3.2	.	.	2.20	.77	1.23	1.60
AS129	-10.52	8.41	3.55	14.96	45.52	.	.	.	.
AS131	-13.43	6.46	3.4	.	.	2.19	.68	1.02	1.51
AS135	d	.	.	.	.	2.22	.66	.57	.87

continued on next page

Burial	$\delta^{13}C$	$\delta^{15}N$	C/N	%C	%N	Ca/P	Sr/Ca	Ba/Ca	Ba/Sr
Itzan									
IT1	-9.10	7.10	3.11	16.36	43.68	2.21	.17	.15	.88
IT2	d	.	.	.	.	2.11	.20	.08	.41
IT5	-8.70	8.92	3.3	.	.	2.15	.19	.09	.48
IT6	-9.46	9.12	3.2	15.89	43.54	2.26	.31	.21	.68
IT7	-9.18	7.30	3.16	16.33	44.18	2.17	.20	.13	.63
IT8	-9.39	7.36	3.2	.	.	2.21	.15	.28	1.81
Seibal									
SE1	-11.20	8.81	3.3	.	.	2.20	.31	.34	1.09
SE2	-8.47	7.38	3.04	17.41	45.40	2.24	.39	.41	1.06
SE4-3	-8.65	7.21	3.14	16.29	43.80	2.19	.39	.31	.79
SE4a	-9.32	9.94	3.17	17.31	46.99	2.21	.39	.35	.89
SE4b	-10.30	10.84	3.16	17.09	46.29	2.17	.39	.38	.97
SE4c	-7.44	10.00	3.15	16.55	44.69	2.17	.26	.26	.99
SE5	-10.10	10.32	3.2	.	.	2.21	2.93	.84	.29
SE6	-9.22	9.87	3.0	.	.	.	.	.	.
SE7	-10.63	10.46	3.09	16.31	43.22	2.24	.56	.60	1.07
SE9	-9.04	8.90	3.07	16.50	43.46	.	.	.	.
SE11	-8.61	9.29	3.0	.	.	2.27	.42	.47	1.13
SE14	-8.22	9.26	3.1	16.40	43.66	2.21	.32	.29	.90
SE15	-10.81	8.27	3.09	16.52	43.80	2.20	.38	.19	.50
SE16	-8.10	9.91	3.08	17.74	46.86	2.22	.34	.36	1.04
SE17	-8.52	9.14	3.2	.	.	2.19	.31	.36	1.18
SE18	-9.38	10.95	3.3	.	.	2.21	.23	.13	.58
SE20	-7.97	8.55	3.09	16.37	43.36	2.27	.29	.15	.53
SE22	-10.39	8.88	3.5	.	.	2.23	.26	.17	.68
SE23	-8.68	9.46	3.11	16.37	43.71	2.25	.76	.42	.56
SE24	-10.37	10.15	4.2	.	.	2.24	.99	.69	.69
SE25	-9.33	9.31	3.08	16.49	43.55	2.18	.71	.37	.52
SE26	-9.32	8.98	3.09	16.67	44.10	2.21	.72	.51	.71
SE28	-10.00	8.43	3.2	.	.	2.27	.38	.19	.49
SE29	-8.25	9.65	3.10	16.18	43.01	2.23	.26	.37	1.42
SE30	-10.03	9.85	3.4	.	.	2.26	.28	.27	.95
SE31	-8.62	8.69	3.3	.	.	2.22	.19	.16	.85
SE32	-12.86	10.17	4.4	.	.	2.15	.26	.21	.82
SE34	-9.22	8.32	3.25	15.72	43.79	2.19	.21	.16	.77
SE35	-11.09	9.63	3.4	.	.	2.26	.36	.38	1.05
SE36	-7.88	11.32	3.19	15.89	43.51	2.25	.84	.34	.41
SE37	d	.	.	.	.	2.23	.71	.16	.23
SE38	-8.76	9.49	3.3	.	.	2.19	.34	.31	.91
SE39	-10.32	8.83	3.55	14.62	44.54	2.16	.23	.22	.96
SE40	-11.84	9.62	3.18	16.08	43.82	2.19	.49	.33	.68
SE41	-8.02	11.43	3.14	17.34	46.70	2.19	.19	.12	.65
SE42	-10.65	8.66	3.4	.	.	2.22	.28	.17	.59
SE43	-11.40	9.71	3.2	.	.	2.26	.44	.17	.40

continued on next page

Burial	$\delta^{13}C$	$\delta^{15}N$	C/N	%C	%N	Ca/P	Sr/Ca	Ba/Ca	Ba/Sr
Aguateca									
AG1	-9.87	9.06	3.15	16.07	43.43	2.16	.24	.14	.61
AG5A	-8.78	7.98	3.06	16.60	43.61	2.20	.13	.15	1.11
AG5B	-9.34	9.13	3.15	16.35	44.19	.	.	.	.
QCH1#21	-9.20	10.60	3.01	16.45	42.45	.	.	.	.
QCH1#35	-9.20	10.70	3.08	17.29	45.71	2.23	.18	.23	1.26
QCH5	-9.90	7.90	*	.	.	2.22	.17	.09	.52
QCH6	-11.0	10.10	*	.	.	2.26	.21	.15	.72
QCH7	d		.	.	.	.	.	.	.
QCH9	-9.20	*	*	.	.	2.21	.18	.16	.93
CCH1	-9.11	10.19	2.91						
Dos Pilas									
DP1	-7.04	9.31	3.14	17.87	48.06	2.19	.33	.37	1.13
DP2	-8.94	8.69	3.15						
DP3	-8.20	8.22	3.17	15.95	43.32	2.14	.31	.13	.42
DP4	-9.07	9.67	3.17	17.30	47.02	2.16	.30	.18	.58
DP5	-8.58	7.66	3.3	.	.	2.10	.28	.15	.54
DP6	d	.	.	.	.	2.29	.37	.38	1.04
DP8	d	.	.	.	.	2.32	.40	.30	.75
DP9	-9.59	9.46	3.14						
DP10A	-8.62	11.63	3.15						
DP10B	-8.95	9.08	3.13						
DP12	-7.82	12.36	3.13						
DP13	-9.84	9.13	3.17	15.64	42.55	2.16	.30	.23	.76
DP16	-9.72	7.50	3.19	15.17	41.45	.	.	.	.
DP17	-9.65	10.3	3.2	.	.	.	.	.	.
DP20	-9.60	11.00	3.09	16.73	44.34	2.19	.37	.17	.47
DP22	-7.70	10.6	3.12	17.36	46.38	2.15	.30	.15	.49
DP25	-22.19	14.47	*	.	.	2.19	.19	.12	.62
DP26	-9.23	9.88	3.39	15.73	45.69	2.09	.19	.08	.43
DP29	-9.70	10.15	3.21	13.97	38.40	2.08	.23	.09	.40
DP30	-8.53	8.90	3.16	16.13	43.65	2.11	.40	.22	.55
DP33	-9.50	8.34	3.26	15.51	43.28	2.15	.27	.18	.67
DP34	-25.04	16.50	*	.	.	2.19	.23	.13	.55
DP35	d	.	.	.	.	2.14	.25	.08	.33
DP38	d	.	.	.	.	2.11	.16	.06	.36
DP43	-8.60	10.10	3.3	.	.	2.17	.29	.14	.49
DP44	-11.30	10.20	3.1	.	.	.	.	.	.
DP45	-8.20	10.30	3.08	16.27	42.99	2.15	.26	.09	.34
DP47	-8.30	11.10	3.2	.	.	.	.	.	.
DP49	-10.10	9.90	3.0	.	.	2.21	.16	.12	.75
DP50	-9.10	9.70	3.18	16.12	43.91	.	.	.	.
DP51	d	.	.	.	.	2.10	.21	.05	.22
DP52	-8.64	10.52	3.09						
DP55	-8.64	10.08	3.16						

continued on next page

Burial	$\delta^{13}C$	$\delta^{15}N$	C/N	%C	%N	Ca/P	Sr/Ca	Ba/Ca	Ba/Sr
DP-PD1A	-8.35	11.56	3.31						
PD-PD1B	-11.29	9.57	1.86						
DP-PD1E	-12.03	12.69	2.83						
DP-PD1G	-11.16	9.70	3.31						
DP-PD1H	-8.62	9.11	3.05						
DP-PD1I	-8.81	10.42	3.08						
Tamarindito									
TA1A	-9.30	8.10	*						
TA2	-13.00	8.20	*						
TA4	-9.08	9.77	3.20						
TA6	-8.91	10.23	3.28						
TA8	d	.	.						
TR3-1	-12.59	8.79	3.21						
TR3-2	-9.72	10.88	3.28						
Arroyo de Piedra									
AP4	-9.69	2.34	3.20						
AP5	d	.	.						
La Paciencia									
LP1	-10.28	9.59	3.15						
Punta de Chimino									
PC1	d	.	.						
PC2	-8.40	10.50	3.11						

An asterisk indicates that C/N ratios or $\delta^{15}N$ could not be measured due to insufficient sample. A "d" indicates that sample dissolved entirely.

limits. In the human samples, %C ranges between 38.4 and 48.37% (mean = 44.59, s.d. = 1.83), which is very close to values for pure collagen of bovine tendon (47.6%; Ambrose 1990:438). Likewise, %N ranges between 13.97 and 18.41% (mean = 16.54, s.d. = 0.84), again similar to bovine tendon (16.0%; Ambrose 1990:437). The Pasión archaeological fauna (n = 6) show comparable values (%C = 43.51 to 45.99; %N= 15.71 to 17.65).

These results suggest that the pseudomorphs consist of almost pure collagen. These concentrations are higher than those obtained on most archaeological material (Ambrose 1990). However, a number of human samples from lower Central America analyzed by Norr (1991) are comparable (especially those from El Molino and Nacascolo). Preparation technique may play a role. Ambrose (1990:445–46) suggests that low concentrations of C and N in archaeological collagen may be due to incomplete removal of clay minerals and salts from collagen. It is possible that EDTA extraction used here eliminated these contaminants more successfully, producing a purer product. The modern fauna show lower %C and %N than archaeological specimens, in line with other results (Ambrose 1990), and were prepared by HCl "chunk" extraction instead of EDTA. Perhaps methanol/chloroform treatment did not remove all the lipids from these samples. The concentration of C and N reported by Ambrose (1990) and Norr (1991) were obtained from HCl extractions of ground bone. The whole-bone preparation used here is preferred because "collagen" is not lost on the filter, and more collagen fragments of higher molecular weight are retained (Schoeninger et al. 1989; Schwarcz and Schoeninger 1991:293). Schwarcz and Schoeninger recommend EDTA preparation for samples suspected to have low collagen yields

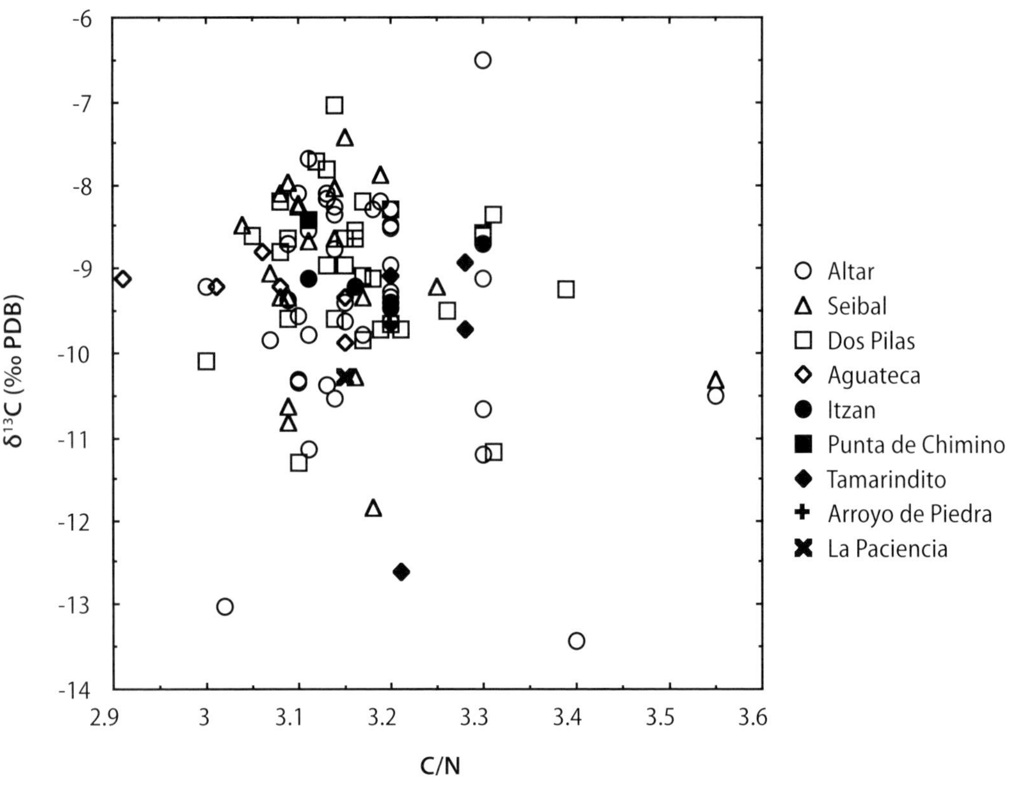

Figure 7.1. Relationship between atomic C/N ratios and δ^{13}C in bone collagen from Pasión archaeological skeletons

because it is able to recover more collagen. These differences may account for the high C and N concentrations obtained here in archaeological bone.

It has been suggested that "collagen" C/N ratios within the range of 3.4 to 3.6 may be slightly contaminated by C3 humic acids and lipids (Ambrose 1993; Kennedy 1988; Schoeninger et al. 1989). Here, three samples show slightly high C/N ratios (SE22 = 3.50, SE39 = 3.55, AS129 = 3.55) and five others have C/N of 3.4, so δ^{13}C for these samples may also be unreliable. It may be significant to note that over half of these are from Preclassic skeletons, which we expect to show poorest preservation due to the longer period of interment. White and Schwarcz (personal communication 1993) have had difficulty obtaining collagen from Preclassic skeletons in Belize. Percent C and %N for the two samples with C/N of 3.55 (SE39, AS129) are well within acceptable levels for collagen preservation, as is that of DP26. Percent C is within the range of the other samples. The %N of SE39 and AS129 is at the low end of the range, producing the higher C/N. Percent C and %N were not measured for the other five samples. Since collagen preservation cannot be fully evaluated for all of these samples, I decided to selectively eliminate only those samples that appear to be outliers relative to the variation in δ^{13}C and δ^{15}N in their respective chronological/site series. Most are clearly within the range of other data in each series, so were retained for statistical analysis and diet reconstruction. Only AS131, a Preclassic sample with δ^{13}C of −13.43‰, is an outlier and probably affected by noncollagen organic contamination. One Early Classic sample, AS55, shows an acceptable C/N of 3.02 and typical Pasión %C and %N, but it is definitely an outlier relative to other data from this series. Since postmortem contamination of isotopic signals cannot be excluded for these two individuals and it is better to err on the side of caution, these data are excluded from statistical evaluation of dietary differences between samples but are still shown in the graphs.

Alkaline Earth Elements

Calcium and phosphorus levels and the Ca/P ratio provide some indications of the composition of bone mineral. Well-preserved bone mineral should have a Ca/P ratio similar to the theoretical value for hydroxyapatite, 2.15, and be composed of approximately 39.9% Ca and 18.5% P (White and Hannus 1983). Mean Ca and P levels and Ca/P ratios for human bone at each site are in Table 7.2 with descriptive statistics for elemental abundances. Overall, skeletal Ca/P ratios range from 2.08 to 2.32 (Table 7.1), very close to the theoretical value for hydroxyapatite and to values measured in the modern vertebrate bones sampled (mean = 2.15). Archaeological fauna show mean Ca/P at 2.21. Concentrations of Ca and P are also close to the theoretical values. Superficially, these are biologically acceptable values. Acid treatment appears to have removed calcite that might crystallize in bone pores (Parker and Toots 1980; Pate and Brown 1985).

Soil pH levels measured in burials from the Petexbatun excavations were generally slightly basic and often produced a color reaction that was more basic than that given for the highest pH illustrated in the kit, pH 7.5. In laboratory tests, Dunning (personal communication 1991) has found soil pH across the region to range from 6.0 to 8.5. These values should be conducive to good bone preservation (Gordon and Buikstra 1981) because hydroxyapatite is insoluble above pH 6.5; yet the skeletons are very fragmentary and preservation of trabecular elements is rare. Above pH 6.9, hydroxyapatite crystallizes in soil solutions (Lindsay 1979), so recrystallized diagenetic hydroxyapatite would not be distinguishable from biogenic mineral by its Ca/P value. Yet, collagen degradation by microorganisms, which must be responsible for decay of the missing elements, would produce local acidity in the microenvironment of the bone (White and Hannus 1983) and would contribute more significantly to bone mineral diagenesis than would total soil pH. In addition, soil Ca/P values are several orders of magnitude higher than that of bone mineral, because P is very efficiently recycled in tropical rain forests and bound up in vegetation (Golley 1983; Jordan 1984). It is likely that mineral recovered is largely biogenic.

Elemental relationships within the archaeological bones provide another means to evaluate diagenetic changes. Table 7.2 also contains descriptive statistics by site for each element in human bones. Raw data for elements in human bone ash for each burial are in Wright (1994). At each site, kurtosis and skewness are large for most elements, indicating that the data are not normally distributed and that nonparametric statistics are appropriate. Levels of elements that have been identified in other studies (Lambert et al. 1984, 1983) as soil contaminants (Al, Fe, K, Mn) are low, indicating that the affect of soil contamination was minimized by surface cleaning and acid soaking. These elements also show large standard deviations, being inconsistently represented within sites. Strontium and Ba are present in low concentrations, but differ in abundance in different sites. In contrast, the metabolically regulated elements (Mg, Na, Zn) are present in roughly comparable levels in all sites.

Correlation matrices for elements were calculated for Altar, Seibal, and Dos Pilas (Table 7.3). In order to maximize the data employed, the calculation used pairwise deletion to deal with missing data for burials from which collagen was not preserved. To minimize Type I error, I consider correlations to be significant when $p < 0.01$ rather than $p < 0.05$. Sample sizes from Aguateca and Itzan are too small to obtain significant correlations. Isotopic data are included in these matrices to examine their correlation with elements that potentially discriminate dietarily. In previous studies, Pearson's r has been applied directly to elemental data (Ezzo 1992b) or to log-transformed data (Buikstra et al. 1989). Concentrations of major elements may often be log-normally distributed in large samples (Bishop et al. 1982). There is some evidence that dietary elements are also log-normally distributed in very large samples of bones (Jim Burton, unpublished data). I attempted several different manipulations, all of which gave similar results, both in terms of correlation and principle component loadings. As the sample sizes are small, I

Table 7.2. Descriptive statistics for elemental concentrations (ppm) in human bone ash by site

Element	Mean	s.d.	Kurtosis	Skew	Element	Mean	s.d.	Kurtosis	Skew
Altar de Sacrificios (n=40)					**Seibal (n=37)**				
Al	421	244	.97	1.18	Al	399	212	6.18	2.28
Ba	305	135	1.34	.88	Ba	130	65	.91	1.04
Ca (%)	39.1	0.5	3.13	-.77	Ca (%)	39.3	0.5	-.63	-.31
Fe	131	180	5.47	2.35	Fe	62	100	7.36	2.79
K	213	64	.86	.57	K	267	71	1.21	1.12
Mg	1256	235	.18	.26	Mg	1077	189	1.89	1.06
Mn	49	120	11.22	3.39	Mn	2	18	23.58	4.79
Na	3313	591	.29	.98	Na	3430	463	.79	.52
P (%)	17.7	0.3	.92	.86	P (%)	17.7	0.2	-.05	-.08
Sr	227	81	1.86	1.21	Sr	189	177	20.19	4.29
Zn	157	44	.38	.65	Zn	123	28	.22	.89
Ca/P	2.21				Ca/P	2.22			
Dos Pilas (n=26)					**Aguateca (n=9)**				
Al	688	322	2.62	1.29	Al	674	184	-.35	1.03
Ba	66	35	.94	1.12	Ba	66	23	.22	.89
Ca (%)	39.2	0.6	-.52	5.67	Ca (%)	39.9	0.5	-.61	-.22
Fe	172	226	12.94	3.45	Fe	178	206	-.90	.85
K	184	108	-.70	.54	K	125	102	-1.05	-.77
Mg	1374	291	-.03	.22	Mg	1457	228	.01	-.28
Mn	43	75	6.87	2.79	Mn	24	49	3.88	2.38
Na	3356	756	.51	1.08	Na	3253	232	-1.49	.02
P (%)	18.2	0.4	-.32	-.67	P (%)	18.0	0.3	-.66	-.27
Sr	112	28	-.88	-.01	Sr	72	12	-.27	.57
Zn	123	32	1.36	-.84	Zn	130	22	-1.18	.39
Ca/P	2.16				Ca/P	2.20			
Itzan (n=6)									
Al	231	87	.38	1.24					
Ba	61	30	-.41	.86					
Ca (%)	39.2	1.7	.65	-1.48					
Fe	13	11	-.36	.78					
K	115	57	-1.01	.70					
Mg	1003	247	-.18	.91					
Mn	9	12	.32	1.31					
Na	3534	310	-.99	-.22					
P (%)	17.9	1.1	.68	-1.52					
Sr	79	17	.07	1.07					
Zn	110	18	-1.01	.61					
Ca/P	2.18								

Table 7.3. Pearson's r correlation matrices for elemental and isotopic ratios in human bone

Element	Al	Ba	Ca	Fe	K	Mg	Mn	Na	P	Sr	Zn	$\delta^{13}C$	$\delta^{15}N$
(a) Altar de Sacrificios (n=40)													
Ba	-.145	1											
Ca	-.272	.348	1										
Fe	**.857**	.017	-.175	1									
K	**.676**	-.135	-.187	**.580**	1								
Mg	-.195	.151	-.112	-.120	-.092	1							
Mn	**.605**	.027	-.099	**.828**	**.506**	-.235	1						
Na	**-.410**	.037	.097	-.303	-.146	.222	-.210	1					
P	-.345	-.226	.060	-.159	**-.429**	-.085	-.057	.342	1				
Sr	.062	.245	.092	.027	.127	.124	-.051	-.147	-.217	1			
Zn	**.472**	-.381	-.153	.334	**.525**	-.158	.348	-.372	-.123	.016	1		
$\delta^{13}C$	-.052	**-.399**	-.061	-.006	.111	-.097	-.155	-.132	.174	.126	.072	1	
$\delta^{15}N$	-.147	-.050	.237	-.025	.053	.059	.019	.300	.082	-.037	-.001	.056	1
(b) Seibal (n=37)													
Ba	.340	1											
Ca	-.024	-.214	1										
Fe	**.852**	**.475**	-.239	1									
K	**.695**	.348	-.096	**.616**	1								
Mg	.250	.016	.006	.289	-.027	1							
Mn	.235	**.503**	-.268	**.496**	.189	.025	1						
Na	.084	-.026	.252	-.082	.102	.106	-.051	1					
P	-.183	-.307	.178	-.131	-.125	-.036	-.303	-.023	1				
Sr	.119	**.672**	-.163	.312	.200	-.158	**.820**	-.065	-.289	1			
Zn	.083	**.443**	-.200	.333	-.046	.025	.350	-.207	.145	.400	1		
$\delta^{13}C$	-.017	-.025	.235	-.094	-.074	.133	-.065	.348	.233	-.105	-.034	1	
$\delta^{15}N$	-.008	.182	.022	.034	.002	.074	.043	-.129	.101	.219	.140	.055	1
(c) Dos Pilas (n=26)													
Ba	.283	1											
Ca	.009	**.651**	1										
Fe	**.884**	.213	-.178	1									
K	.339	.348	.130	.154	1								
Mg	-.221	.286	.319	-.232	.078	1							
Mn	**.532**	.179	-.183	**.544**	.453	-.069	1						
Na	-.018	**.561**	**.584**	-.129	**.494**	.256	-.236	1					
P	-.410	-.327	.084	-.403	**-.652**	-.175	-.364	-.402	1				
Sr	.233	**.743**	.346	.094	.385	.396	.253	.266	-.264	1			
Zn	.191	-.086	.003	.063	-.174	.185	.335	**-.589**	.247	.128	1		
$\delta^{13}C$	-.383	.145	.272	**-.540**	.032	.041	-.418	.341	.305	.189	-.005	1	
$\delta^{15}N$	.147	-.214	-.229	.052	.514	-.239	.302	.310	-.439	-.192	-.173	-.036	1

Values of r in bold are significant at the $p = 0.01$ level of confidence.

did not log-transform the data. Although the data are non-normal, Pearson's r is more likely to reject H_0 than Spearman's Rho; thus, Pearson's r is used here.

Among Altar burials, high positive correlations are observed among soil contaminant elements: Al, Fe, K, and Mn. Barium is positively correlated with Sr and negatively with $\delta^{13}C$ as predicted by dietary discrimination of these elements. Ba is not correlated with Mn, indicating that it does not occur in microbial manganese oxides (Parker and Toots 1980). Instead, Ba is negatively correlated with $\delta^{13}C$, reflecting the dietary incorporation of both elements. Among Seibal burials, soil elements are also highly intercorrelated. Sr and Ba are positively correlated with each other and are also correlated with Mn, suggesting some oxide contamination. Ba is also correlated with Zn and Fe, indicating that it may be more severely affected by diagenesis than Sr. Among Dos Pilas burials, the familiar intercorrelation of soil elements occurs, as well as the Ba-Sr correlation, and the Mn-Ba correlation is insignificant, suggesting better maintenance of biological levels than at Seibal.

I conducted principle components factor analysis on these correlation matrices to identify groups of covarying elements. Principle components factor analysis is appropriate for use here since it makes no distributional assumptions about the data (Krzanowski 1988:488). Thus, extended consideration of the distribution of the data is not imperative (as in Buikstra et al. 1989:192–94). For the same reason it is not necessary to log-transform the data before analysis. The analysis extracted factors with eigenvalues greater than 1, and the resulting factors were rotated according to the varimax orthogonal transformation in order to maximize the variance accounted for by the factors. Rotated factor matrices are in Table 7.4 for Altar, Seibal, and Dos Pilas.

For Altar, the first principle factor (PF1) documents the coocurrence of soil contaminants (Al, Fe, K, and Mn). Ba and Sr show very low loadings on PF1, indicating that their concentration is not linked to soil contamination. PF2 documents the inverse dietary relationship between Ba and $\delta^{13}C$ which is related to maize consumption. PF3 documents a relationship between Sr and P that is insignificant. Na and $\delta^{15}N$ load enigmatically on PF4, but r is insignificant for this pair. The association between Ca and Mg is similarly insignificant, so PF3, PF4, and PF5 can be considered as specific factors reflecting dietary (PF4) or metabolic processes (PF3, PF5).

For Seibal, PF1 documents insidious contamination by microbial oxides that bind Ba and Mn. Sr also appears to be affected by this process. PF2 documents soil contamination by Al, Fe, and K. Bone mineral components are linked with dietary isotopes on the following two factors, although the correlations that produced these combinations are generally insignificant: Ca, Na, and $\delta^{13}C$ on PF3 and P, Zn, and $\delta^{15}N$ on PF4. The final factor is specific to Mg. The association of Ca and Na on PF3 may indicate diagenetic substitution of Na^{+} for Ca^{++} (Buikstra et al. 1989:203), although the correlation is positive. Overall, soil contamination plays a greater role than diet in structuring elemental relationships in Seibal bone—a stark contrast to Altar patterns.

At Dos Pilas, PF1 again reflects the contributions of soil contaminants, and the loading of $\delta^{13}C$ here is due to a low correlation. PF2 describes the fundamental relationship between alkaline earth elements, reflecting their similar chemical properties and dietary behavior. Na also loads heavily here so may indicate diagenetic substitution for alkaline earth elements. PF3 suggests that K contamination is related to lower concentration of P, that is, loss of bone mineral. The association of $\delta^{15}N$ here is insignificant and obscure. PF4 describes antagonistic relationships between Na and Zn, while PF5 is specific to Mg.

In sum, these patterns suggest some contamination of archaeological bone by soil elements at all sites. Dietarily informative elements covary with these contaminants only at Seibal. At Altar and Dos Pilas, manganese oxides that form on bone surfaces may have been effectively removed by surface abrasion, as Ba content is not related to Mn, but this treatment was apparently inadequate to remove oxide contamination at Seibal. For Seibal the data are suspect, but these results

Table 7.4. Varimax rotated principle components matrices for elemental and isotopic data in human bone

	Element	PF 1	PF 2	PF 3	PF 4	PF 5
(a) Altar de Sacrificios	Al	**.881**	.054	.100	-.238	-.046
(n=40)	Ba	-.105	**-.796**	.375	.037	.166
	Ca	-.219	-.259	.229	.379	**.674**
	Fe	**.906**	-.086	-.001	-.043	.046
	K	**.781**	.209	.285	.104	-.152
	Mg	-.206	-.183	.244	.236	**-.730**
	Mn	**.850**	-.176	-.160	.025	.171
	Na	-.291	-.189	-.331	**.647**	-.274
	P	-.287	.187	**-.637**	.224	.210
	Sr	-.034	.049	**.789**	.024	.043
	Zn	**.566**	.450	.067	-.105	.022
	$\delta^{13}C$	-.109	**.790**	.156	.065	.134
	$\delta^{15}N$	.060	.109	.020	**.851**	.086
b) Seibal	Al	.107	**.922**	.030	-.045	.195
(n=37)	Ba	**.762**	.315	-.030	.127	.004
	Ca	-.255	-.027	**.622**	.097	-.192
	Fe	.329	**.823**	-.175	.107	.295
	K	.108	**.882**	.036	-.088	-.204
	Mg	-.063	.123	.084	.001	**.925**
	Mn	**.851**	.145	-.094	-.031	.079
	Na	.039	.059	**.772**	-.300	.075
	P	-.448	-.049	.147	**.705**	-.078
	Sr	**.923**	.067	-.040	.096	-.184
	Zn	.470	.020	-.235	**.588**	.161
	$\delta^{13}C$	-.004	-.082	**.732**	.237	.216
	$\delta^{15}N$	.170	-.014	.036	**.579**	-.006
c) Dos Pilas	Al	**.828**	.236	.204	.165	-.260
(n=26)	Ba	.223	**.907**	.070	-.092	.131
	Ca	-.167	**.803**	-.139	-.147	.029
	Fe	**.939**	.053	.062	.048	-.166
	K	.134	.315	**.848**	-.038	.057
	Mg	-.186	.305	-.019	.086	**.870**
	Mn	**.560**	.008	.472	.516	.030
	Na	-.187	.580	.408	**-.638**	.054
	P	-.453	-.101	**-.664**	.265	-.348
	Sr	.105	**.749**	.165	.259	.280
	Zn	.025	.017	-.142	**.915**	.071
	$\delta^{13}C$	**-.748**	.403	.062	.061	-.313
	$\delta^{15}N$	-.031	-.274	**.848**	-.111	-.210

Heavy loadings are indicated in **bold**.

provide little indication that Ba and Sr concentrations in bone are not essentially biogenic at Dos Pilas and Altar.

Elemental values in archaeological human bones can be assumed to represent biogenic mineral if archaeological animal bones are found to have values comparable to modern animals of the same species. Although archaeological faunal collections are limited, I sampled a few bones from species for which modern specimens were also available. A few faunal bones were obtained from excavations at Dos Pilas and Aguateca; most are from Punta de Chimino, which is hydrologically similar to Altar. Figure 7.2 illustrates Ba/Ca and Sr/Ca in modern and archaeological fauna from the Petexbatun region. As noted above, archaeological fauna show Ca/P values that approximate those of modern fauna, indicating that bone mineral consists largely of hydroxyapatite.

Ba/Ca values for archaeological deer and agouti are bracketed by the modern values, demonstrating that they are largely biogenic. Turtle values are also comparable. However, prehistoric peccary Ba/Ca is higher than the modern data, implying Ba enrichment. Archaeological felid values bracket the modern value but indicate a broad distribution. For one of the prehistoric peccaries, Mn and Fe concentrations are very high, as are Mn, Fe, and Al concentrations for the high-Ba prehistoric cat, indicating that anomalous Ba/Ca in these two specimens is due to soil contamination. The crocodile also shows moderately high Al, suggesting that its Ba/Ca may also be diagenetic. Although no modern value is available, the carnivorous crocodile should have Ba/Ca similar to felids.

The Sr/Ca values may be less affected by diagenesis, as the archaeological values correspond closely to modern data for all species. A single Punta de Chimino turtle specimen is somewhat high in Sr/Ca and also shows an elevated Mn concentration implying contamination. The crocodile Sr/Ca is similar to that of terrestrial fauna and lower than the turtle, which is consistent with that expected for a carnivore feeding on freshwater foods of high Sr/Ca.

These data indicate that bone composition of archaeological fauna closely resembles that of its modern counterparts. Although some specimens suffer demonstrable diagenesis, these can be identified by their high levels of soil contaminants. Only one specimen, a peccary mandible from Punta de Chimino, shows Ba enrichment that would not be detected by soil contaminant levels. Furthermore, many of these bones are superficially less well preserved than the human material and include elements with thin cortices and trabecular bone that should be subject to more severe diagenetic change than human long bones.

Diagenesis can be further investigated by examining elemental concentrations of soils at each site. Table 7.5 lists Spearman rank-order correlations for elemental concentrations in bone ash with the relative elemental concentration of soils in direct contact with bone for each site from which soil samples were obtained (Nelson and Sauer 1984; White 1986). At Altar, no correlations were significant, but Rho for Ba approaches significance. At Dos Pilas, a significant correlation was observed only for Na, but the value for P also approaches significance. There are no significant correlations at Aguateca or Itzan, perhaps due to the small sample sizes.

Among Petexbatun burials, bone-soil dynamics can be further investigated in the multiple samples collected from many burials. As soil characteristics for Aguateca and Dos Pilas are largely similar, the two sites are pooled for this comparison (only two burials for Aguateca). Because soil elements are not normally distributed, I use the nonparametric Mann-Whitney U test to compare soil samples. Test results are in Table 7.6. The Mann-Whitney test failed to detect a significant difference for any element between samples adjacent to bone and those located at 10 or 20 cm from the bone. This result indicates that elemental transport between bone and soil was not sufficient to affect soil concentrations or that chemical dynamics between bone and soil have already reached equilibrium over a large horizontal distance.

In addition to examining correlations for each element between bone and soil, the relationship between Ca content of soils with Sr and Ba content, described above, can be used to address diagenetic issues. If bone levels of Sr and Ba reflect diagenetic alteration, they should be posi-

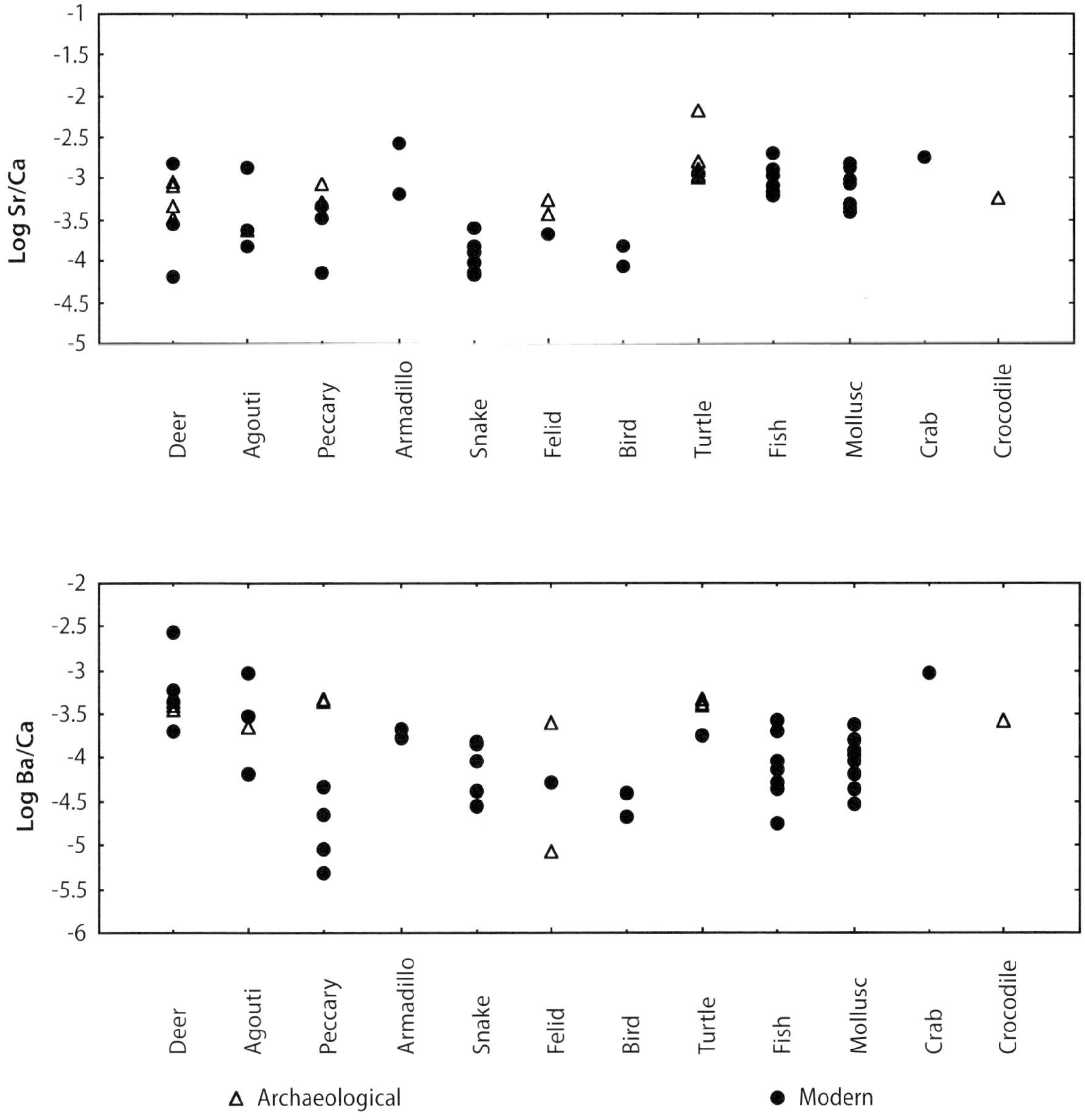

Figure 7.2. Ba/Ca and Sr/Ca ratios in modern and archaeological fauna from the Pasión region

tively and negatively correlated with Ca content of adjacent soils, respectively. For Altar and the small Itzan sample, no relationship is apparent for either element (Altar, $n = 17$, Sr: Rho = 0.00, $p = 1.00$; Ba: Rho = 0.04, $p = 0.89$; Itzan, $n = 5$, Sr: Rho = −0.10, $p = 0.84$; Ba: Rho = −.10, $p = .84$). At Aguateca, the correlation of Ca with bone Sr is insignificant ($n = 7$, Rho = −0.11, $p = 0.79$), but bone Ba approaches a significant positive correlation with soil Ca (Rho = 0.74, $p = 0.07$). This is opposite to that expected if bone mineral reflects diagenetic recrystallization, but a biological explanation is also obscure. The small sample size might be responsible. For Dos Pilas, soil elements differ in hydrologically distinct areas of the site, but, overall, no relationship is noted between bone Sr or Ba levels and soil Ca (Sr: Rho = −0.07, $p = 0.78$; Ba: Rho = −0.18, $p = 0.46$). Moreover, Mann-Whitney U tests reveal no significant differences

Table 7.5. Spearman's Rho for correlations of elemental concentrations in bone ash with adjacent soil

	Altar (N=17)		Dos Pilas (N=19)		Aguateca (N=7)		Itzan (N=5)	
Element	Rho	p	Rho	p	Rho	p	Rho	p
Al	-.037	.88	.268	.25	-.270	.51	.205	.68
Ba	.426	.08	.114	.63	.126	.76	-.051	.92
Ca	.315	.21	-.071	.76	.234	.57	-.100	.84
Fe	.213	.39	.354	.13	.595	.14	.500	.32
K	-.068	.79	.112	.63	-.414	.31	.300	.55
Mg	.203	.42	.405	.08	.306	.45	.100	.84
Mn	.249	.32	.341	.15	.577	.16	.000	1.00
Na	.346	.17	**.475**	.04	-.018	.96	-.500	.32
P	.179	.47	.398	.09	-.018	.96	.300	.55
Sr	.049	.84	-.113	.63	.000	1.00	.600	.23
Zn	.151	.55	.167	.48	-.649	.11	.800	.11

Values of Rho in bold are significant at $p \leq 0.05$.

Table 7.6. Mann-Whitney U test comparisons of elemental concentrations in soil adjacent to bone with elemental concentrations in soil at 10 and 20 cm from bone, for Dos Pilas and Aguateca combined

	0 cm vs. 10 cm (n=17)				0 cm vs. 20 cm (n=10)			
Element	U	U′	Z	p	U	U′	Z	p
Al	139	150	-.19	.85	46	54	-.30	.76
Ba	139	150	-.19	.85	50	50	.00	1.00
Ca	142	147	-.09	.93	48	52	-.15	.88
Fe	134	155	-.36	.72	46	54	-.30	.76
K	139	150	-.19	.85	49.5	50.5	-.04	.97
Mg	134	155	-.36	.72	49	51	-.08	.94
Mn	143	147	-.05	.96	45	55	-.39	.70
Na	138.5	150.5	-.21	.84	41	59	-.68	.49
P	101	188	-1.49	.13	29	71	-1.59	.11
Sr	144.5	144.5	.00	1.00	47	53	-.23	.82
Ti	142	147	-.09	.93	48.5	51.5	-.11	.91
Zn	142.5	146.5	-.07	.95	49	51	-.08	.94

Only burials with multiple samples are considered in each case.

in bone Sr and Ba between Dos Pilas burials interred in soil with less than 8% Ca and those interred in greater than 8% Ca (Sr: $U = 29$, $U' = 55$, $z = -1.10$, $p = 0.27$; Ba: $U' = 26$, $U' = 58$, $z = -1.35$, $p = 0.18$, $n = 19$).

Despite these indications that most Pasión bone mineral is biogenic, a few burials show anomalous levels of several elements. The comparison of modern and archaeological fauna illustrated that diagenetic enrichment of Ba/Ca was also heralded by high levels of soil contaminant elements. In order to minimize possible effects of diagenesis on human bone, I discarded data for samples that showed high levels of contaminants. I chose these contaminant cutoff levels by examining the distribution of each element to identify outliers. I excluded samples that showed more than 900 ppm Al, 300 ppm Fe, 400 ppm K, or 100 ppm Mn. Most of the data discarded exceed two or more of these limits. In all, elemental data for 14 samples are excluded from the dietary reconstruction that follows: Burials AS41, AS70, AS92, AS129, AG5B, QCH1B, QCH7, DP16, DP17, DP44, DP47, DP20, SE6, and SE9. Excluding these data, I recalculated the elemental correlations and repeated the principle components factor analysis for the samples from Altar de Sacrificios, Seibal, and Dos Pilas (Table 7.7).

For Altar de Sacrificios, exclusion of four burials that show soil contamination divided the soil elements into two groups. Contamination by Al and Fe, indicated on PF1, remains a significant factor in total sample variability, but K, Mn, and Zn contamination now fall on PF3, indicating that such contamination is governed by a different process than that governing Al and Fe and that it is relatively less important. PF2 describes the functional relationship between Ba and Ca in bone mineral. $\delta^{13}C$ is separated from Ba onto PF5, indicating that the dietary information imparted by the two measures is not entirely congruent. In the edited data, the correlation of Ba with $\delta^{13}C$ is slightly lower, −0.378, and significant only at $p < 0.05$. PF4 retains the Na-$\delta^{15}N$ relationship initially observed, while PF5 combines Sr with P and Mg, suggesting that Sr variability is not strictly tied to diet in this sample.

The edited data show a dramatic change in elemental relationships among Seibal bones with the data from three contaminated bones discarded. No longer dominated by soil and oxide contamination, Sr and Ba account for most of the variability, falling on PF1. The loading of Mn on this factor is very low, suggesting that oxide contamination does not affect the remainder of the sample significantly and should not cause undue alarm. This is because the correlations of Mn with Ba (−0.008) and Sr (−0.099) are extremely low. Apparently the three discarded samples were responsible for the patterns seen in the unedited factor matrix. PF2 and PF3 also describe bone elements, linking Ca, Na, and $\delta^{13}C$ on PF2, and P and Zn on PF3. As noted previously, Na loading on PF2 may suggest some diagenesis. Soil elements account for little variability in the data, and load on PF5 and PF6. At Dos Pilas, elimination of data from five contaminated samples resulted in the loading of dietary (alkaline earth) elements Ba, Ca, Sr, and $\delta^{13}C$ on PF1. The association of $\delta^{15}N$, P, Na, and K falls now on PF2. Soil contamination is less important in explaining variation in the sample, with the elements indicating contamination loading on PF3 and PF5. PF4 records Mg, which was similarly isolated in other samples. Thus, elimination of a few contaminated samples substantially changed the structure of the Dos Pilas data set so that dietary factors explain most of the variation and soil contamination is relatively unimportant.

To summarize, archaeological human bone from the Pasión region does not appear to have suffered severe diagenetic effects. Although slight diagenetic effects are suggested by various avenues of investigation, these results do not generally confirm each other. Ca/P ratios indicate that archaeological bone mineral consists essentially of hydroxyapatite. Altar and Seibal bones may show low P indicating elevated levels of foreign mineral, but they still have Ca/P within an acceptable biogenic range. Deviations from expected levels were easily identified by soil contaminant concentrations, suggesting that screening of human samples for contaminants could minimize this bias. Correlation and principle components analysis indicate that the distribution of dietary elements in human bone mineral is not closely linked to that of soil

Table 7.7. Varimax rotated principle components matrices for edited elemental and isotopic data in human bone

(a) Altar de Sacrificios (n=36)

Element	PF 1	PF 2	PF 3	PF 4	PF 5	PF 6
Al	**.827**	-.258	.192	-.191	.074	.159
Ba	.098	**.682**	-.235	-.093	-.494	.246
Ca	-.171	**.831**	.056	.174	.055	-.094
Fe	**.922**	.077	-.027	.002	.105	.020
K	.435	-.092	**.630**	.228	.067	.408
Mg	-.163	-.155	-.335	.267	-.242	**.601**
Mn	.063	.239	**.748**	-.051	-.251	-.237
Na	-.217	.003	-.199	**.714**	-.293	-.143
P	-.336	.043	-.202	.153	.184	**-.709**
Sr	.074	.385	-.017	-.196	.358	**.622**
Zn	-.014	-.234	**.811**	-.081	.229	.088
$\delta^{13}C$	.145	-.048	-.001	.019	**.856**	-.070
$\delta^{15}N$	.040	.120	.108	**.848**	.233	.046
(b) Seibal (n=34)						
Al	.065	.078	-.204	**.846**	-.021	.201
Ba	.908	-.001	.013	.061	.015	-.010
Ca	.063	**.662**	.053	.370	.242	.125
Fe	.015	-.394	.307	**.774**	-.224	-.007
K	.033	.061	-.271	.257	.108	**.748**
Mg	-.188	.121	-.175	.005	.212	**-.812**
Mn	.010	.114	-.019	.295	**-.782**	-.093
Na	.006	**.735**	-.254	-.108	-.153	.019
P	-.341	.184	**.787**	-.054	.219	.139
Sr	**.803**	.120	-.023	.011	.171	.398
Zn	.379	-.173	**.734**	.018	-.024	-.222
$\delta^{13}C$	.018	**.749**	.222	-.193	-.062	-.160
$\delta^{15}N$	.131	.047	.102	.115	**.780**	-.163

continued

contaminants once burials with particularly high contamination are eliminated, although contamination initially appeared to be a significant problem for Seibal. Soil contamination is a substantial factor in the distribution of elements only in the samples from Altar but does not appear to have strong influence over Sr or Ba distribution in any sample once contaminated samples are excluded. Prehistoric faunal bone composition closely parallels modern trophic-level relationships and absolute elemental abundances. Soil comparisons indicate no Ba or Sr correlations between bone and soil, and no gradients in elemental distribution in grave soils, with the exception of P. At Dos Pilas the demonstration that bone levels do not mimic properties of two disparate soils supports the conclusion that archaeological bone mineral is largely biogenic.

(c) Dos Pilas (n=21)

Element	PF 1	PF 2	PF 3	PF 4	PF 5
Al	.250	.224	**.876**	.047	.198
Ba	**.929**	.099	.161	-.106	.050
Ca	**.700**	.148	.110	-.085	.080
Fe	.108	-.160	**.953**	-.002	-.004
K	.347	**.798**	.110	-.048	.124
Mg	.357	-.067	-.064	**-.826**	.002
Mn	.210	.160	.077	.128	**.884**
Na	.530	**.766**	.170	-.036	-.242
P	-.188	**-.572**	-.408	.538	.129
Sr	**.822**	.015	.134	-.168	.124
Zn	-.019	-.554	.109	-.159	**.738**
$\delta^{13}C$	**.627**	.054	.070	.606	.034
$\delta^{15}N$	-.243	**.893**	-.184	.123	.017

Heavy loadings are indicated in **bold**.

This conclusion is surprising, given the poor overall preservation of bone. Bone is clearly decaying significantly, yet the chemical composition is not markedly altered from the expected biogenic pattern. A clue may lie in the nature of wet tropical soils. Tropical ecosystems differ from the temperate ones in which most trace element studies have been conducted to date. Heavy rainfall and constant high temperatures support high rates of soil respiration. Resulting carbonic acid releases cations from clays and, presumably, interred bone; those cations are rapidly leached away by heavy rainfall. Carbonic acid also binds free P, so that plants have developed elaborate mechanisms to efficiently cycle soil P (Jordan 1984). Could it be that the heavy leaching of Ca^{++} and P-cycling removed decaying bone mineral and local soil cations from the microenvironment of the bone, preempting recrystallization of hydroxyapatite that would differ from the original bone composition? The high Sr/Ca in the freshwater ecosystem indicates that Sr is rapidly and differentially leached, supporting this idea. Although diagenetic alteration of the human material is not conclusively demonstrated, it remains possible, and diagenesis will be kept in mind as a possible influence in the ensuing investigation of dietary patterns in Pasión prehistory.

Paleodietary Interpretations

Results of intersample comparisons in isotopic and elemental bone composition are in Table 7.8. The Mann-Whitney U test was used to evaluate intersample chemical differences instead of the parametric ANOVA used by many bone chemists, because of the deviations from normality and small sample sizes. Moreover, the presence of distinct social heterogeneity within samples indicates that the assumptions of the ANOVA are violated in these data. I consider the results of intersample comparisons below with respect to chronological and intersite trends. In subsequent sections, I discuss sexual and mortuary differences in consumption and reevaluate the broader trends in light of these social patterns.

Chronological and Spatial Trends

ALTAR DE SACRIFICIOS

At Altar de Sacrificios, which has the most complete chronological record, several trends occur in both isotopic and elemental results. Figure 7.3 shows the isotopic and elemental composition of Altar bone collagen for all periods. The most obvious pattern in the isotopic data is a shift toward heavier $\delta^{13}C$ over time. $\delta^{13}C$ rises from a Preclassic low to a high in the Late Classic period.

Terminal Classic $\delta^{13}C$ drops slightly, to a level equivalent to the Early Classic period. The $\delta^{13}C$ rise is statistically significant at $p < 0.05$ for comparisons between Preclassic and all later periods (Table 7.8). Between the Early and Late Classic samples the rise approaches significance ($p = 0.12$; $p = 0.06$ if outlying AS55 is included). The Terminal Classic drop is not statistically significant when compared with the Late Classic, but neither is it different from the Early Classic, supporting the interpretation of slightly decreased $\delta^{13}C$ in the final occupation. The nitrogen isotopic composition of Altar bones does not show any chronological trends, and samples from all periods are not statistically different for any pairwise comparison. The Preclassic and Early Classic data are more tightly clustered than the Late or Terminal Classic data, which show considerable dietary diversity.

This pattern is best interpreted to indicate a change in the relative consumption of maize versus other plant foods. Although increasing consumption of animal protein could also raise $\delta^{13}C$ levels, it would result in concomitant $\delta^{15}N$ increases, which are not detected. Accordingly, maize consumption probably increased at Altar over the span of the Classic period. In the Late Classic, $\delta^{13}C$ levels (mean = −8.34‰) approach the predicted value for a diet based entirely on maize (−5‰, assuming +5‰ enrichment between diet and collagen). However, the lowest $\delta^{15}N$ measured in Late Classic collagen (7.9‰) is about 2‰ heavier than herbivore collagen, a value close to the diet-collagen enrichment factor for $\delta^{15}N$ (+3‰), indicating that substantial C4-meat consumption contributes to the high $\delta^{13}C$ in this period. The slight decrease in $\delta^{13}C$ of Terminal Classic collagen indicates a decline in maize consumption during the final occupation of the site after the elite collapse, with no change in animal protein consumed.

The elemental composition of Altar bones shows a similar picture (Figure 7.3). Preclassic bone mineral contains the most Ba, and Ba/Ca declines from Preclassic through Terminal Classic samples, though the Early and Late Classic samples are highly variable. Only the distinction between Preclassic and Terminal Classic Ba/Ca is statistically significant; however, the Preclassic to Early Classic rise approaches significance ($p = 0.09$). For Sr/Ca, a similar trend is visible in the graph but does not attain statistical significance for any intersample comparison. The paucity of significant differences in elemental data highlights the relative degree of variability in elemental ratios between periods. Both the Preclassic and Terminal Classic samples show fairly tight clustering of alkaline earth ratios. In contrast, the Early Classic and Late Classic samples show much broader variation, with lower means, but broadly overlap the range of other periods. Most periods show a fairly tight linear relationship between Ba/Ca and Sr/Ca; however, a few Late Classic samples deviate from this trend toward higher Sr, perhaps due to freshwater protein consumption or a change in maize preparation, though diagenetic enrichment cannot be excluded.

The parallel trend observed in Ba/Ca and $\delta^{13}C$ at Altar reflects the negative correlation between these two dietary measures, which approaches significance (Rho = −0.33, $p = 0.07$, $n = 32$). Since no difference in $\delta^{15}N$ is substantiated, trends in Ba/Ca are best attributed to changes in the relative contribution of maize to the diet, mirroring the isotopic results. If maize were untreated or treated with plant ashes that have little effect on the total Ca content of maize, this result would be due to the greater visibility of meat signals in the total diet. Moreover, if shifting herbivore ranges average alkaline earth ratios and fauna were hunted off the alluvial plain of the Pasión, then meat eaten at Altar might have had disproportionately low Ba/Ca with respect to local agricultural plants (which are higher in Ba/Ca at Altar than at other sites). This greater divergence would accentuate the trophic effect of Ba/Ca more than Sr/Ca and could contribute to the Ba/Ca-$\delta^{13}C$ correlation.

Ba/Sr also shows a significant negative correlation with $\delta^{13}C$ at Altar (Rho = −0.51, $p = 0.004$) that is largely attributed to the Ba/Ca correlation. This pattern hints that maize might have been prepared with snail-shell lime at Altar. However, Sr/Ca shows no correlation with $\delta^{13}C$ overall (Rho = 0.16, $p = 0.36$), and snail-lime processing would be more likely to produce an increase in Sr/Ca than a decline of Ba/Ca. This might be seen in a few Late Classic samples, that deviate toward higher Sr and bias the Ba/Sr cor-

Table 7.8. Mann-Whitney U statistics for intersample dietary comparisons

(a) $\delta^{13}C$

Sample	Mean	N	AS TC	AS LC	AS EC	AS PC	SE TC	SE LC	SE PC	DP TC	DP LC	AG LC	IT LC
AS TC	-9.01	16											
AS LC	-8.32	7	-1.24										
AS EC	-9.10	5	-0.33	-1.54									
AS PC	-10.36	8	**-3.00**	**-3.01**	**-2.93**								
SE TC	-9.36	16	-0.83	**-1.74**	-0.21	**-2.21**							
SE LC	-9.35	11	-0.32	-1.31	-0.40	-1.82	-0.27						
SE PC	-9.61	7	-1.34	**-2.11**	-1.22	-1.39	-0.54	-0.77					
DP TC	-9.44	15	-1.15	-1.80	-0.31	**-2.00**	-0.17	-0.34	-0.53				
DP LC	-8.93	17	-0.14	-1.18	-0.59	**-3.20**	-1.04	-0.69	-1.52	-1.06			
AG LC	-9.51	9	-1.47	**-2.55**	-0.88	**-2.11**	-0.49	-0.70	-0.58	-0.80	-1.85		
IT LC	-9.18	5	-0.74	**-1.71**	-0.10	**-2.93**	0.00	-0.62	-0.98	-0.04	-0.94	-0.96	
TA LC	-10.00	5	**-2.03**	**-2.03**	-0.52	-1.46	-0.66	-1.08	-0.24	-0.92	-1.61	-0.07	-0.52

(b) $\delta^{15}N$

Sample	Mean	N	AS TC	AS LC	AS EC	AS PC	SE TC	SE LC	SE PC	DP TC	DP LC	AG LC	
AS TC	8.78	16											
AS LC	8.99	7	-0.40										
AS EC	8.18	5	-0.99	-1.38									
AS PC	8.40	8	-0.74	-1.16	-0.15								
SE TC	8.91	16	-0.45	-0.13	-1.65	-1.47							
SE LC	9.87	11	-2.81	-1.77	-3.12	-3.06	-2.49						
SE PC	9.69	7	**-1.91**	-1.47	**-2.52**	**-2.55**	-1.80	-0.23					
DP TC	9.96	15	**-2.33**	-1.44	**-2.49**	**-2.45**	-1.87	-0.28	-0.18				
DP LC	9.84	17	**-2.70**	-1.62	**-2.78**	**-3.09**	**-2.85**	-0.68	-0.67	-0.34			
AG LC	9.45	8	-1.10	-0.58	**-2.03**	-1.62	-0.87	-1.01	-0.45	-0.61	-0.55		
IT LC	7.96	5	-1.32	-1.54	-0.52	-1.17	-1.53	**-2.89**	**-2.28**	**-2.53**	**-2.86**	**-1.95**	
TA LC	9.44	5	-.59	-0.57	-1.78	-1.46	-0.66	-0.40	-0.57	-0.57	-0.59	-0.29	-1.78

continued on next page

(c) Ba/Ca

Sample	Mean	N	AS TC	AS LC	AS EC	AS PC	SE TC	SE LC	SE PC	DP TC	DP LC	AG LC
AS TC	0.64	14										
AS LC	0.73	7	-0.08									
AS EC	0.76	7	-0.82	-0.19								
AS PC	1.10	8	**-3.00**	-1.27	-1.62							
SE TC	0.28	17	**-4.33**	**-2.70**	**-3.08**	**-3.96**						
SE LC	0.36	11	**-3.18**	**-2.04**	**-2.40**	**-3.47**	-1.15					
SE PC	0.34	7	**-2.39**	**-1.98**	**-2.24**	**-3.01**	-0.03	-0.50				
DP TC	0.26	4	**-2.76**	**-1.89**	**-2.27**	**-2.09**	-0.27	-1.38	-0.19			
DP LC	0.14	17	**-4.68**	**-3.59**	**-3.72**	**-3.96**	**-4.01**	**-3.12**	**-2.51**	**-2.15**		
AG LC	0.15	6	**3.46**	**-2.86**	**-2.88**	**-3.00**	**-2.94**	**-2.61**	**-2.00**	-1.28	-0.91	
IT LC	0.16	6	**-3.46**	**-2.72**	**-2.72**	**-3.00**	**-2.66**	**-2.51**	-1.85	-1.71	-0.42	-0.48

(d) Sr/Ca

Sample	Mean	N	AS TC	AS LC	AS EC	AS PC	SE TC	SE LC	SE PC	DP TC	DP LC	AG LC
AS TC	0.59	14										
AS LC	0.64	7	-0.08									
AS EC	0.51	6	-1.04	-0.45								
AS PC	0.60	8	-0.82	0.12	-1.04							
SE TC	0.34	17	**-3.73**	**-2.38**	**-2.38**	-3.50						
SE LC	0.57	11	-0.06	-0.50	-0.68	0.00	**-2.19**					
SE PC	0.68	7	**-2.39**	-1.60	-1.73	**-2.32**	-0.15	-1.40				
DP TC	0.35	4	**-2.55**	-1.51	-1.51	**-2.09**	-0.45	-1.18	-0.76			
DP LC	0.26	17	**-4.56**	**-3.21**	**-3.33**	**-3.96**	**-2.36**	**-3.22**	-1.49	**-2.15**		
AG LC	0.18	6	**-3.46**	**-3.00**	**-2.88**	**-3.00**	**-3.29**	**-3.11**	**-2.86**	**-2.56**	**-2.38**	
IT LC	0.20	6	**-3.46**	**-2.86**	**-2.72**	**-3.00**	**-3.01**	**-2.92**	**-2.43**	**-2.35**	-1.75	-0.48

(e) Ba/Sr

Sample	Mean	N	AS TC	AS LC	AS EC	AS PC	SE TC	SE LC	SE PC	DP TC	DP LC	AG LC
AS TC	1.19	14										
AS LC	1.24	7	-0.22									
AS EC	1.47	7	-1.34	-0.70								
AS PC	1.87	8	**-2.46**	-1.74	-1.39							
SE TC	0.84	17	**-2.54**	-1.81	**-3.08**	**-3.44**						
SE LC	0.71	11	**-2.63**	-1.77	**-2.94**	**-3.38**	-1.39					
SE PC	0.75	7	**-2.31**	-1.60	**-2.75**	**-2.89**	-0.54	-0.32				
DP TC	0.74	4	**-1.91**	-1.32	**-2.45**	**-2.09**	-1.08	0.00	-0.19			
DP LC	0.52	17	**-3.89**	**-2.44**	**-3.72**	**-3.90**	**-3.63**	-1.48	-1.87	-1.70		
AG LC	0.86	6	-1.48	-1.29	**-2.40**	**-2.57**	-0.21	-1.01	-0.57	-0.43	**-2.45**	
IT LC	0.82	6	-1.65	-1.00	-1.76	**-2.43**	-1.40	-0.20	-0.29	-0.43	-1.61	-0.80

Values in bold indicate a significant difference at the $p \leq 0.05$ level of confidence.

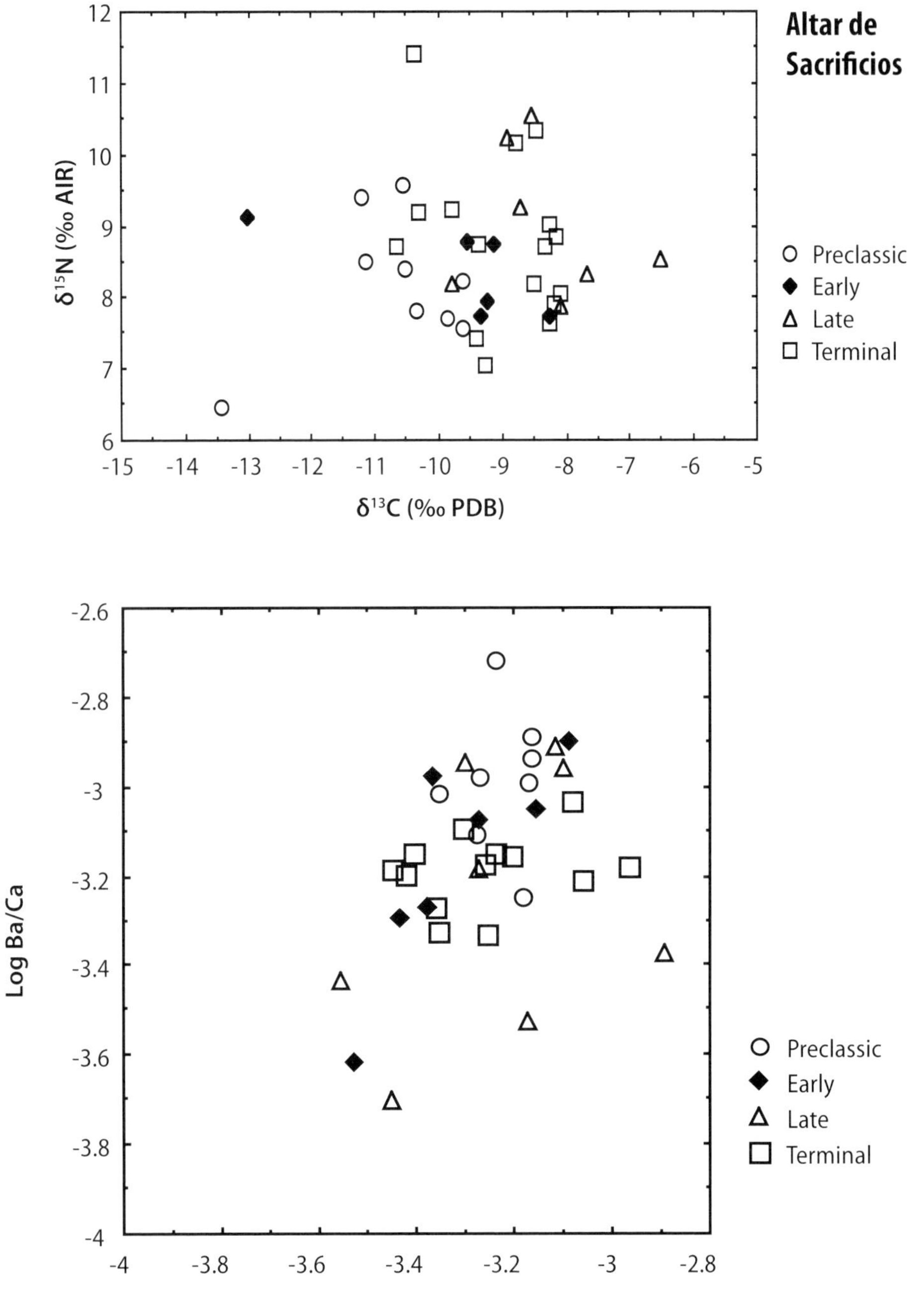

Figure 7.3. Chronological patterns in isotopic and elemental composition of bone from Altar de Sacrificios

relation with $\delta^{13}C$. With no change in meat consumption (terrestrial or aquatic) indicated by $\delta^{15}N$, perhaps changes in Ba/Sr are a result of Late Classic Sr enrichment from greater consumption of maize treated with snail lime relative to other plant foods. If limestone was used to treat maize and raised maize Ca to the level of other plants, we would expect maize and C3 plants to have similar Ba/Sr ratios, so $\delta^{13}C$ would show no trends with elemental ratios. Given the absence of local limestone at Altar, it is not surprising that alternate sources of lime might have been sought, though limestone could have been obtained several kilometers away. The most conservative hypothesis is that plant ashes were the primary source of alkali at Altar; however, heterogeneity in alkaline processing methods over time and among subpopulations cannot be excluded.

SEIBAL

Very different trends are found in the samples from Seibal. Bone collagen shows no chronological trends in $\delta^{13}C$, and the Mann-Whitney test identifies no significant differences between samples in $\delta^{13}C$ (Figure 7.4; Table 7.8). However, nitrogen isotopes do differ. Terminal Classic collagen shows lower $\delta^{15}N$ than Preclassic and Late Classic collagen. This difference is significant only for the Late-Terminal comparison but approaches significance for the Preclassic-Terminal Classic comparison ($p = 0.07$). This pattern indicates that the relative contribution of maize to Seibal diet changed little over time but that meat or fish consumption possibly declined during the Terminal Classic period.

Elemental data complements this interpretation (Figure 7.4). No correlations are found between $\delta^{13}C$ and any elemental measures, indicating either that maize did not differ in elemental content from other plant foods or that the Ca increment from maize processing dominates elemental signatures. This result probably means that alkali was obtained from the locally abundant limestone, in contrast to the plant ash that may have been used at Altar. The lower Ba/Ca of Seibal bone implies cultivation of upland areas and a lesser trophic distinction between agricultural products and herbivore bone than at Altar. Given the narrow range of $\delta^{13}C$, this smaller trophic effect may account for the absence of correlation between isotopic and elemental data at Seibal, unlike the result at Altar.

Late Classic Seibal alkaline earth ratios are more variable than in earlier or later periods, indicating greater culinary heterogeneity. Samples from the Preclassic and Terminal Classic periods show a high linear correlation between Ba/Ca and Sr/Ca, but the Late Classic samples lie further to the right, with higher Sr/Ca paralleling the Altar pattern. They contain significantly more Sr than Terminal Classic bone mineral does (Table 7.8). Freshwater protein consumption or a shift to *Pachychilus* as a source of alkali might account for this difference, as the distribution parallels the distinction between the linear correlation of terrestrial resources with the Sr enrichment of the aquatic ecosystem. However, diagenetic Sr elevation of Late Classic burials cannot be excluded from consideration.

But the nitrogen isotopic composition of Late Classic collagen is quite high (mean = 9.90‰) and could be enriched from fish consumption. In conjunction with the isotopic data, this result might be interpreted in terms of exploitation of terrestrial protein sources in the Preclassic and Terminal Classic periods, with a Late Classic shift to aquatic protein consumption at the expense of some terrestrial faunal protein. Alternately, a shift from limestone to molluscan lime for maize processing in the Late Classic, with no change in menu selection, could potentially account for the high Sr in Late Classic Seibal bones. The lower $\delta^{15}N$ of the Terminal Classic burials, which show elemental composition similar to that of Preclassic bones, suggests a reduction in consumption of high trophic-level aquatic protein, perhaps offset by legume consumption at the expense of other C4 plants and renewed exploitation of terrestrial fauna. Nonetheless, the mean $\delta^{15}N$ of the Terminal Classic remains 2 to 3‰ heavier than herbivore signatures, indicating that meat supplies were not severely limited.

DOS PILAS

At Dos Pilas, few statistical differences for either isotopic or elementary signals are detected

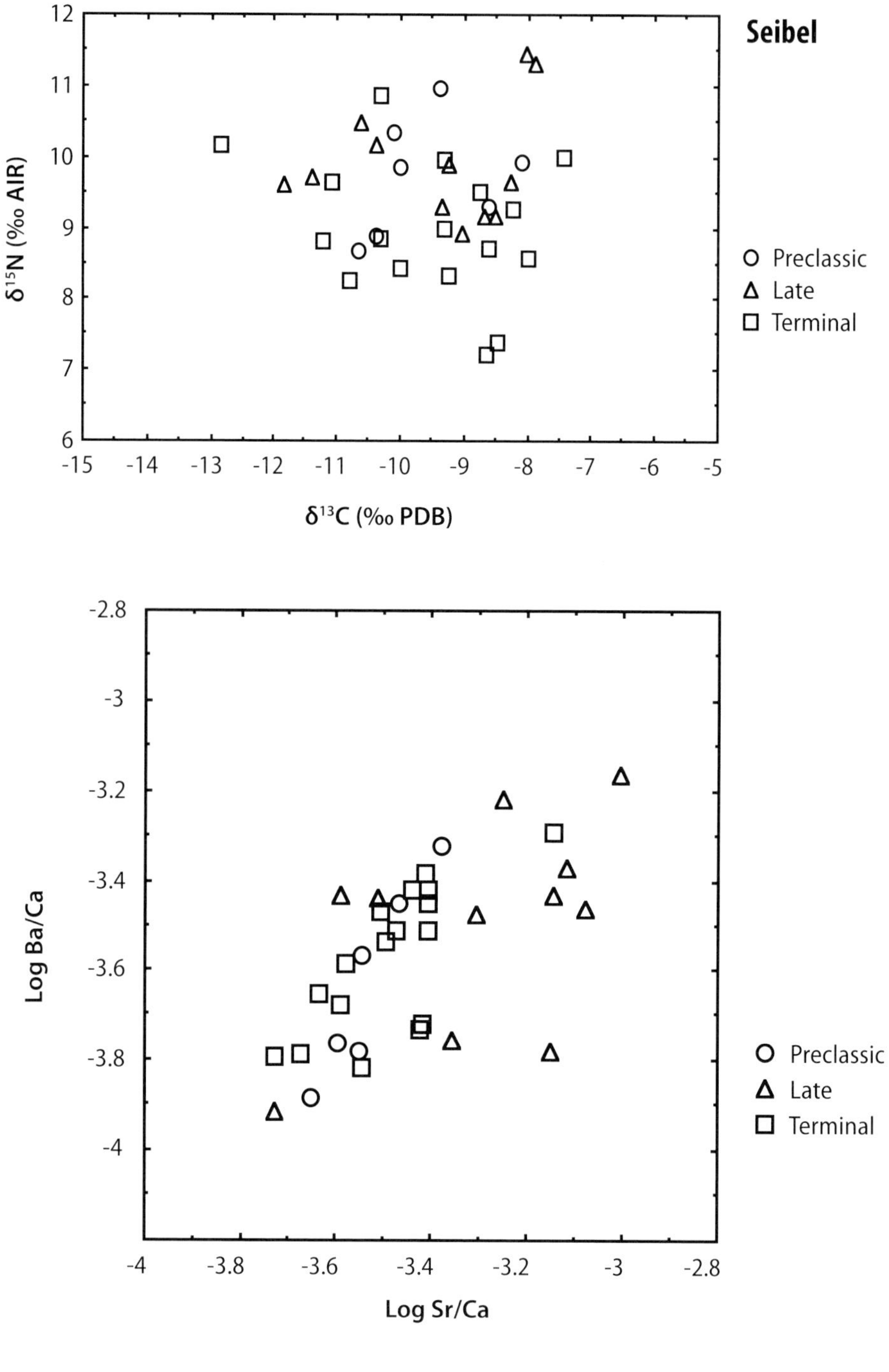

Figure 7.4. Chronological patterns in isotopic and elemental composition of bone from Seibal

between the Late and Terminal Classic skeletons (Figure 7.5; Table 7.8). The isotopic dataset is substantially larger than the elemental dataset since several Terminal Classic decapitated crania were sampled for isotopic analysis after the elemental analysis had been completed.

The elemental sample, which contains only primary burials for the Terminal Classic period, hints at some dietary differences between the occupations (Figure 7.5). These Terminal Classic bones contain significantly more Ba and Sr relative to Ca than many Late Classic Dos Pilas bones. When the decapitated crania are excluded from consideration, the Terminal Classic primary burials appear to lie toward the light end of the $\delta^{13}C$ range, and are somewhat light in $\delta^{15}N$. This might imply a greater emphasis on C3 plants in the small population that remained at the site after the elite withdrawal, an interpretation that may be consistent with the elemental data. C3 plants could have contributed more Ca to the Terminal Classic diet than to the Late Classic diet, if maize contained less Ca than other plants. Like Seibal, no correlations obtain between $\delta^{13}C$ and elemental ratios at Dos Pilas, so it is unlikely that aquatic lime sources were used. Uncertainty about the prehistoric maize processing techniques makes it different to interpret these results with respect to the maize/meat confound; herbivore elemental values are only slightly lower than local flora so a parallel distinction might not be found anyway.

INTERSITE PATTERNS

These chronological patterns attain greater relevance when differences between sites are also evaluated (Table 7.8). Intersite comparisons are strictly valid only for isotopic data, as the isotopic composition of food resources is not expected to vary systematically between sites. In contrast, differences in the Ba/Ca ratio in ground water hinder intersite comparisons of elemental ratios. Soil differences are of a magnitude that confounds with the range of dietary variability documented over time. Were differences greater, Ba/Ca ratios might be useful in evaluating shifts in agricultural land use patterns, particularly at sites (e.g., Seibal) with access to soils of differing elemental composition. In the present case, however, this does not appear to be feasible.

Isotopic analyses reveal dramatic differences between the two key sites occupied during the Preclassic period (Figure 7.6). Seibal Preclassic burials are heavier in both C and N isotopic composition than Altar Preclassic burials. The difference is significant only for $\delta^{15}N$, suggesting greater consumption of faunal protein at Seibal than Altar, which would also contribute to the $\delta^{13}C$ trend. The single Preclassic burial excavated from the rural site, Bayak, by the Petexbatun Project is most similar to the Preclassic Altar skeletons. The Early Classic Altar sample is similar in $\delta^{13}C$ to Preclassic Seibal but significantly lower in $\delta^{15}N$, again indicating differences in faunal protein consumption between sites.

For the Late Classic sites a broad similarity in collagen composition occurs across the region, but some intersite patterns are statistically significant (Figure 7.7). The samples from Altar, Seibal, and Dos Pilas show a similar spread of $\delta^{13}C$ and are not statistically distinguishable. Late Classic collagen from Itzan, Tamarindito, and Aguateca is significantly different from Altar collagen, showing lower $\delta^{13}C$ and, therefore, less maize consumption. Seibal collagen is statistically heavier in $\delta^{15}N$ than Itzan, and perhaps Altar ($p = 0.08$), possibly reflecting greater freshwater protein consumption at Seibal. The Itzan samples are the lightest in $\delta^{15}N$, being significantly lighter than contemporary Seibal, Dos Pilas, and Aguateca, a trend that might result from less animal protein consumption because of the "lower" status of these "suburban" individuals. Regardless, Itzan $\delta^{15}N$ remains 1 to 2‰ higher than herbivore values. Dos Pilas samples are intermediate and not significantly different from any of the other Late Classic sites for either C or N isotopes.

Among Terminal Classic sites, diets continue to illustrate broad isotopic ranges due to substantial dietary diversity within each site (Figure 7.8). Collagen from Terminal Classic samples from Altar and Seibal is comparable in both C and N isotopic composition; no significant differences can be detected among them. Also, the ranges covered in each of the samples are very similar, indicating

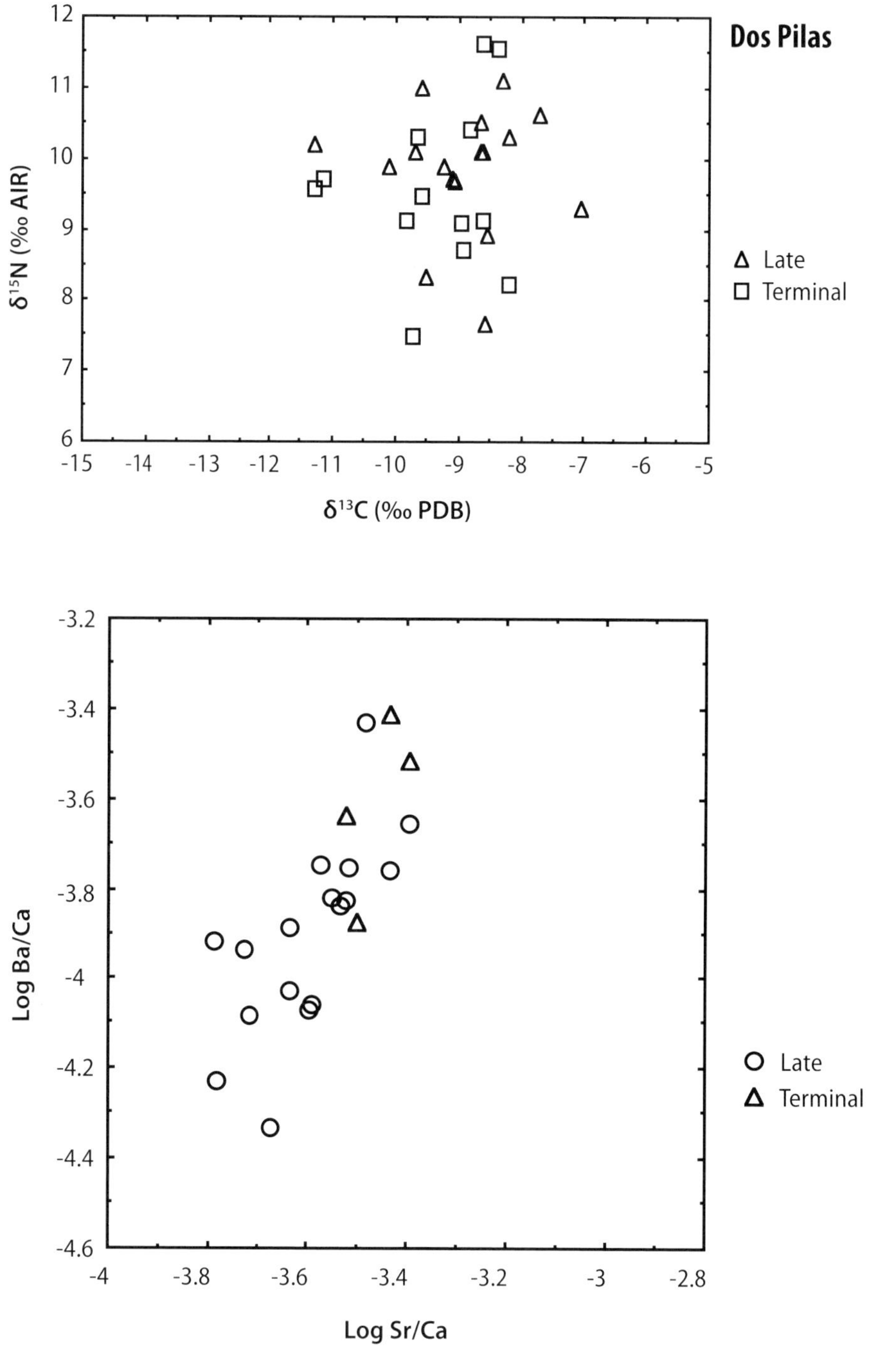

Figure 7.5. Chronological patterns in isotopic and elemental composition of bone from Dos Pilas

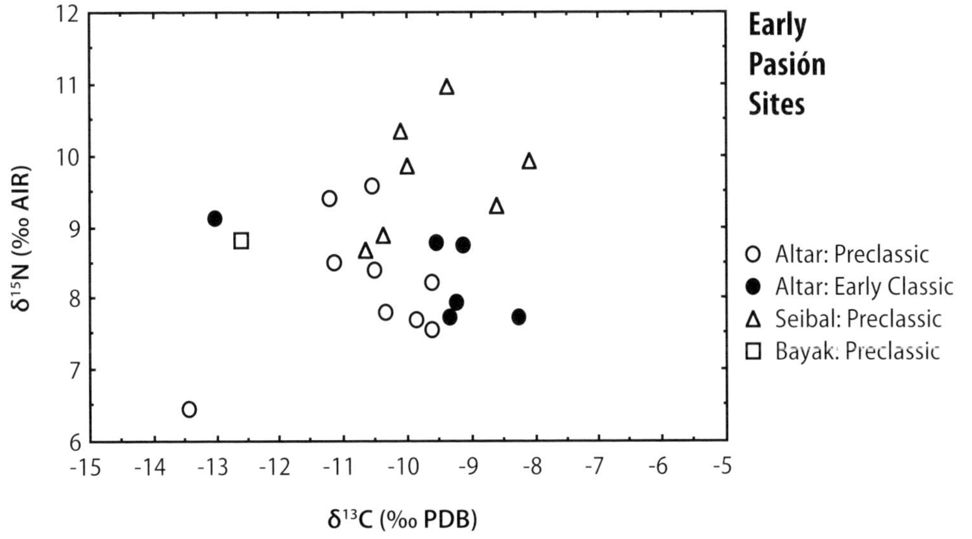

Figure 7.6. Intersite patterns in isotopic composition of bone during the Preclassic and Early Classic Periods

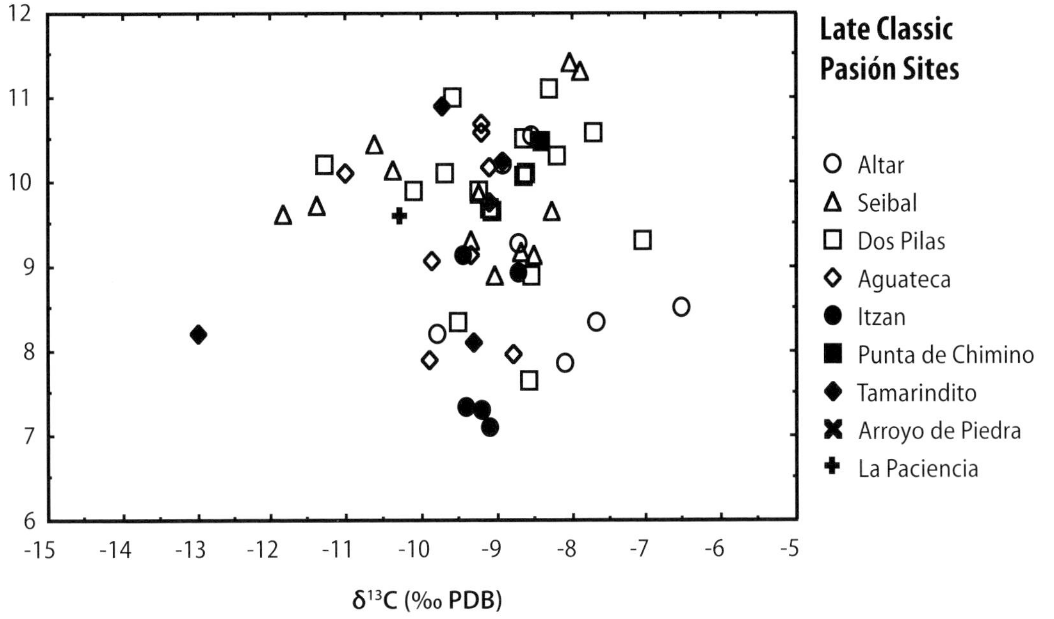

Figure 7.7. Intersite patterns in isotopic composition of bone during the Late Classic Period

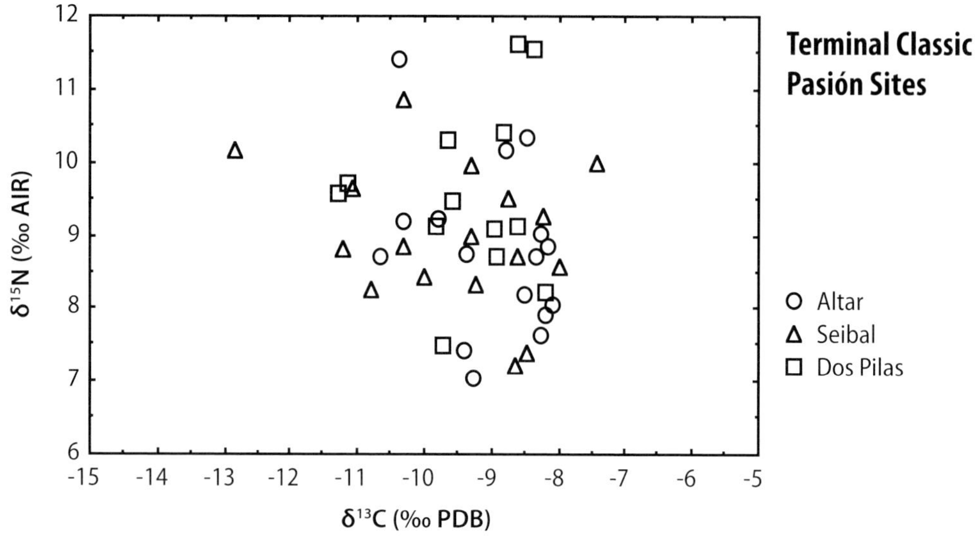

Figure 7.8. Intersite patterns in isotopic composition of bone during the Terminal Classic Period

comparable intrasample variability in bone collagen isotopes from this period. Terminal Classic Dos Pilas collagen is similar to Altar and Seibal collagen in $\delta^{13}C$ but is significantly more enriched in ^{15}N than Altar, presumably due to greater carnivory. The average $\delta^{15}N$ is also a full permil higher than coeval Seibal, although the difference is not statistically significant.

Social Patterning

Intrasample variability in isotopic and elemental bone composition is illustrated in the ensuing figures with respect to the mortuary clusters defined statistically for each sample and the sex of the skeleton. Because small numbers of graves from each cluster were analyzed chemically, statistical evaluation of mortuary partitioning of diet is not feasible. Therefore, interpretation incorporates the obvious statistical caveats, but a number of patterns are apparent, and probably real. Sexual differences in bone chemistry are tested with the Mann-Whitney U test (Table 7.9) because of the small samples, non-normality, and mortuary heterogeneity that crosscuts the sexual divisions.

Social differences are evident in a number of samples. In some cases isotopic data show social patterning, while in others, elemental data are more revealing. This might at first seem contradictory but probably is a reflection of the different dietary processes underlying each technique. For instance, relative changes in consumption of different plant foods characterized under the isotopic umbrella "C3" can affect elemental ratios with little isotopic impact, as Ca content is not related to isotopic discrimination. Likewise, social differences in food preparation methods would also be more likely to affect elemental ratios than isotopic ones. In some cases a lack of elemental difference between clusters might be a consequence of diagenetic averaging—a possibility that cannot be excluded for any sample.

ALTAR DE SACRIFICIOS

Dietary variability among Preclassic Altar de Sacrificios burials is illustrated in Figure 7.9. Isotopic analysis finds little difference between the two burial clusters from which bone samples could be analyzed, and sexual distinctions are not significant. The data are tightly clustered, suggesting a fairly homogeneous diet. Recall that AS131 with $\delta^{13}C$ of −13.3‰ is an outlier possibly affected by diagenesis. This homogeneous pattern is contradicted by the elemental data, which shows a clear division of the two clusters, with higher ratios in Cluster D (in domestic architecture) than C (in public architecture). This would suggest greater

Table 7.9. Mann-Whitney U statistics for comparisons between the sexes

Sample	Males			Females			Mann-Whitney	
	N	Mean	s.d.	N	Mean	s.d.	z	p
(a) $\delta^{13}C$								
AS TC	8	-8.8	0.87	6	-9.6	0.74	-1.62	0.11
AS LC	4	-8.0	1.36	3	-8.6	0.42	-0.89	0.37
AS EC	3	-10.3	2.40	3	-9.2	0.10	-0.66	0.51
AS PC	7	-10.7	1.34	2	-10.5	0.00	-0.30	0.77
SE TC	10	-8.9	1.07	5	-10.1	0.86	**-2.21**	**0.03**
SE LC	10	-9.4	1.42	1	-9.0	-	0.00	1.00
SE PC	5	-9.9	0.81	2	-8.8	0.92	-1.55	0.12
DP TC	12	-9.4	1.35	3	-9.4	0.67	-0.43	0.66
DP LC	8	-8.5	0.91	8	-9.4	0.82	-1.78	0.07
AG LC	4	-9.8	0.85	4	-9.3	0.45	-0.89	0.37
IT LC	2	-9.1	0.49	3	-9.2	0.21	-0.58	0.56
TA LC	4	-9.2	0.35	1	-13.0	-	-1.41	0.16
(b) $\delta^{15}N$								
AS TC	8	8.7	1.06	6	9.0	1.42	-0.65	0.52
AS LC	4	8.2	0.25	3	9.5	0.67	**-2.12**	**0.03**
AS EC	3	8.5	0.74	3	8.1	0.53	-0.89	0.38
AS PC	7	8.0	0.89	2	9.0	0.85	-1.46	0.14
SE TC	10	8.7	0.92	5	8.9	0.64	-0.12	0.90
SE LC	10	10.0	0.83	1	8.9	-	-1.59	0.11
SE PC	5	9.4	0.67	2	10.4	0.78	-1.37	0.17
DP TC	12	10.3	1.45	3	8.6	0.93	-1.73	0.08
DP LC	8	10.0	0.70	7	9.7	1.13	-0.21	0.83
AG LC	4	9.8	1.31	3	8.7	0.64	-1.06	0.29
IT LC	2	8.2	1.06	3	7.8	1.10	-0.58	0.56
TA LC	4	9.7	1.12	1	8.2	-	-0.71	0.48
(c) Ba/Ca								
AS TC	7	0.62	0.09	5	0.66	0.12	-0/41	0.68
AS LC	4	0.60	0.40	3	0.63	0.52	0.00	1.00
AS EC	3	1.07	0.18	4	0.53	0.24	**-2.12**	**0.03**
AS PC	7	1.07	0.42	1	1.30	-	-1.09	0.28
SE TC	10	0.27	0.09	6	0.30	0.13	-0.54	0.59
SE LC	11	0.36	0.17	0	-			-
SE PC	5	0.39	0.28	2	0.24	0.16	-0.78	0.44
DP TC	1	0.13	-	1	0.23	-		-
DP LC	10	0.13	0.10	7	0.15	0.03	-1.56	0.12
AG LC	3	0.16	0.07	3	0.15	0.01	-0.22	0.83
IT LC	3	0.15	0.11	3	0.16	0.04	-0.66	0.51

continued on next page

Sample	Males			Females			Mann-Whitney	
	N	Mean	s.d.	N	Mean	s.d.	z	p
(d) Sr/Ca								
AS TC	7	0.52	0.17	5	0.62	0.27	-0.73	0.46
AS LC	4	0.66	0.41	3	0.58	0.26	0.00	1.00
AS EC	3	0.65	0.20	4	0.40	0.10	-1.77	0.07
AS PC	7	0.58	0.09	1	0.68	-	-1.53	0.13
SE TC	10	0.30	0.07	6	0.41	0.16	-1.52	0.13
SE LC	11	0.57	0.26	0	-			-
SE PC	5	0.84	1.17	2	0.28	0.08	-0.78	0.44
DP TC	1	0.31		1	0.76			-
DP LC	10	0.25	0.08	7	0.28	0.05	-1.27	0.20
AG LC	3	0.19	0.02	3	0.18	0.05	-0.22	0.33
IT LC	3	0.18	0.02	3	0.23	0.07	-1.09	0.28
(e) Ba/Ca								
AS TC	7	1.28	0.37	5	1.21	0.52	-0.41	0.68
AS LC	4	1.10	0.86	3	1.12	0.60	-0.35	0.72
AS EC	3	1.75	0.62	4	1.26	0.32	-0.71	0.48
AS PC	7	1.87	0.77	1	1.91	-	-0.22	0.83
SE TC	10	0.88	0.16	6	0.75	0.23	-1.30	0.19
SE LC	11	0.71	0.37	0	-			-
SE PC	5	0.73	-.33	2	0.81	0.32	0.00	1.00
DP TC	1	0.42		1	0.76			-
DP LC	10	0.52	0.26	7	0.53	0.08	-0.68	0.49
AG LC	3	0.83	0.39	3	0.88	0.25	-0.22	0.83
IT LC	3	0.90	0.79	3	0.73	0.13	-0.66	0.51

Values in bold indicate a significant difference at the $p \leq 0.05$ level of confidence.

consumption of high-Ca (mostly C3) plants by Cluster D individuals. Since $\delta^{13}C$ and $\delta^{15}N$ indicate no discrepancies between clusters, this difference is unlikely to be due to differential meat consumption. Sex differences in isotopic and elemental content cannot be evaluated in the small sample.

In the Early Classic Altar sample, there is also little isotopic distinction between clusters or sexes (Figure 7.10). It is difficult to evaluate status differences in this sample due to the small number of skeletons analyzed. The single male sample from Cluster A (AS55) is very low in $\delta^{13}C$, which may be a social difference as this grave is the only one interred in public architecture analyzed from this period; but it is also an outlier and may be an artifact of poor collagen quality, so I excluded it from statistical evaluation. The elemental data contrasts males and females from the domestic burials of Cluster B, with females perhaps consuming more meat than males did, given the lack of $\delta^{13}C$ differences.

Late Classic Altar shows a different pattern. Although the sample is small, isotopic analysis suggests distinctions in meat consumption (Figure 7.11). Both sampled skeletons from Cluster D are very high in $\delta^{15}N$, indicating greater meat consumption by those individuals than by the rest of the sample. Since these two graves (AS128, AS88) represent a superordinate status dimension—perhaps royalty—it is reasonable to suggest that high-status individuals were afforded greater access to meat than low-status individuals at Late Classic Altar. Systematic differences among the remaining

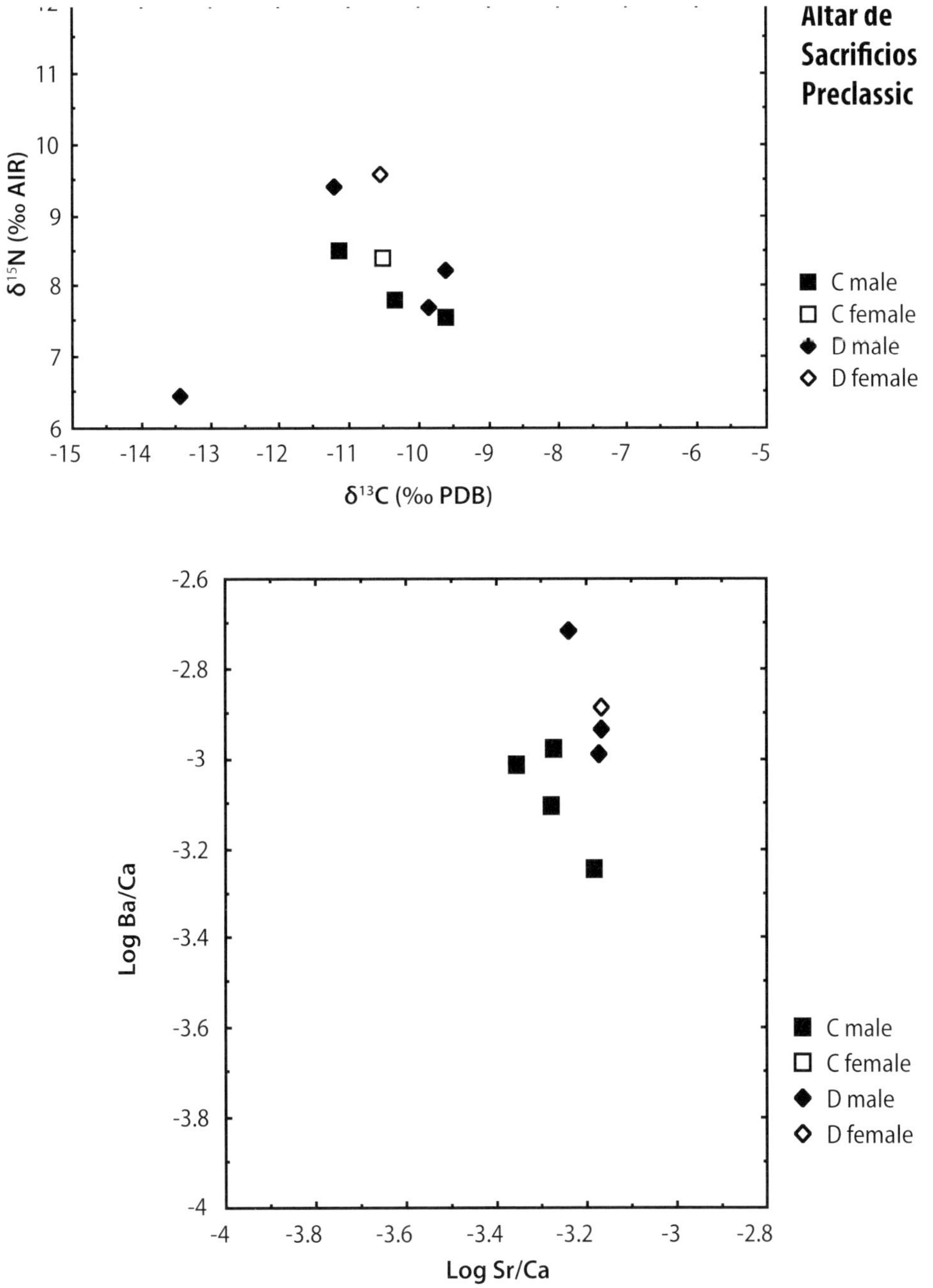

Figure 7.9. Isotopic and elemental patterning between sexes and among mortuary clusters at Preclassic Altar de Sacrificios

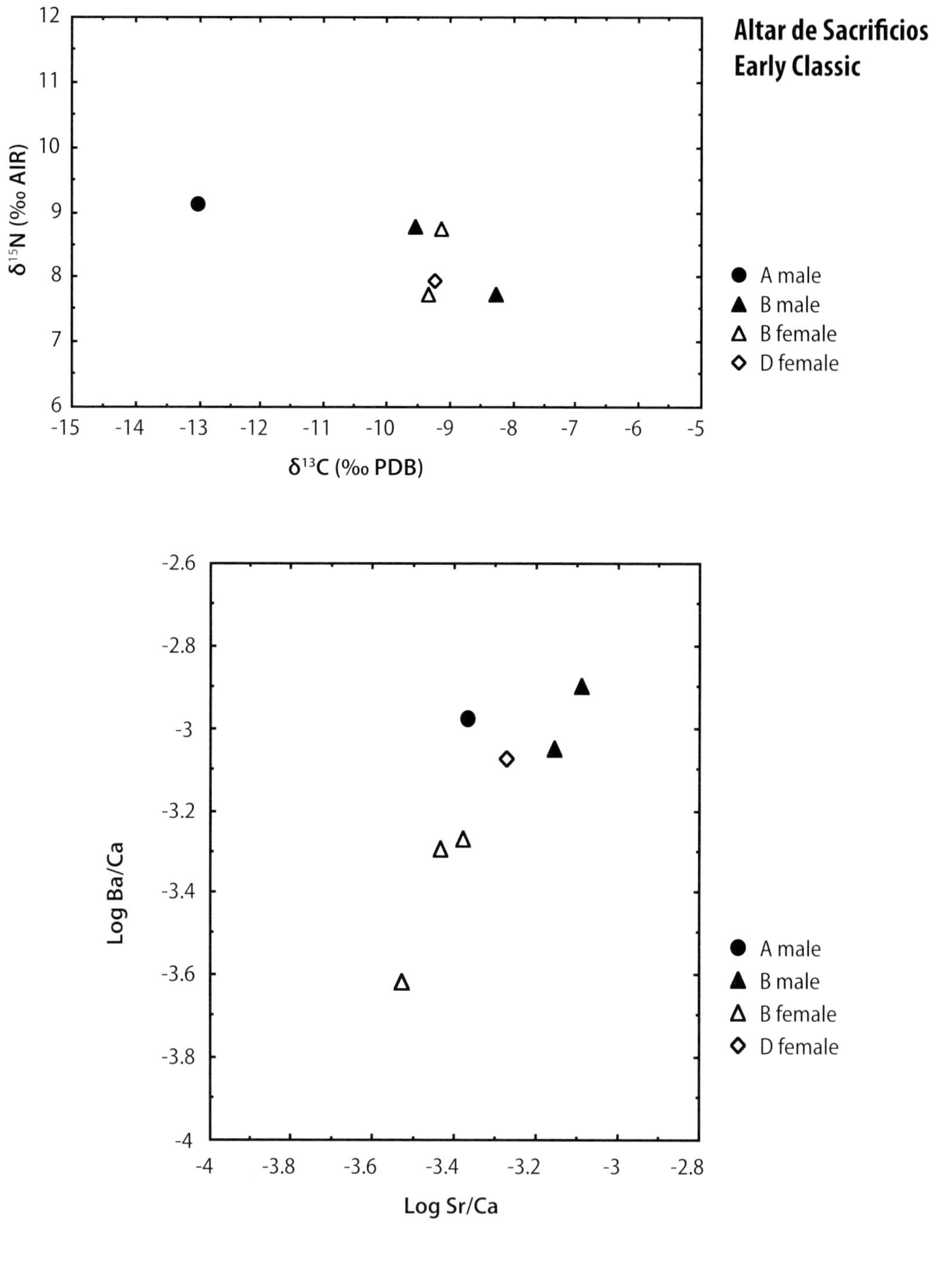

Figure 7.10. Isotopic and elemental patterning between sexes and among mortuary clusters at Early Classic Altar de Sacrificios

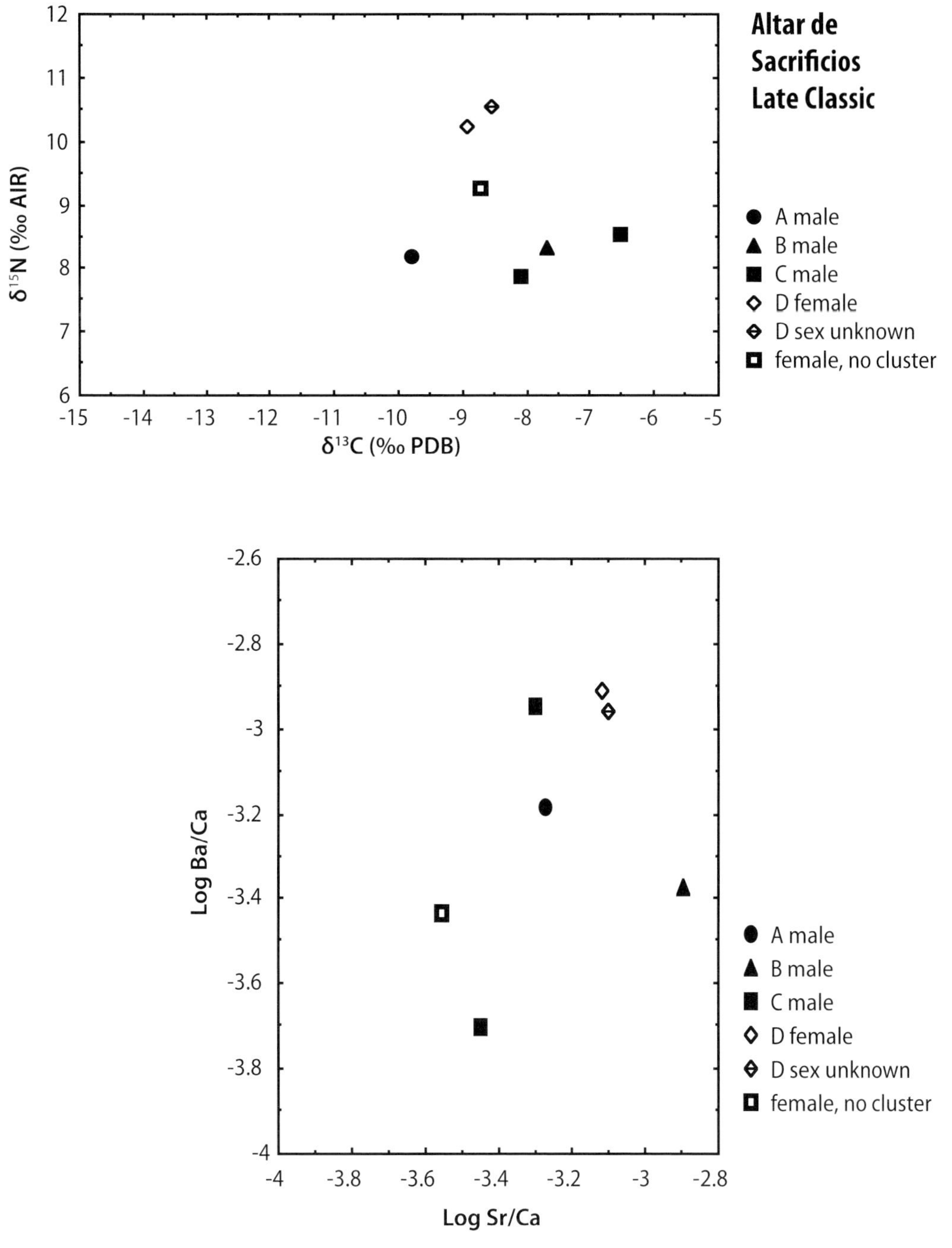

Figure 7.11. Isotopic and elemental patterning between sexes and among mortuary clusters at Late Classic Altar de Sacrificios

clusters are not evident, perhaps due to the small number of burials sampled.

Elemental data is somewhat at odds with this isotopic characterization (Figure 7.11). The two elite Cluster D skeletons are at the high end of the range, reflecting a plant signature rather than a meat signature. This might be taken to indicate either greater consumption of Ca-rich plant foods by the Cluster D individuals or differences in alkali processing methods. Alternately, it might indicate that agricultural products consumed by this group were grown only on the local floodplain, while lower-status groups might have fed on products from *milpas* farther afield on rendzina soils that would produce lower Ba/Ca ratios. The subordinate-status samples show diverse elemental compositions with little patterning.

In the Terminal Classic Altar de Sacrificios occupation, there are no distinct groupings of bone-collagen isotopic signatures by mortuary cluster (Figure 7.12). All clusters show a very broad diversity of isotopic ratios, indicating extreme dietary variability. This result parallels the observation that mortuary clusters are less distinct or less formally constituted in this sample than in previous occupations at the site. The lack of isotopic differences indicates that mortuary clusters do not define groups of individuals that differed from other groups in dietary access. There appears to be a slight difference between the sexes in this sample overall. Male collagen tends toward heavier $\delta^{13}C$ than does female collagen; however, this difference is not statistically confirmed.

The elemental data also show little distinction among mortuary groups (Figure 7.12). There is no patterning in Ba/Ca or Sr/Ca between either mortuary clusters or sexes in this sample. Together with the isotopic data, these patterns indicate that following the collapse of elite authority at Altar there was a breakdown in the formality of social-class distinctions in both the organization of funerary features and the nature of dietary differences between social groups.

SEIBAL

Social distinctions are also difficult to discern in the small Preclassic sample from Seibal. Clusters A and D may differ slightly in N isotopic ratios, but this is difficult to evaluate with only two graves per cluster (Figure 7.13). Seibal females are about 1‰ heavier in $\delta^{13}C$ than males, but the difference does not reach statistical significance in this small sample. Elemental signatures do not show any patterning with respect to either burial cluster or sex. These results are similar to those from Preclassic Altar, in which clear social patterning was not apparent in bone-chemistry signatures.

The Late Classic sample from Seibal is not useful for evaluating sexual differences since it contains but a single female skeleton. The isotopic data show little distinct patterning between burial clusters (Figure 7.14). This contrasts with the pattern observed in the Altar Late Classic sample but might be explained by the absence of burials from a superordinate-status dimension from this sample. This lack is easily attributed to excavation bias, since few ceremonial buildings were probed from this period. The sex ratio is clear evidence of this bias. If the skeletons recovered are not representative of a broad cross-section of Seibal society, the mortuary divisions may be finer in scale than those represented in the Altar sample.

More differentiation is visible among the elemental signatures (Figure 7.14). Cluster A males contain the most Ba and Sr, with a single outlier having low values. This would suggest greater high-Ca plant consumption in this subsample. It might also reflect differences in soils exploited agriculturally by individuals in each cluster. Given the narrow floodplain at Seibal, the population probably exploited soils of differing signatures. It is conceivable that the rich floodplain soils might have been cultivated for use by a restricted social group, while others farmed karstic uplands to the east and west. The three Cluster C males are somewhat shifted toward high Sr/Ca, perhaps indicating more freshwater protein consumption, but this is difficult to evaluate given the sample size. As noted above with respect to chronological patterning, the Late Classic Seibal people may have consumed more freshwater protein than at other times and sites. Differences in consumption of mollusks versus plants could account for the small variation observed in elemental content without much

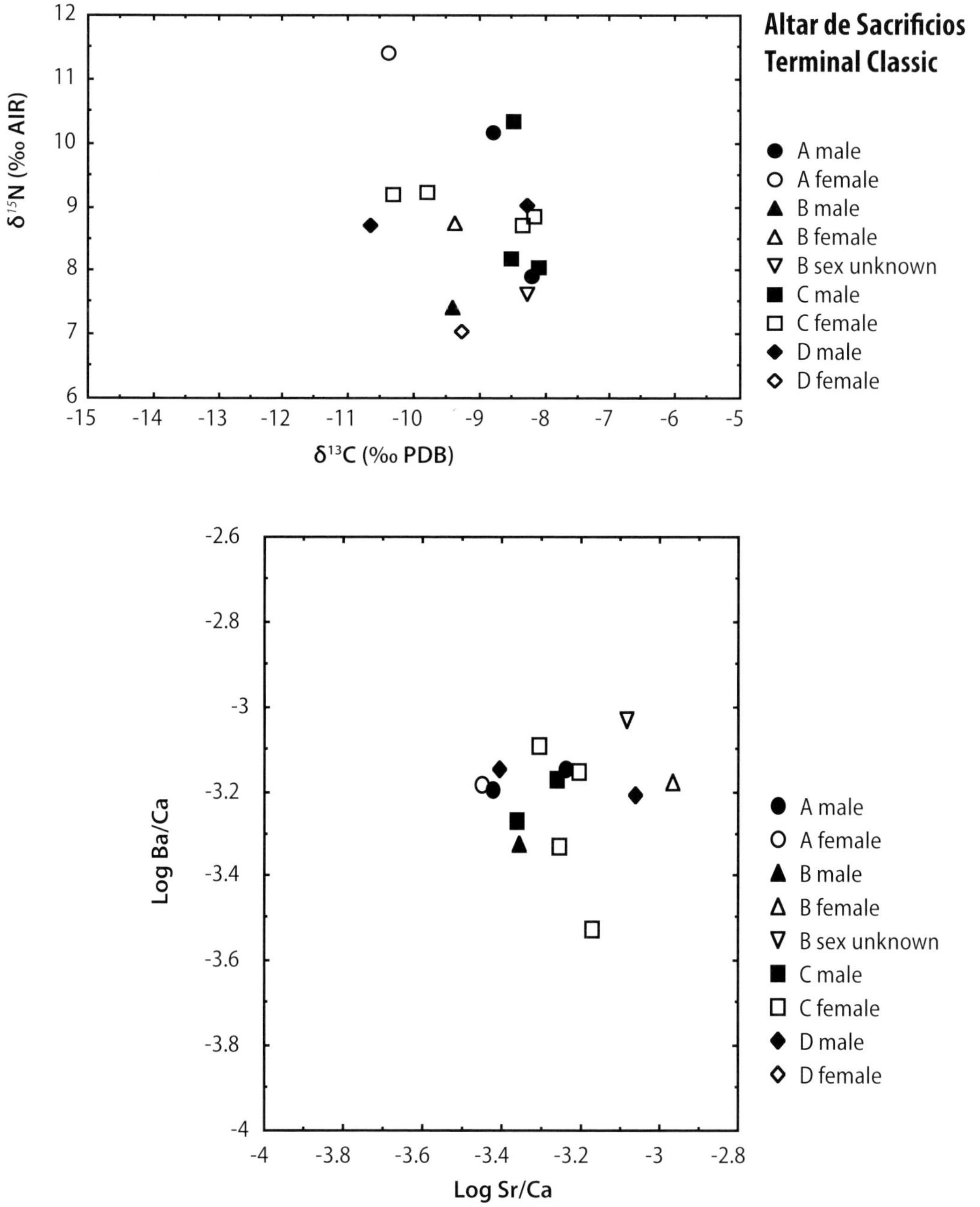

Figure 7.12. Isotopic and elemental patterning between sexes and among mortuary clusters at Terminal Classic Altar de Sacrificios

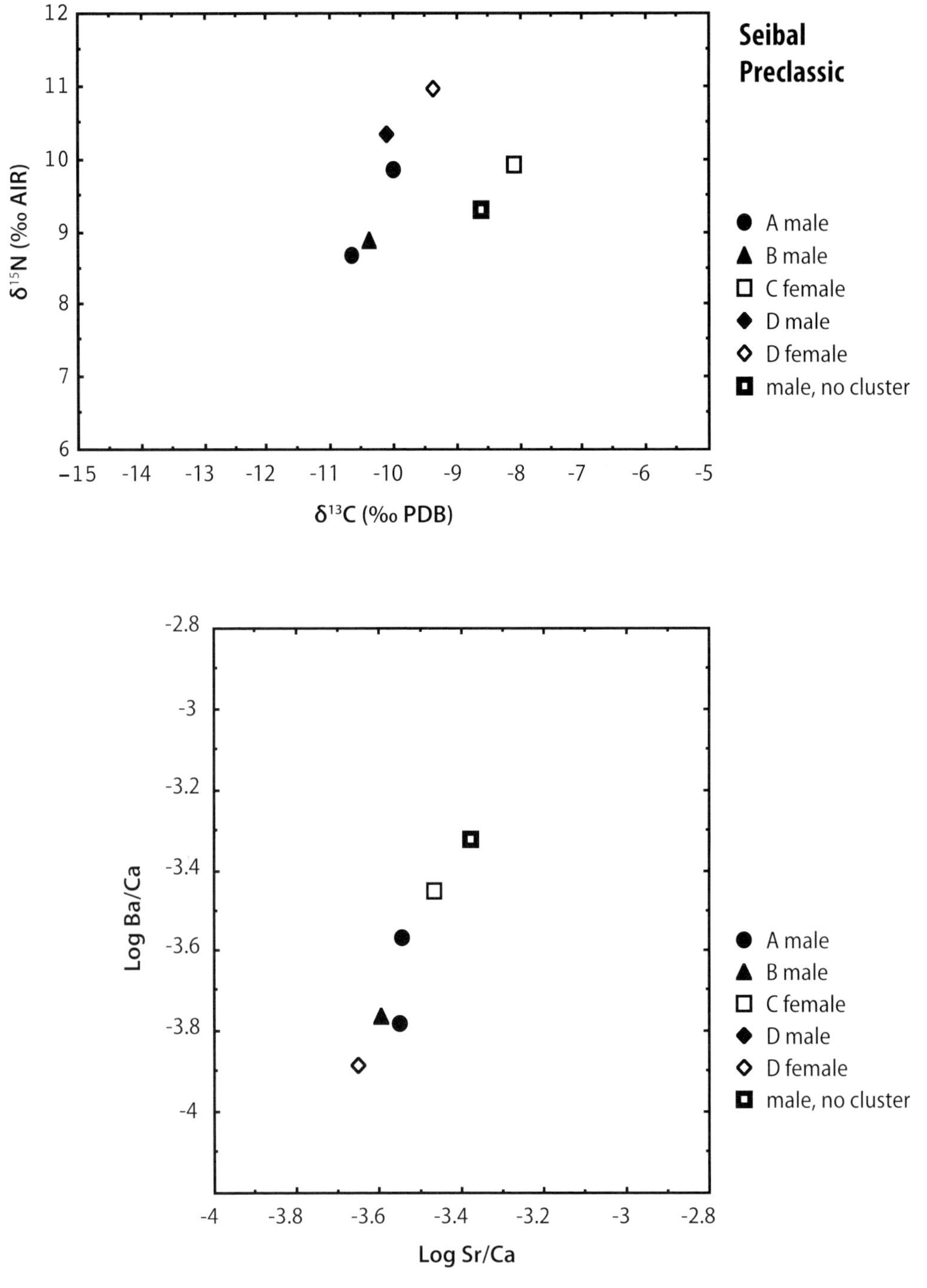

Figure 7.13. Isotopic and elemental patterning between sexes and among mortuary clusters at Preclassic Seibal

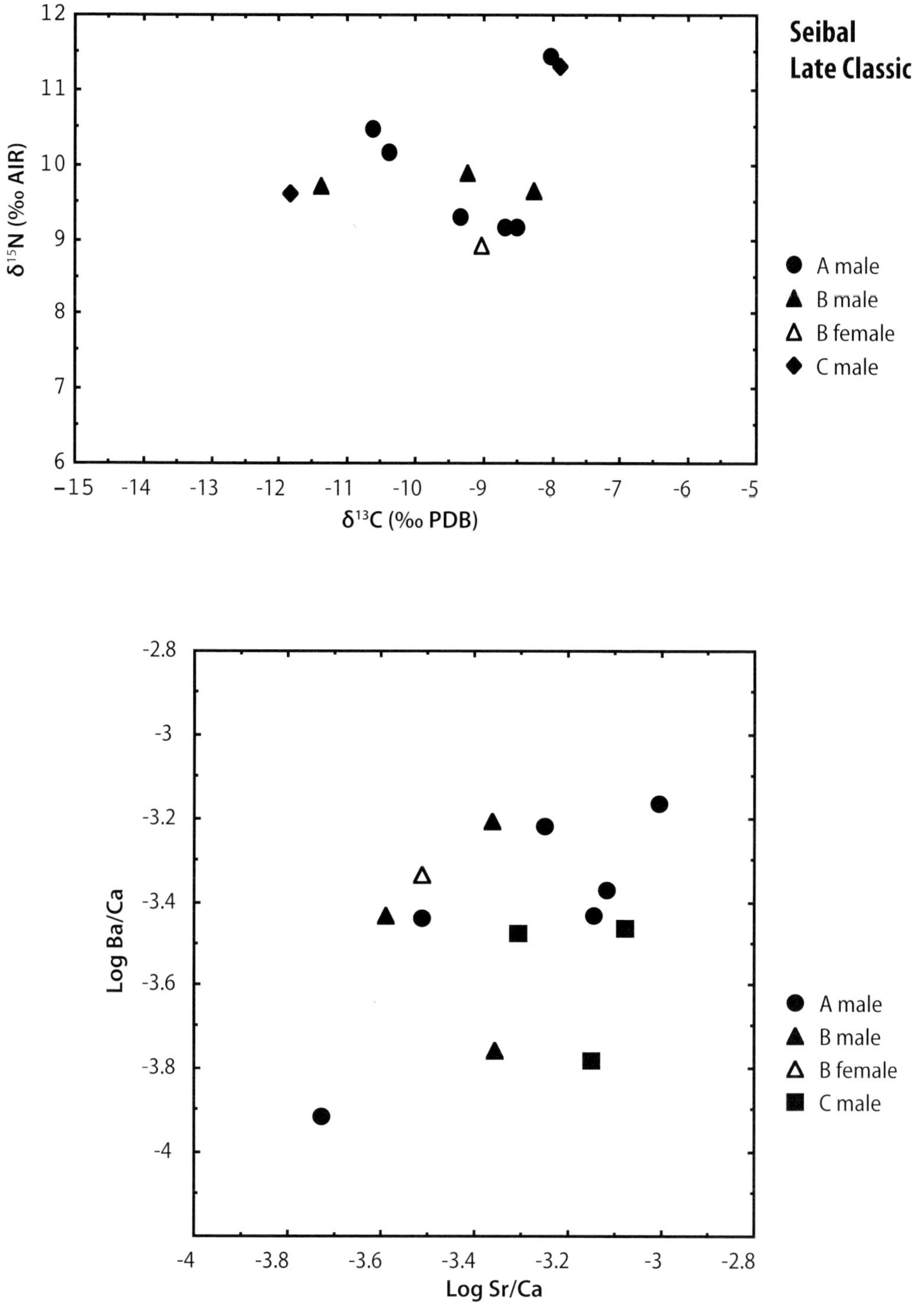

Figure 7.14. Isotopic and elemental patterning between sexes and among mortuary clusters at Late Classic Seibal

overall isotopic change. Yet, the general pattern is not one of large chemical distinctions between groups.

Terminal Classic Seibal samples show clear patterning that contrasts with the earlier picture. Isotopic distinctions between mortuary clusters are not apparent, but the sexes differ significantly in $\delta^{13}C$ (Table 7.9, Figure 7.15). Females are isotopically lighter, indicating greater consumption of C3 plants at the expense of maize. Nitrogen isotopes do not differ between the sexes, so greater meat consumption does not contribute to the lower $\delta^{13}C$ of females. Moreover, this sexual trend crosscuts social divisions in mortuary treatment. The single female burial that can be categorized as illustrating a superordinate-status dimension (Cluster A) shows the lightest $\delta^{13}C$, which might reflect dietary access, but it clearly resembles other female samples, so it cannot be considered as evidence for dietary distinction of this individual.

The elemental data do not reveal such a distinct sexual pattern, nor do they differentiate between mortuary traits (Figure 7.15). Sexual differences are not statistically significant for either Ba/Ca or Sr/Ca. The Cluster A female falls squarely in the range of other samples, further documenting the lack of social dietary distinctions in the final occupation of Seibal.

DOS PILAS

Quite distinct elemental and isotopic patterns can be seen among Late Classic Dos Pilas skeletons (Figure 7.16). Nitrogen isotopes differentiate Cluster C from other burials. These burials were interred in simple graves, flexed, with few offerings, all attributes generally interpreted as reflecting low status. Lower $\delta^{15}N$ in these skeletons may confirm the pattern observed at Altar that meat consumption was linked to status. Interestingly, the female DP20 of Cluster E contains high $\delta^{15}N$, mirroring the elite meat consumption observed at Altar. But surprisingly, the male DP30 is chemically more akin to the simple, low-status graves of Cluster C. Burials in crypts with ceramic vessels, Clusters A and D, span a broad range of $\delta^{13}C$ and do not differ systematically. They also show quite restricted range of $\delta^{15}N$. Overall, Dos Pilas males have statistically heavier $\delta^{13}C$ than females, which may be due to a consistent difference crosscutting clusters. Each cluster contains both sexes.

In contrast, social distinctions are more evident in Dos Pilas elemental data (Figure 7.16). The elite Cluster E graves contain high elemental ratios, indicating a large contribution by plant foods to the Ca ingested. The female (DP20) is shown here despite high Mn since it does not seem to have anomalous alkaline earth composition. Cluster E graves are chemically similar to the simpler Cluster C graves and distinct from the crypt clusters. The latter burials show some distinctions between clusters, with Cluster D having the lowest alkaline earth ratios. Since these skeletons tend toward higher $\delta^{13}C$ than Cluster A skeletons, the lower elemental ratios might reflect this difference rather than discrepancies in meat consumption. One Cluster A male falls with the Cluster E graves, instead of with other Cluster A graves. It may be significant to note that the clustering of this grave (DP50) in Cluster A may be artificial since it lacked grave ceramics (scored as missing data), which were probably removed in antiquity along with the skull and major long bones. Other indications, such as grave form, jade, and location in vaulted architecture, suggest a fairly high status for this individual. Since soil characteristics are more homogeneous near Dos Pilas, status differences in land use are unlikely explanations for the elemental pattern. The similarity of this result to the Altar data also suggests that dietary menu choices or preparation methods, not geographical factors, are responsible for intrasample variability at Altar.

The Terminal Classic sample from Dos Pilas (Figure 7.17) shows isotopic differences between the decapitated crania of Cluster C and the primary burials (Clusters B and D). The decapitated crania are more enriched in $\delta^{15}N$ than are the majority of primary burials. As there are only four primary burials, the crania were not analyzed for elemental signatures, and they derive from a single domestic group, the elemental data for Terminal Classic Dos Pilas is insufficient to evaluate social differences in diet.

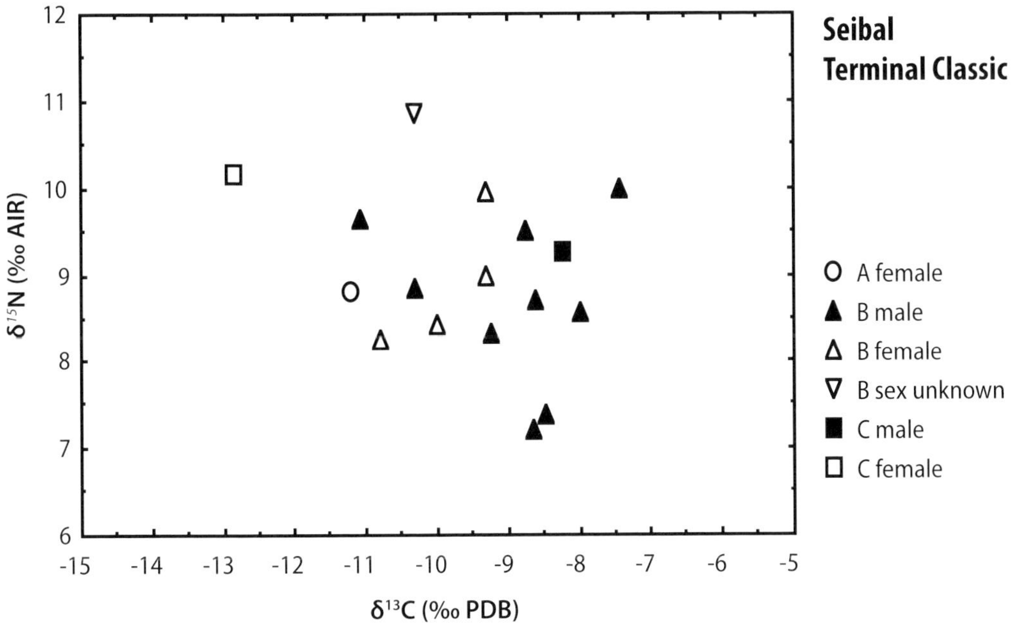

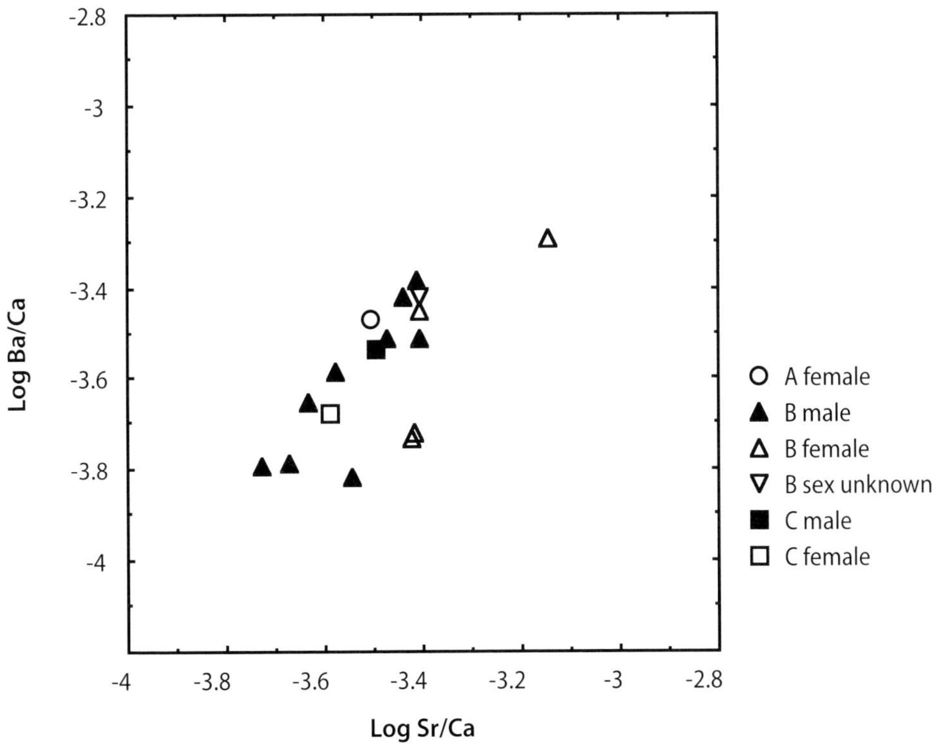

Figure 7.15. Isotopic and elemental patterning between sexes and among mortuary clusters at Terminal Classic Seibal

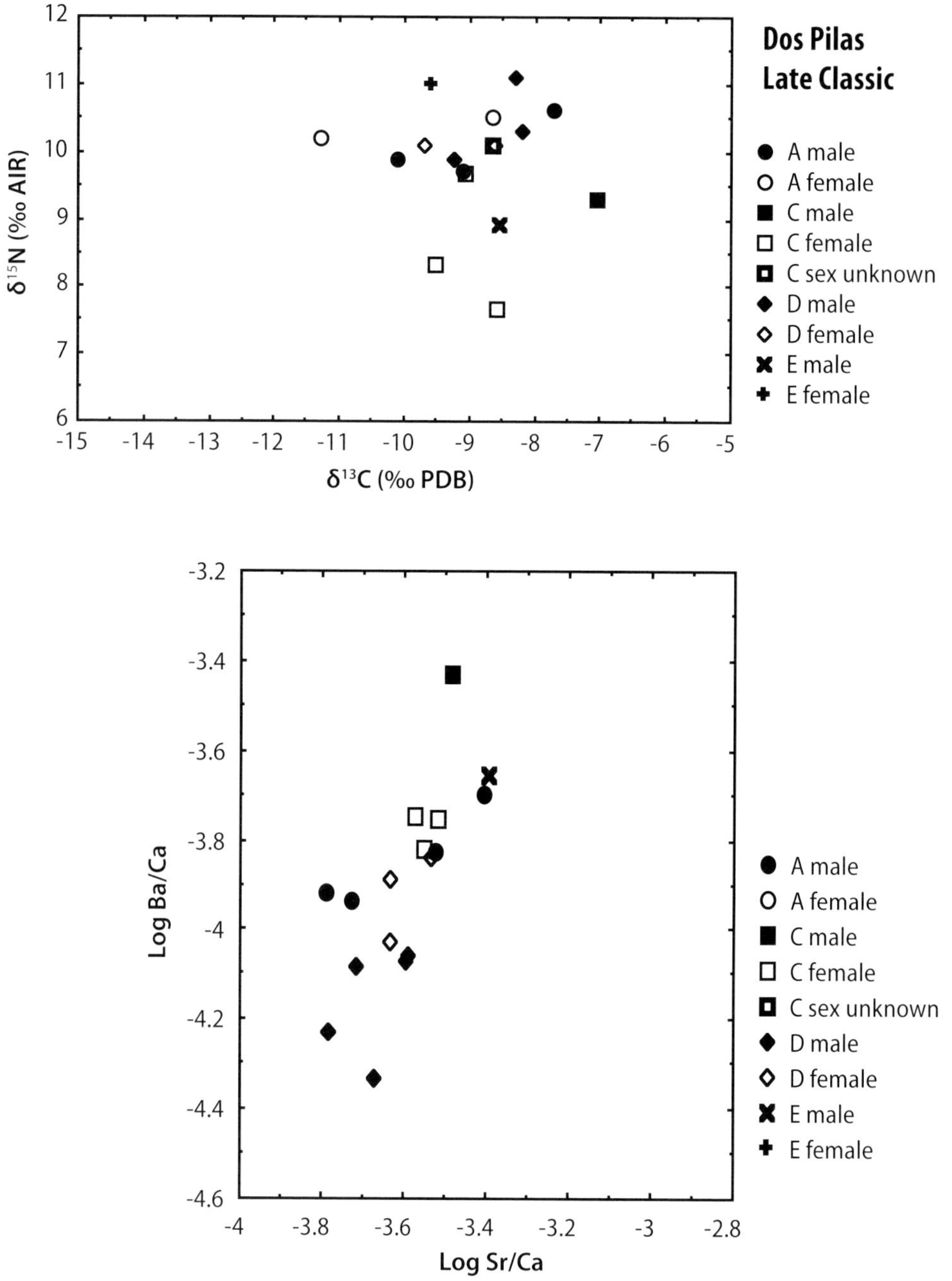

Figure 7.16. Isotopic and elemental patterning between sexes and among mortuary clusters at Late Classic Dos Pilas

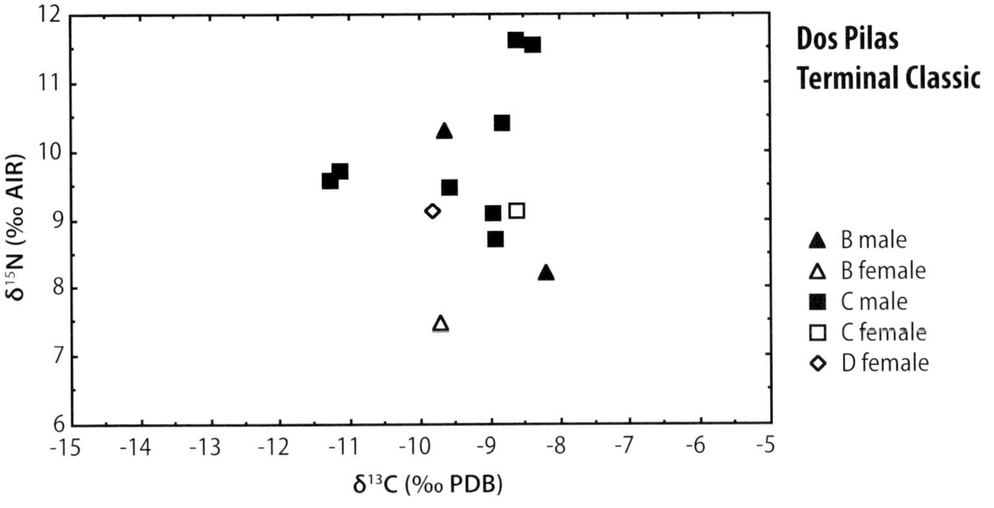

Figure 7.17. Isotopic patterning between sexes and among mortuary clusters at Terminal Classic Dos Pilas

ITZAN

The Late Classic sample from Itzan is also small, and the isotopic data are fairly concentrated (Figure 7.18). It is interesting to note that the burials from Clusters A and B are both higher in $\delta^{15}N$ and lower in Ba/Ca, suggesting a greater emphasis on plant proteins in these clusters than in burials from Clusters C and D. No sexual differences can be detected. Beyond this minimal distinction, the few data points allow little speculation.

AGUATECA, TAMARINDITO, AND THE PETEXBATUN

At Aguateca, sexes show no isotopic distinctions, but it is interesting to note that three female skeletons from central Aguateca, Cluster D, show lower $\delta^{15}N$ than Clusters C and E males from the suburban Quim Chi Hilan and the unclustered adolescent (possible male) from the Cerro de Cheyo (Figure 7.19). Likewise, elemental ratios show little patterning, but homogeneity of Ba/Ca ratios from Cluster D is striking.

The five burials sampled for isotopic analysis from Tamarindito do not constitute a large enough series to identify social patterns in diet, especially since only one burial was sampled from each cluster. The only female analyzed is much lighter in $\delta^{13}C$ than are the male skeletons. Viewed from the perspective of all Late Classic skeletons from the Petexbatun region (Figure 7.20), it is an outlier and possibly affected by diagenesis.

Given the proximity of all the Petexbatun sites and their political interconnections, it seems reasonable to consider the possibility of social distinctions in diet on the regional scale. At Dos Pilas, Tamarindito, and Altar, Late Classic superordinate-status dimensions were indicated by a common set of mortuary variables. As discussed in Chapter 4, the following burials can be interpreted as of superordinate status: DP30, DP20, DP54, TA6, and LP1. On the regional level (Figure 7.20), these burials lie in the center of the $\delta^{13}C$ range, indicating that there was no systematic differences in maize consumption between royalty and the rest of the population. But, all of them fall in the upper part of the $\delta^{15}N$ range, suggesting greater meat consumption than some, but not all, members of the population.

Sampling Bias and Dietary Trends

The temporal and spatial trends in Pasión dietary chemistry outlined above are biased by social patterns described above, which in turn are affected by sampling differences. In addition to sampling

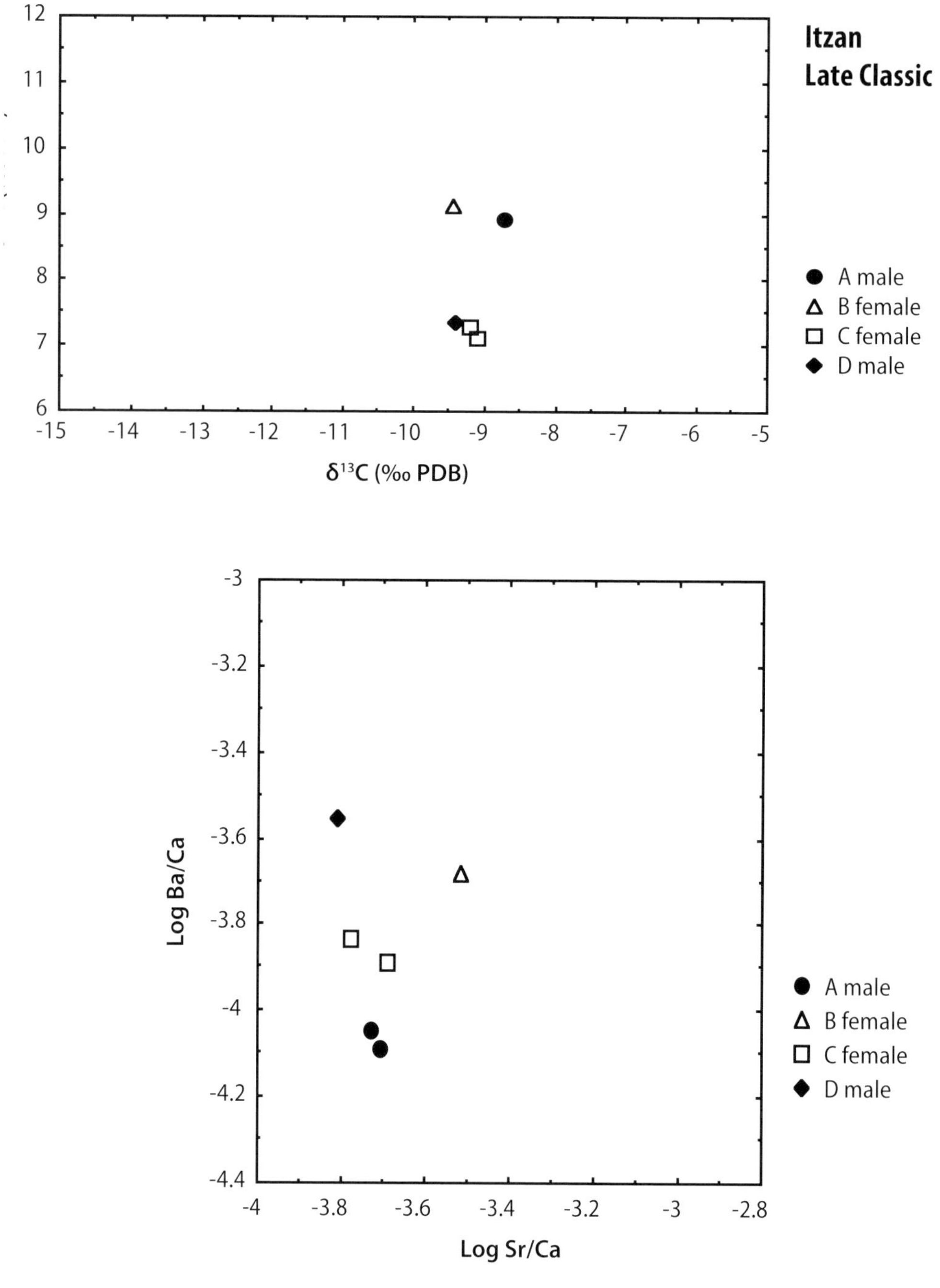

Figure 7.18. Isotopic and elemental patterning between sexes and among mortuary clusters at Late Classic Itzán

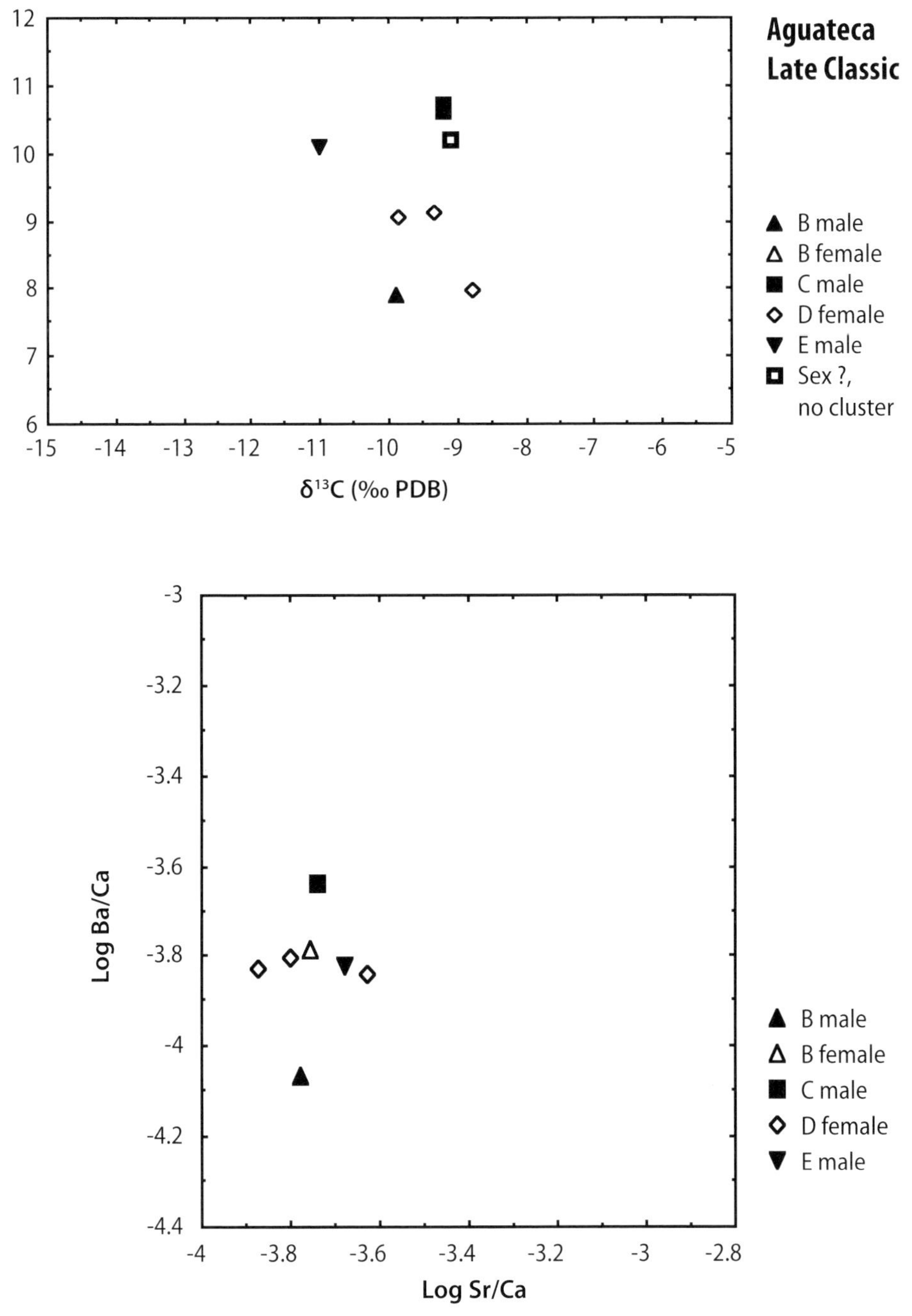

Figure 7.19. Isotopic and elemental patterning between sexes and among mortuary clusters at Late Classic Aguateca

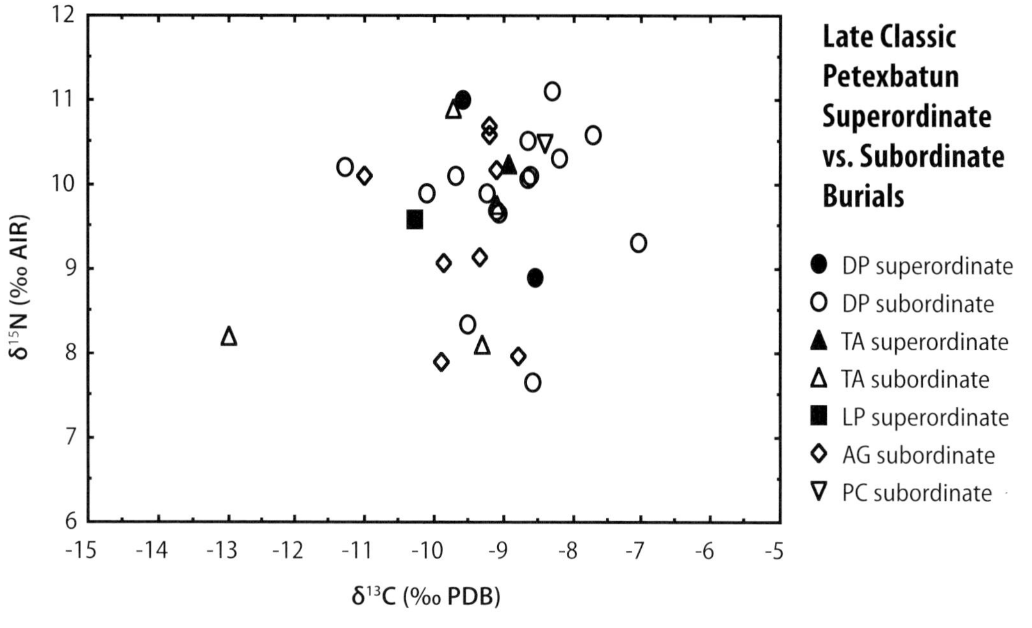

Figure 7.20. Isotopic patterning among status levels in the Late Classic Petexbatun region.

bias introduced by differing excavation strategies between sites, differential preservation of the remains recovered further limited chemical sampling. Chronological differences in diet within the temporal spans delineated here might also influence the results.

Excavation strategies that produced the Preclassic and Early Classic samples at Altar and Seibal were comparable—deep plaza tests and architectural trenching—so the intersite differences documented are probably real. Social distinctions cannot be identified at either site because of the small sample sizes. In comparison to later times, however, both samples show relatively homogeneous diets, with little intrasample variability. This trend of slight social and sexual differences is continued in the Early Classic sample from Altar.

The Late Classic series differ radically in excavation biases, with Petexbatun Project and Seibal excavations concentrated in domestic architecture, and Altar represented by more excavation of public architecture. Domestic architectural contexts were most broadly sampled at Dos Pilas, and this sample provides the best indication of status differences among burial clusters. These differences include both isotopic and elemental distinctions relevant to differences in both plant and meat consumption between groups. At Seibal, the superordinate cluster is not represented. Moreover, the lack of female burials suggests that sampling was further biased away from contexts in which females might have been interred. Given this, it is possible that the minimal status distinctions observed in this series are not necessarily due to a lack of social restrictions to diet, but may indicate bias toward greater social homogeneity within both the mortuary and the chemical sample. In contrast, the Altar series includes burials of more diverse social origins, with burials from both public and domestic contexts. The sample is small and shows little distinction among subordinate clusters, perhaps because many of these are underrepresented in the chemical sample.

To what extent these differences bias comparisons of diet across sites and chronological periods is difficult to assess. The greatest distinction between Late Classic sites is the underrepresentation of elite graves at Seibal and of domestic ones at Altar. At Altar the elite graves have distinctly different $\delta^{15}N$ than subelites, but the analogous cluster is not so distinguished isotopically at Dos Pilas. At other Petexbatun sites, superordinate burials tend to the heavier part of the nitrogen isotope range, but many other burials show similar ratios. This result indicates that dietary status distinctions were not defined by identical mechanisms at each site. Eliminating these superordinate burials for the purpose of intersite isotopic comparison would lower the $\delta^{15}N$ of the Altar sample but have little effect on the mean values of Late Classic Dos Pilas. Moreover, this would not change the significance of $\delta^{15}N$ stability over time at Altar and would accentuate the observed difference between Altar and Seibal Late Classic $\delta^{15}N$. The bias against females in the Seibal Late Classic sample might cause artificial characterization of this sample. This is most likely to affect $\delta^{13}C$, given the Late Classic sex difference at Dos Pilas, but Seibal $\delta^{13}C$ is not anomalously high. If only males are considered, the $\delta^{15}N$ distinction of this sample also holds with respect to both Late Classic Altar (M-W $z = -2.83$, $p = 0.005$) and Terminal Classic Seibal (M-W $z = -2.65$, $p = 0.008$). Recall that the heavy-$\delta^{15}N$ elites at Altar are female and of indeterminate sex, and the female DP20 is more enriched in ^{15}N than the male DP30.

In sum, social differences in diet appear to be independently constituted at each Late Classic polity. In itself, this is a significant finding, as it indicates considerable but highly structured diversity in culinary behavior at this time. Moreover, it contrasts with both the similar patterning within Preclassic samples at Altar and Seibal (despite gross differences in the mean composition of Preclassic diets) and the homogeneity of Terminal Classic diets across the region. Given these patterns, there is little justification for selectively eliminating burials from the samples for evaluation of regional trends. With the exception of the decapitated skulls from Dos Pilas, mortuary patterning is absent from the Terminal Classic samples, so excavation bias is unlikely to obscure the nature of dietary comparisons involving these samples. The Terminal Classic samples are undoubtedly the most representative of chronological samples at Seibal, and probably also at Altar, both because they are the largest samples and because they contain burials from a diversity of contexts. As these series show the most balanced representation of the sexes, sexual distinctions are unlikely to be a source of error. With these caveats in mind, I consider the data set in its entirety in evaluating trends that might shed light on the nature of the collapse.

Recalling the hypothesized dietary changes that characterize environmental models of the collapse, it is evident that the Pasión data do not entirely follow the expected pattern caused by dietary crisis. The models call for increasing maize reliance and decreasing consumption of animal protein over time. The isotopic and elemental data from Altar lend some support to this model, with greatest maize consumption in the Late Classic. However, the Terminal Classic decline in $\delta^{13}C$ at Altar implies dietary improvement rather than deterioration. At Dos Pilas, if the decapitated crania are excluded, the Terminal Classic also shows a slight, though nonsignificant, decline in $\delta^{13}C$. Finally, stability of $\delta^{13}C$ at Seibal demonstrates considerable agricultural continuity in the face of dramatic changes in population density. Trends in protein consumption also fail to aid the environmental models. In particular, nitrogen isotope trends are absent at Altar, despite maintenance of a large population in Terminal Classic times. At Dos Pilas, the Terminal Classic decapitated crania are the most enriched subgroup among all burials analyzed, but the local population, represented by the four primary burials, shows a slight decline, like that at Altar. The decline in Terminal Classic nitrogen isotope ratios at Seibal indicates that fish consumption declined, making the diet generally more similar to that at other sites. It does not indicate a crisis in protein availability. $\delta^{15}N$ values at all sites are heavy enough to indicate that sufficient high-trophic-order protein was available for collagen synthesis.

Instead, the chemical data suggest changes in the way foods were distributed across the spectrum of ancient Maya society. The early periods are distinctive for the tight clustering of the data, which contrasts with the broader ranges of later periods. Late Classic diets were highly variable and differed systematically between social groups that were distinguished in mortuary ritual. Although this suggests a highly structured social environment, the dietary distinctions were constituted differently at each site, as indeed were the elements of mortuary ritual.

The structured character of Late Classic diets is not apparent in the Terminal Classic samples but is replaced by sexual difference in maize consumption that is shared across the region. Mortuary differences are absent from both Terminal Classic Altar and Seibal diets, indicating a loss of economic diversity shown in Late Classic diet-status patterning. The sexual difference in $\delta^{13}C$ shown at Seibal is suggested but not statistically confirmed at Altar. If these two samples are combined, the sex difference is reconfirmed (M-W $z = -2.52$, $p = 0.01$, $n = 34$) at a higher level of confidence, demonstrating that it is indeed a broad regional trend. Such lumping is justified, given the broad overlap of isotopic signatures at this time and lack of systematic social differences. This sexual distinction appears to carry over from the Late Classic period (where it was documented at Dos Pilas). Indeed, greater maize consumption by males has been noted at Late Classic Copan (Reed 1999).

Rather than supporting environmental models of collapse, the chemical data reveal changes in social dynamics of economic inequality within Maya society over time. The decline of systematic social distinctions in diet occurred at the end of the Classic period concurrently at Altar, which experienced an early elite collapse, and at Seibal, which maintained centralized political authority through the Terminal Classic period. This pattern indicates that this process was deeply rooted and may reflect broad changes that were remodeling the structure of Maya society in the Pasión as a whole, independent of the political history of individual sites.

CHAPTER 8
Enamel Hypoplasia

Dental Records of Childhood Health

Dental tissues are unique among skeletal structures in that they provide a mineralized record of their developmental history that is not remodeled during later life. Variations and upsets in the development of a tooth produce characteristic features that are preserved in tooth structure. In enamel, temporary growth arrest is indicated by the presence of circumferential bands of deficient enamel, known as enamel hypoplasias (Plate 8.1). Hypoplastic enamel can be caused by a variety of disease and nutritional factors but is best interpreted as a response to nonspecific systemic stress.

Enamel is the product of secretory cells called ameloblasts, and it is deposited in apposition to dentin-producing odontoblasts along the dento-enamel junction (DEJ) of the embryonic dental papilla. Enamel formation, or amelogenesis, is initiated at what is to become the cusp of the tooth, where epithelial cells of the dental papilla first differentiate to become ameloblasts. Successively, more cervical cells differentiate and commence secretion so that the layer of secretory ameloblasts gradually moves cervically as amelogenesis proceeds. The ameloblasts secrete a protein matrix in which hydroxyapatite crystallizes to form characteristic enamel prisms. Pressure generated by the secreted product against the dentin pushes the ameloblasts away from the DEJ. When the cells reach the location of the future tooth surface, secretion stops, and the cells are reorganized to a maturative state in which they act to resorb excess protein matrix and control mineral flow to the maturing enamel (Osborn 1973).

Together, the cervical progress of ameloblast differentiation and the retreat of secretory ameloblasts from the DEJ are responsible for a tangential orientation of the secretory front to the DEJ at any given time. Any variation in the rate of ameloblastic secretion causes a synchronous shift in cellular positions that is recorded in mature enamel as a stria marking the location of the secretory front at that time. Slight undulations in prism width at 4 μm intervals, known as cross striations, are thought to reflect diurnal variation in the rate of ameloblastic secretion.

More pronounced variation in ameloblastic activity leads to hypoplasia formation. Metabolic disturbance of ameloblasts may cause a decreased rate of matrix secretion, slowing down ameloblastic movement. This results in a decrease of enamel thickness for that portion of enamel under formation at the time of insult. An extreme disturbance might cause ameloblasts to terminate their secretion prematurely. With the resumption of normal conditions, more cervical ameloblasts would differentiate, resume secretion, and leave a zone of markedly deficient enamel thickness. The age at which the defect formed can then be estimated from the relative location of the hypoplasia on the tooth crown.

Enamel hypoplasias occur commonly in association with a number of specific diseases, including metabolic conditions (phenylketonurea, erythropoietic porphyria, vitamin D-dependency rickets), infectious diseases (rubella, syphilis, tetanus), endocrinopathies (hypothyroidism, hypoparathyroidism, diabetes), and neonatal disturbances (hypocalcemia, haemolytic anemia) (Nikiforuk and Fraser 1981; Pindborg 1982). However, hypoplasias are also abundant in malnourished children in many impoverished countries. For instance, Sweeney and Leon (1971) report much

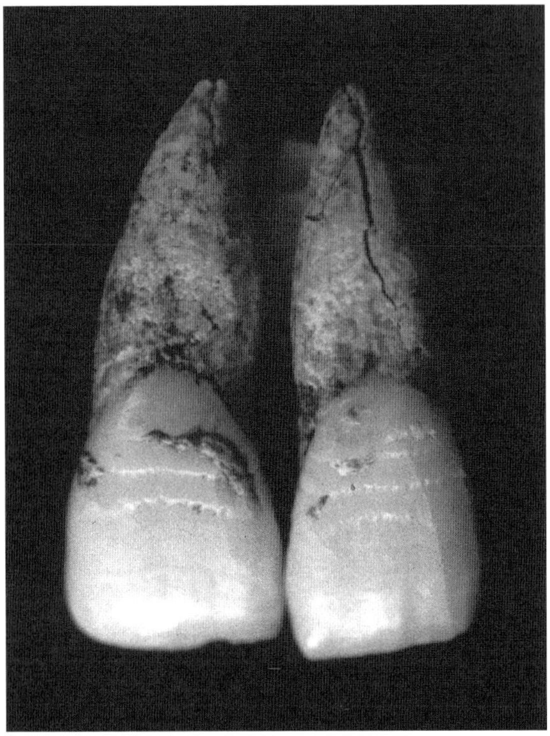

Plate 8.1. Enamel hypoplasias on the maxillary central incisors of burial DP-PD1A.

higher prevalence of hypoplasias in Guatemalan children suffering third-degree malnutrition than those with second-degree malnutrition. Similar patterns are described among malnourished versus healthier Nigerian children (Enwonwu 1973; Sawyer and Nwoku 1985). Recently, Goodman et al. (1991) demonstrated that fewer undernourished Mexican children develop hypoplasias when given daily nutritional supplements throughout the period of enamel growth than did unsupplemented children in a control group. A study of malnourished Guatemalan children found similar results (May et al. 1993). Clearly, poor nutritional status can play a role in the development of the lesions.

Many bioarchaeologists have attempted to link the occurrence of hypoplasias with stress encountered at weaning, due to poor weaning diets and weanling diarrhea. Although some congruence between weaning age (historically known or estimated) and the age of hypoplasia development has been found (Corruccini et al. 1985; Goodman et al. 1987; Goodman et al. 1991), it is likely that the chronological distribution of hypoplasias is largely governed by the mechanics of tooth crown architecture (Goodman and Armelagos 1985a, 1985b). Recent work has begun to de-emphasize the role of weaning in hypoplasia formation (Blakey et al. 1994; Katzenberg et al. 1996).

Studies of skeletal samples document that factors contributing to hypoplasias also predispose children to higher mortality, so the defects are significantly more abundant in teeth of subadults than in those who survived to adulthood (Cook 1981; Goodman and Armelagos 1988).

Hypoplasias are best interpreted as responses to systemic stress. Seyle (1956) proposed that physiological disturbances caused by illness, malnutrition, and other stimuli evoke a single biological reaction—stress. Hypoplasias are thought to occur by means of Seyle's General Adaptation Syndrome in which the sympathetico-adrenal medullary and pituitary-adrenal cortical axes are activated, releasing hormones that inhibit protein synthesis, and thereby ameloblastic activity, as well as other physiologic processes in the body (Seyle 1956).

Hypoplasia formation is best understood in terms of a threshold model (Goodman and Rose 1990). Together, nutritional status and illness contribute to a total stress load experienced by a child during the period of tooth formation. Fluctuations in this total stress load over time lead to defect formation when the stress level rises above a threshold for ameloblastic disruption. Since teeth, and indeed individuals, differ in susceptibility to stress, this threshold is specific for each tooth and individual. Unlike the Goodman and Rose model, which implies a constant threshold, I would argue that genetic susceptibility to stress and sensitivity of each specific tooth to metabolic disruption should be incorporated into the position of this threshold. Illness is expected to be the most variable of the stress factors that lead to the formation of defects, though fluctuation in nutritional status could have a similar effect. Given the well-documented synergistic relationship between nutrition and infection, however, it is difficult to separate the relative contribution of these factors to the formation of individual defects. The magnitude and duration of stress fluctuations above this threshold may account for the form and severity of the resulting enamel defect (Condon 1981; Goodman and Rose 1990; Suckling 1989; Wright 1990).

Tooth types appear to vary in susceptibility to hypoplasia. Maxillary central incisors and mandibular canines record the greatest number of lesions. It appears that the polar teeth of developmental fields that are most tightly controlled by developmental genetics are most likely to develop hypoplasias (Goodman and Armelagos 1985a, 1985b). In terms of the threshold model, susceptibility to hypoplasia is lower for posterior teeth such as premolars and molars; the threshold for ameloblastic disturbance is higher, so that only extreme fluctuations rise above the threshold to cause defects. In addition, the differences in developmental chronology between teeth mean that each tooth records stress during a specific childhood period. Study of a number of different teeth can therefore document stress experience over a broad span of childhood.

Enamel hypoplasias have been used to examine the health consequences of human behavior in many prehistoric skeletal samples. Increases in hypoplasia prevalence with the adoption of agriculture occurred in many world areas (Cohen and Armelagos 1984; Cook and Buikstra 1979; Goodman et al. 1980). High levels of stress are indicated by hypoplastic enamel in several historic skeletal series, including Barbados slaves (Corruccini et al. 1985) and American slaves and free blacks (Blakey 1987; Rathbun 1987). Contact with the Spanish led to an increase in the duration of stress episodes indicated by hypoplasia width in the Santa Catalina de Guale mission population on the Georgia coast (Hutchinson and Larsen 1988). This trend is not paralleled in mission cemeteries at Lamanai and Tipu in Belize (Cohen et al. 1994; White 1986). In Mesoamerica, Hodges (1987) found no difference in hypoplastic prevalence between early and later occupations of the Oaxaca Valley, suggesting little change in health with agricultural intensification.

Here, I employ hypoplasias as indicators of the general quality of childhood health. Changes in diet brought about by agricultural intensification and resource stress might lead to changes in childhood diet that would affect the prevalence and severity of hypoplasias. In addition to dietary change, increased risk of childhood infection due to overpopulation could further raise hypoplastic incidence. Moreover, the overall pattern of defects provides a means to examine the timing of childhood stress. Because subadult skeletons are largely missing from the Pasión skeletal series, the examination of hypoplastic patterning provides an alternate approach for examining aspects of demographic processes in the collapse.

Methods

I examined the labial surfaces of all teeth for enamel hypoplasias and scored macroscopic hypoplasias under natural or incandescent lighting, without the aid of any magnifying device. Hypoplasias were scored as linear enamel hypoplasia (LEH, narrow depressed bands), major growth arrests (MGA, deep acutely depressed bands), shallow broad depressed zones, or linear arrangements of pits, but are treated here as a single class of defects. To record the location of each defect, I measured the distance from the cemento-enamel junction (CEJ) to the midpoint of each hypoplasia to the nearest 0.02 mm using sliding calipers. In addition, I recorded the height of scorable enamel from the CEJ, to control for cuspal attrition. Dental calculus is slight in this series and generally restricted to a narrow cervical ring, often located on the root apical to the CEJ. Teeth with calculus obscuring the DEJ or labial enamel surface are not considered. For each individual, I consider hypoplastic data for each tooth type. Where both antimeres were present and scorable, the antimere with the greatest hypoplastic expression was selected; or, in cases with disparate degrees of attrition, the antimere with a greater scorable crown height was selected for statistical analysis.

I derived regression formulae to calculate the age of ameloblast arrest using the distance of each defect from the cemento-enamel junction (Table 8.1), using the methodology described in Wright (1997b). The formulae incorporate mean total crown heights of unworn teeth. In the Pasión series, initial calculations showed that Pasión tooth height is greater than that of the usual published standards (Goodman and Rose 1990; Hodges and

Wilkinson 1990; Swärdstedt 1966). Ages for the initiation and completion of enamel formation generally follow those of Massler (Goodman et al. 1980; Massler et al. 1941) except that I assumed crown completion for the mandibular canine to be complete by age 4.5 years rather than 6.5 years. The earlier age appears to be more accurate for Amerindians (Anderson et al. 1976; Fanning and Brown 1971; Skinner and Goodman 1992; Ubelaker 1978), producing better correspondence between hypoplastic age distributions of the mandibular canine and central maxillary incisor (Norr 1991). The initial period of enamel formation is not expressed on the tooth surface but is buried below the cusp, shortening the developmental period observed. Skinner and Goodman (1992) suggest that this "buried" enamel accounts for one-quarter to one-third of the developmental span of a tooth, or 0.9 to 2.0 years for different teeth. Because these values are not well documented, I consider the first year of development to be "buried" for all tooth types. Using these parameters, the linear regression formulae in Table 8.1 assume a constant enamel growth rate as recommended by Goodman and Rose (1990).

Using the same formulae, I calculated the youngest age of scorable enamel present for each tooth from the scorable crown height measurements. To control for differential attrition in sample prevalence and age comparisons, a minimum age of enamel development was chosen for each tooth type. Data for enamel cuspal to this limit is excluded from the study. I selected this minimum enamel age limit to include all teeth scored and the youngest possible enamel age, excluding as few hypoplasias as possible. Scorable age limits considered in statistical analysis are in Table 8.1.

An inverse relationship is documented between the prevalence of enamel hypoplasias and age-at-death (Cook 1981; Goodman and Armelagos 1988). To minimize bias in hypoplastic prevalence that might be introduced by different age structures of the samples, I consider only data from adult skeletons. Among adults, chi-square tests show no differences in the proportion of young, middle, and old adults affected by hypoplasia for the maxillary central incisor (I^1) ($p = 0.27$), maxillary lateral incisor (I^2) ($p = 0.14$), maxillary canine (C^1) ($p = 0.43$), and mandibular canine (C_1) ($p = 0.44$) (Wright 1997b). Therefore, adults of all ages are pooled. Since evaluation of site specific patterning would be prone to Type I error, I do not attempt to examine chronological trends within sites.

Statistical analyses of hypoplasias were performed at the level of each tooth. As the tooth positions scorable for each skeleton are highly variable in this series, I made no attempt to compile hypoplasias across teeth to a single scale of stress experience as has been done by other researchers (e.g., Goodman et al. 1980). Pasión dentitions are variably affected by a high degree of antemortem loss, artificial mutilation, calculus deposits, and inconsistency of collection or curation. I scored anterior teeth that are mutilated only when a broad continuous segment of enamel was unaffected, the height of which was also recorded. Many mutilated teeth from Altar de Sacrificios and Seibal were separated from the skeletal collections for study (Smith 1972) and are not available. Furthermore, although relatively good correlation has been reported between the mandibular canine and maxillary central incisor, developmental standards are not adequate to ensure accurate identification of coeval defects across teeth. I compared the proportion of teeth affected by hypoplasias, the mean number of hypoplasias per tooth, and the mean age of hypoplasias across samples for each tooth using the chi-square test and Student's t-test. Differences between samples were accepted as statistically significant when $p \leq 0.10$ was attained.

Results

Hypoplasias are common on Pasión teeth but are seldom severe in extent. Most lesions are classified as LEH and consist of shallow, narrow depressed bands. Broad, shallow hypoplasias also occur but are generally not extensive. Pitted hypoplasias are rare and often consist of a single pit or pair of pits, rather than a continuous line of pits. Very few hypoplasias could be classed as MGA. Since no statistical differences are found between the relative abundance of hypoplasia types between time periods for either the maxillary central incisor ($X^2 = 0.08$, $p = 0.78$), mandibular canine ($X^2 = 0.73$,

Table 8.1. Regression equations used to estimate age of hypoplasia formation

Tooth	Unworn crown height Mean	Unworn crown height s.d.	N	Developmental age at Cusp	Developmental age at CEJ	Regression equations[2]	Minimum scorable age limit
Maxillary							
I^1	11.14[1]	0.64	8	1.0	4.5	Age = -0.307x + 4.5	2.5
I^2	10.49	0.82	13	2.0	4.5	Age = -0.238x + 4.5	3.0
C^1	11.18	1.34	17	1.0	6.0	Age = -0.313x + 6.0	3.5
P^3	8.40	0.78	17	3.0	6.0	Age = -0.357x + 6.0	4.0
P^4	7.39	0.71	16	3.5	6.0	Age = -0.338x + 6.0	4.0
M^1	7.32	0.78	8	1.0	3.5	Age = -0.342x + 3.5	2.0
M^2	7.29	0.56	12	4.0	7.5	Age = -0.480x + 7.5	5.0
Mandibular							
I_1	9.86	0.89	10	1.0	4.0	Age = -0.304x + 4.0	2.5
I_2	9.74	0.77	17	1.0	4.0	Age = -0.308x + 4.0	2.5
C_1	11.61	1.45	11	1.5	4.5	Age = -0.258x + 4.5	2.5
P_3	8.28	0.67	20	2.0	6.0	Age = -0.483x + 6.0	3.5
P_4	7.64	0.56	19	3.0	7.0	Age = -0.524x + 7.0	4.5
M_1	7.69	0.73	9	1.0	3.5	Age = -0.325x + 3.5	2.0
M_2	7.5	0.76	8	4.0	7.0	Age = -0.400x + 7.0	5.5

[1] All measurements are taken in mm, and ages calculated in years.
[2] Where x equals the distance of the hypoplasia from the cemento-enamel junction.

$p = 0.39$), or maxillary canine ($X^2 = 2.68$, $p = 0.10$), all types are pooled in the following analyses.

The majority of hypoplasias are found on mandibular and maxillary canines, but the defects are also common on the maxillary central and lateral incisors. Given the variability of tooth representation, it is difficult to estimate the overall percentage of individuals affected by hypoplasia, but 59% of mandibular canines (59 of 100 scorable teeth) show at least one defect in the age range that I considered for prevalence comparisons. Because hypoplasias occasionally occur on other teeth when absent from the canine, it is likely that the true prevalence of hypoplasia for the population is slightly higher than 60%.

Chronological patterns in the prevalence of hypoplasias are apparent for several teeth. Table 8.2 gives the proportion of teeth affected by hypoplasias by chronological period for all sites pooled and the results of chi-square tests for chronological comparisons. For the 2 x 2 tables, Yate's-corrected values are given. These data are illustrated in Figure 8.1. Because of its small sample size, the Early Classic sample from Altar de Sacrificios is pooled with the Preclassic samples. When all three time periods are considered together, five teeth show chronological differences in the proportion of individuals affected: P^3, I_2, P_3, P_4, and M_2. No statistical differences are detected between the Preclassic/Early Classic samples and Late Classic period for any teeth. Significantly more Terminal Classic P^3, I_2, and P_4 show hypoplasias than do the Late Classic teeth, however, fewer Terminal Classic M_2 show hypoplasias.

Interestingly, the teeth that show these statistical differences are those with low overall hypoplastic expression. No temporal differences are evident for the I^1, C^1, or C_1, which are commonly the exclusive focus of study. Differences in susceptibility to stress has been proposed to account for

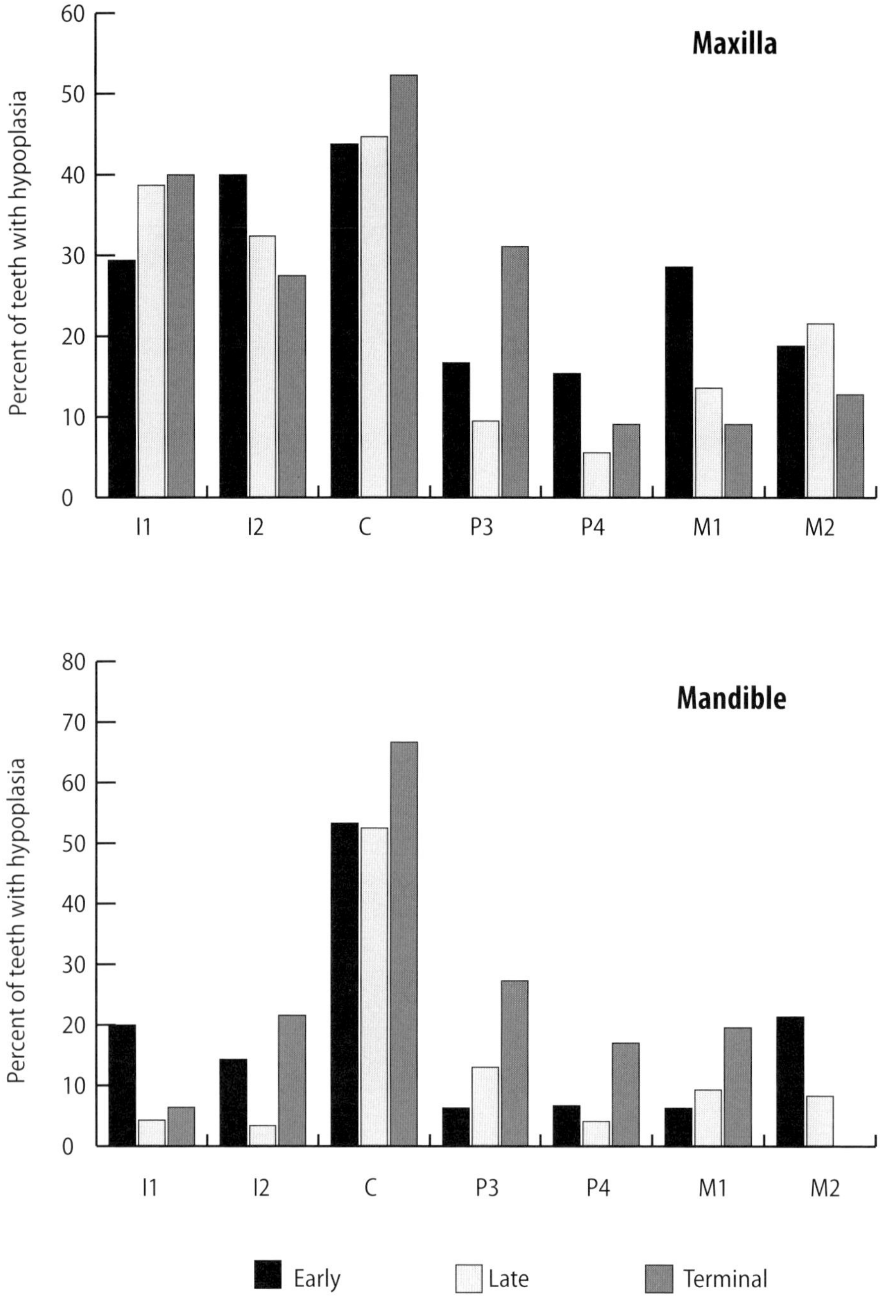

Figure 8.1. Proportion of teeth showing hypoplasias

Table 8.2. Chi-square test for chronological comparisons of the proportion of teeth affected by hypoplasia, by tooth

	"Early"		Late Classic		Terminal Classic		All three periods d.f. = 2		Early–Late d.f. = 1		Late–Terminal d.f. = 1	
Tooth	+	N	+	N	+	N	X^2	p	X^2 (Yates)	p	X^2 (Yates)	p
Maxillary												
I^1	5	17	12	31	16	40	0.60	0.74	0.11	0.74	0.02	0.89
I^2	4	10	11	34	11	40	0.64	0.73	0.00	0.94	0.04	0.84
C^1	7	16	21	47	23	44	0.64	0.73	0.05	0.82	0.26	0.61
P^3	2	12	4	42	14	45	**6.39**	**0.04**	0.03	0.86	**4.92**	**0.03**
P^4	2	13	2	36	4	44	1.20	0.55	0.27	0.60	0.03	0.86
M^1	4	14	6	44	4	44	3.40	0.18	0.78	0.38	0.11	0.74
M^2	3	16	8	37	6	47	1.19	0.55	0.02	0.89	0.62	0.43
Mandibular												
I_1	2	10	1	23	2	31	2.52	0.28	0.61	0.44	0.07	0.79
I_2	2	14	1	29	8	37	**4.53**	**0.10**	0.45	0.50	**3.15**	**0.07**
C_1	8	15	21	40	30	45	1.99	0.37	0.06	0.80	1.23	0.27
P_3	1	16	6	46	12	44	**4.84**	**0.09**	0.08	0.78	2.21	0.16
P_4	1	15	2	49	8	47	**4.70**	**0.09**	0.08	0.78	**3.03**	**0.08**
M_1	1	16	4	43	9	46	2.84	0.24	0.02	0.88	1.14	0.28
M_2	3	14	3	36	0	40	**7.92**	**0.02**	0.63	0.43	1.62	0.20

+ = number of individuals affected by hypoplasia on a given tooth, N = number of scorable individuals.
Values of X^2 in **bold** are significant at $p \leq 0.10$.
Values of X^2 in **underlined bold** also attain significance at $p \leq 0.05$.

discrepancies in hypoplastic expression between tooth types (Goodman and Armelagos 1985a, 1985b). Maxillary central incisors and mandibular canines are the most sensitive and record many stress episodes. The threshold for hypoplastic formation appears to be higher for other teeth, since all teeth developing at the same time do not show precisely corresponding hypoplasias. The absence of incisor and canine differences in the Pasión series suggests little change in the total occurrence of stress episodes but that a change in the nature or severity of stressors produced the observed intertooth pattern.

As an additional avenue to examine these trends, Table 8.3 presents the mean number of hypoplasias per tooth for the four anterior teeth most commonly affected. These trends are illustrated in Figure 8.2. Since the chi-square tests show most differences between Late and Terminal Classic occupations and these samples are the largest, only this time frame is examined. Student's t-tests confirm that hypoplasias are not more common in the susceptible anterior teeth (I^1, C^1, or C_1) of later occupants of the region. They also confirm that Terminal Classic I_2 and P_4 average more hypoplasias than Late Classic ones. The t-test also shows a significantly lower hypoplasia prevalence on Terminal Classic M_2. While both second molars show fewer hypoplasias in the Terminal Classic period, it is not significant for the M^2. This M_2 difference likely contributes to the significant chi-square for the M_2 across all three time periods. Although not

Table 8.3. Student's t-test comparing the mean number of hypoplasias per tooth between Late and Terminal Classic occupations at all sites, combined

	Late Classic		Terminal Classic		Student's t	
Tooth	mean	N	mean	N	t	p
Maxillary						
I^1	.42	31	.50	40	-.483	.63
I^2	.35	34	.30	40	.429	.67
C^1	.53	47	.59	44	-.440	.66
P^3	.19	42	.33	45	-1.077	.28
P^4	.14	36	.11	44	.208	.84
M^1	.14	44	.09	44	.666	.51
M^2	.30	37	.13	47	1.399	.16
Mandibular						
I_1	.04	23	.10	31	-.328	.74
I_2	.03	29	.30	37	**-2.211**	**.03**
C_1	.65	40	.76	45	-1.211	.23
P_3	.17	46	.30	37	-1.109	.27
P_4	.04	49	.23	48	**-2.270**	**.02**
M_1	.09	43	.20	46	-1.369	.17
M_2	.08	36	.00	40	**1.882**	**.06**

Values of t in **bold** are significant at $p \leq 0.10$.

significant, note that both the proportion of teeth affected and the mean prevalence of hypoplasias is also lower for the M^2 from the Terminal Classic than for the Late Classic period.

Because teeth develop at different times, thereby recording stress for different phases of childhood, these intertooth patterns have an age component and indicate a change in the developmental age of hypoplasia over time in the Pasión region. The short age ranges for the development of each tooth are further restricted here by the minimum age limits imposed on the data to control for attrition; thus, each tooth details stress events for a specific narrow age span (Table 8.1). For instance, the M_2 records stress from age 5 to 7.5 years. The lower prevalence of hypoplasias on second molars in the Terminal Classic samples indicates a decline in stress at this age. This suggests better childhood health (or at least reduced severity, if not frequency, of stress) during older childhood in the final occupation of the Pasión region.

Increases in hypoplastic prevalence occur for two teeth developing between these two ranges. Hypoplasias are more common on Terminal Classic I_2 and P_4, which record stress between the ages of 3.0–4.5 and 4.5–7.0 years, respectively, than earlier times indicating increased occurrence or severity of hypoplastic stressors between the ages of 3.5 and 6 years. Together, these patterns suggest that, over time, stressors which produce hypoplasias became more concentrated on a narrower age span in the Pasión Region.

To examine this hypothesis further, I calculated the mean age of hypoplasia for each tooth and compared it across chronological periods using Student's t-test (Table 8.4). The small number of hypoplasias observed on the less-sensitive teeth precludes comparison for many teeth. A significant increase of 3.3 months in the mean age of hypoplasia formation is detected only for the maxillary

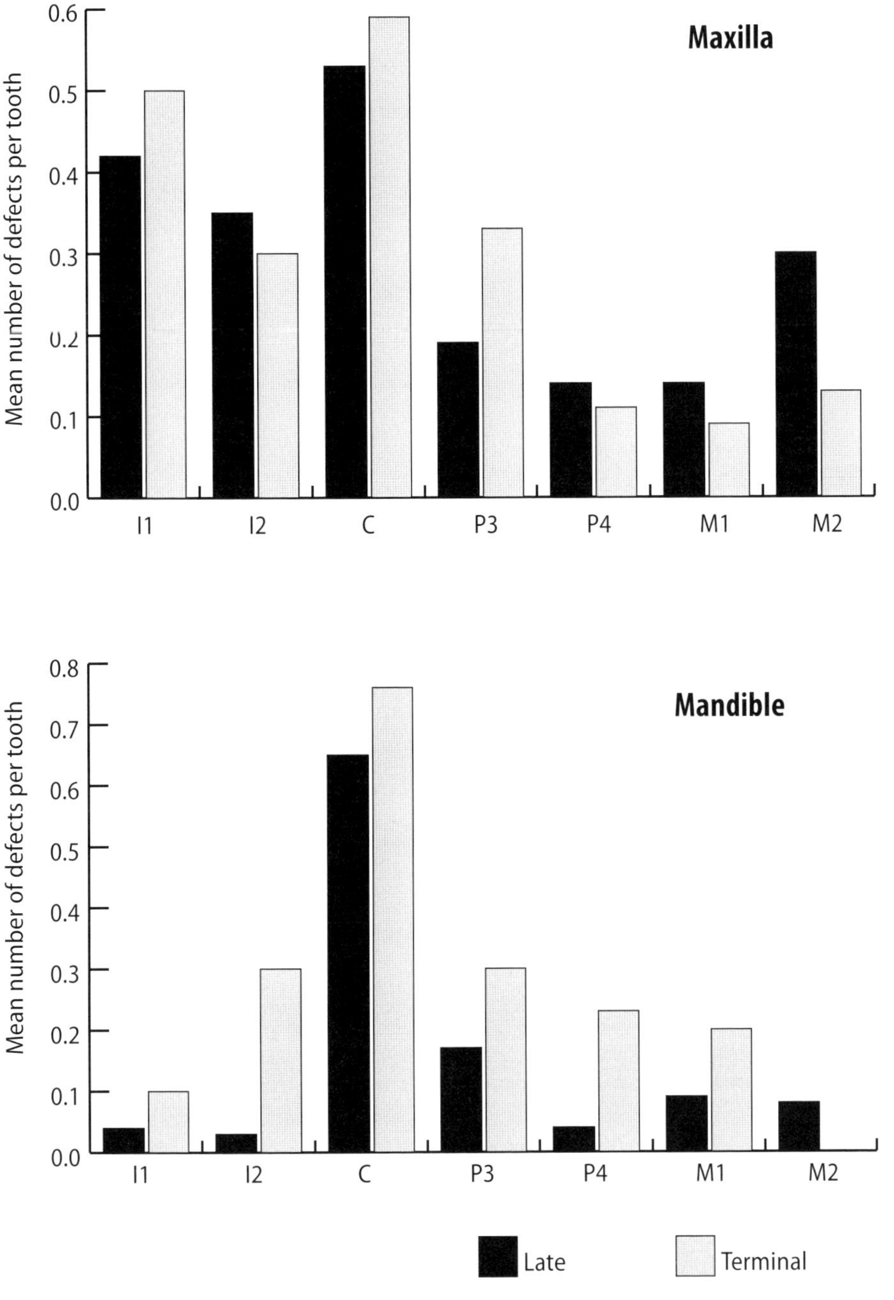

Figure 8.2. Average number of hypoplasias per tooth

Table 8.4. Student's t-test for chronological comparisons of mean age of hypoplasias per tooth

	"Early"		Late		Terminal		"Early"–Late	"Early"–Terminal	Late–Terminal
Tooth	Mean	N	Mean	N	Mean	N	t	t	t
Maxillary									
I^1	3.43	6	3.42	13	3.33	21	.06	.56	.64
I^2	3.65	4	3.81	12	3.78	12	-	-	.20
C^1	4.77	7	5.05	25	4.83	24	**-1.45**[1]	-.26	**2.17**[2]
P^3	5.10	2	4.99	8	4.95	14	-	-	.08
P^4	5.47	2	5.03	5	5.00	5	-	-	.08
M^1	2.73	4	2.88	6	2.82	4	-	-	-
M^2	6.63	4	6.07	11	6.22	6	-	-	-.56
Mandibular									
I_1	3.28	2	3.34	1	3.16	3	-	-	-
I_2	3.06	2	3.45	1	3.02	11	-	-	-
C_1	3.51	11	3.48	26	3.31	34	.17	**1.45**	**1.73**[2]
P_3	4.67	1	4.81	8	4.56	13	-	-	.86
P_4	6.04	1	6.23	3	5.43	10	-	-	**1.85**[2]
M_1	2.60	1	2.71	4	2.81	8	-	-	-
M_2	6.42	3	6.31	3		0	-	-	-

[1] Values of t in **bold** are significant at $p \leq 0.10$ for a one-tailed test.
[2] Values of t are also significant at $p \leq 0.05$ for a one-tailed test.

canine between the Preclassic/Early Classic and the Late Classic periods. Decreases in mean hypoplasia age occur between the Late and Terminal Classic periods for both maxillary and mandibular canines and the P_4. For the canines, this decline is about 2 to 3 months (C^1 = 2.8 mo; C_1 = 2.0 mo), but the P_4 mean age is substantially younger, by 9.6 months. This age change suggests that the Late Classic P_4 hypoplasias record stresses equivalent to those of the second molar hypoplasias. In the Terminal Classic, stress occurs at younger ages, leading to more P hypoplasias, but these stressors do not reach M^2 thresholds and largely predate the M_2 age span.

In summary, the frequency of enamel hypoplasias in Pasión dental remains indicate slight but significant changes in the stress experience of surviving children across both time and space. A lack of statistical differences among samples in the mean number of hypoplasias for the teeth most susceptible to stress (I^1, C_1) indicates that the total abundance of hypoplastic stressors was essentially constant. Less-sensitive teeth illustrate changes in the exposure to and timing of more severe stressors. Stress affecting these teeth appears to have become more concentrated around four years of age.

These shifts in the developmental timing of hypoplastic events are of interest on both bioarchaeological and methodological levels. Methodologically, the results demonstrate that differences in susceptibility to stress among tooth positions are meaningful. They illustrate that studies which concentrate only on anterior teeth may ignore significant changes in stress experience that would be revealed through study of posterior, less-susceptible teeth. In addition, they point to a flaw in methodologies that would unite the occurrence of hypoplasias observed on different teeth into a single scale of stress experience. If any individuals are missing teeth or have teeth that are not scorable, such united scales may misrepresent individual stress experience because of the different thresholds at which tooth positions express hypoplastic lesions.

Bioarchaeolocially, the concentration of defects around four years of age suggests important shifts in the nature of childhood illness in the region. Goodman et al. (1991) found that hypoplasias occur in greater concentration around a central tendency in nutritionally supplemented Mexican children than in nonsupplemented children. By analogy, improved childhood nutrition might be responsible for the changes observed in Pasión hypoplasia chronology. An alternate interpretation, however, is a decrease in the heterogeneity of childhood health among members of the population because of social and dietary practices. This would lead to a greater concentration of stress events around the population central tendency.

Either explicitly or implicitly, the peak age of hypoplasia formation has often been equated with weaning, when children are expected to suffer greatest health and growth stress. However, few researchers have been able to document shifts in timing of hypoplasias in a way that might reflect weaning patterns. This is likely to be because tooth geometry influences hypoplasia expression; the majority of hypoplasias typically occur in the middle third of the enamel for each tooth (Goodman and Armelagos 1985a, 1985b).

Rather than beginning with the elimination of breast milk from the diet, this stress should begin with the feeding of solid foods, which usually occurs long before breastfeeding ends and through which children take in contaminants that may make them ill. Although weaning *per se* is not stressful, after children no longer consume breast milk they do not receive immunological aid to combat these infections. Therefore, the relative timing when solid foods are introduced and when nursing ends (or becomes a rare event) may shape the pattern of early childhood illness. Since these child-care choices are culturally determined, they can vary dramatically among populations or over time in a single population. For instance, under conditions of food scarcity, women may breastfeed children longer than they would in times of abundance, because breastfeeding improves the chances of child survival (Dow 1977; Mølbak et al. 1994).

Hypoplasia data indicates that severe stresses on the Terminal Classic population were more tightly concentrated around four years of age than in the Late Classic. In particular, stress during the later childhood years seems to have shifted to a younger age. This could be caused by a shortened period of post-weanling morbidity or a reduction in variation among subpopulations in the age of weaning. Reduced social variability in economic success might produce this effect. Alternatively, a reduction in weaning age might imply an improved food supply, if women breastfeed children longer during food crises in order to enhance the likelihood of child survival (Dow 1977). Unfortunately, it is difficult to choose between these two hypotheses.

Summary

The enamel hypoplasia data indicate that Pasión Maya children commonly experienced developmental disruptions. However, the abundance of hypoplasias on anterior teeth does not differ among occupations, indicating stability in the total stress load over time. Despite this picture of general stability, childhood stress events that led to hypoplasia formation appear to have become more concentrated around four years of age during the final occupation, perhaps as a result of declining social variability in Terminal Classic weaning practices. This result does not lend support to environmental collapse models that envision increased health stress, especially among children, during the final occupation of the region.

CHAPTER 9

Paleopathology

Skeletal Markers of Disease and Health

In most parts of the world, where soft tissues decay rapidly, investigations of health in prehistoric skeletal remains are necessarily restricted to examining conditions that leave traces in bones and teeth. Although the detection of preserved serum immunoglobulins and pathogen DNA in archaeological bone provides hope that a wider range of diseases might someday be routinely identified in skeletal remains (Ortner et al. 1992; Rogan and Lentz 1994; Salo et al. 1994), at this time gross skeletal pathology provides the most comprehensive data. Pathological change in bone is limited to two processes: the deposition of new bone and the resorption of old bone. Together, the pattern of bone formation and destruction provides clues to the nature of disease entities affecting the skeleton. Additional diagnostic evidence comes from the skeletal distribution of lesions, age, and sex characteristics of affected individuals.

Analyses of skeletal pathology reported here focus on two conditions that occur commonly in archaeological skeletons: periosteal reactions and porotic hyperostosis. The interaction of dietary and health stresses has been implicated in the development of both lesions. Other pathological conditions observed in the Pasión remains, but which occur too infrequently for statistical analysis, are also briefly discussed.

Periosteal Reactions

"Periosteal reaction" is a radiological term given to a new layer of bone material deposited on the surface of the existing bone cortex. Paleopathologists often refer to "periostitis," a term that implies an inflammatory process. As all periosteal new bone is not caused by inflammation, Ortner and Putschar (1985:39) advocate the use of "periostosis" to describe a deposit of unknown origin. Here, periostosis and periosteal reaction will be used interchangeably.

The periosteum, which envelops each bone, consists of an outer fibrous coat and an inner cellular layer that differentiates to form osteoblasts following injury. When the periosteum is lifted from the surface of the bone by inflammation, hemorrhage, or tumor, it responds by producing a thin layer of new bone on the surface of the original cortex. The architecture of the resulting new bone gives some indication of the rate and aggressivity of lesion growth. Chronic benign processes may produce solid periostoses from the gradual deposition of subperiosteal bone. Rapid deposition of new bone forms a layer of woven or fibrous bone that is separated from the underlying cortex by a narrow zone of fibrous tissue. This may occur from many types of disturbance or may be the first of a series of layers deposited in response to repeated injury, producing a lamellated reaction. More rapid processes lead to the formation of spiculated periosteal reactions in which bone is laid down perpendicular to the cortex. If the stimulus of periosteal deposition is removed, the new bone will be gradually remodeled and consolidated into the underlying bone cortex. Given sufficient time to remodel, many periostoses may heal completely, leaving little trace (Edeiken et al. 1966; Ragsdale et al. 1981).

Periosteal reactions may occur in the absence of other osseous changes or may be accompanied by either endosteal resorption or deposition. Without radiographic imaging it may be difficult to evaluate the extent or nature of endosteal involvement. Documentation of the specific location, nature, and extent of periosteal deposits and their relation to endosteal changes is important to diagnosis of disease processes that cause periostoses. Although infection is the most common cause, subperiosteal new bone deposition is a response to many conditions. Here, I consider a few common conditions that may be responsible for periosteal reactions in archaeological samples.

Traumatic damage to the periosteum causing subperiosteal hemorrhage can cause localized periosteal reactions, as may circulatory disturbances such as venous stasis and arterial insufficiency (Resnick and Niwayama 1981:3000). Isolated periostoses may also result from benign tumors such as osteoid osteoma, periosteal osteoblastoma, and chondromyxoid fibroma (Greenfield 1986; Spjut et al. 1971). Malignant tumors of bone typically produce more severe changes that would be easily distinguished from infectious conditions, but Ewing's sarcoma can produce a lamellated periosteal reaction when located in diaphyses (Sherman and Soong 1956). Cancerous periostoses have been documented archaeologically (Ortner and Putschar 1985) but are unlikely to contribute significantly to the overall lesion distribution in a skeletal population because of their rarity.

Inflammation is the typical response to infection and involves the release of fluids, leukocytes, and macrophages to the damaged tissue. This occurs in concert with the proliferation of blood vessels in the area. Fluid and pus at the site of infection separate the periosteum from the surface of the bone, stimulating the deposition of new periosteal bone. Direct infections of bone may be caused by trauma, leading to a single localized periostosis. Alternately, systemic infections may affect bones throughout the skeleton. In archaeological collections, untreated systemic infections can be expected to appear as widespread periostoses and rarely present as solitary periostoses, unless death occurs early in an acute state of infection.

Blood-borne *Staphylococcus aureus* typically localizes in the metaphyses of long bones, causing osteomyelitis. The initial infection produces a small lytic focus known as a Brodie's abscess. Later, cortical necrosis occurs due to obstruction of blood vessels, and new subperiosteal bone forms around the dead tissue as an involucrum. Osteomyelitic infection can be identified by the presence of cloaca through which pus drains and the sequestrum (dead bone) is extruded (Harris and Kirkaldy-Willis 1965; Waldvogel et al. 1970).

A variety of gastrointestinal disturbances may cause systemic periosteal deposition, such as nontropical sprue, Crohn's disease, and chronic ulcerative colitis. Generalized periosteal bone deposition, known as pulmonary hyperotrophic osteoarthropathy, may occur in a number of pulmonary diseases (Greenfield and Schorsch 1967); the extent of periostotic development appears to be related to the duration of the underlying pulmonary condition (Pineda et al. 1987).

Periosteal deposition is common in infection by the spirochete *Treponema*. Four disease syndromes appear to result from infection by the same organism under differing climatic and social conditions (Hudson 1965). In urban and temperate environments, syphilis is transmitted venereally and congenitally to the fetus of an infected mother. However, in warmer climates, direct skin contact between children appears to be the common mode of transmission. In warm, dry climates, the nonvenereal syndrome is known as endemic syphilis, bejel, or treponarid. In more humid tropical climates, yaws occurs. The fourth syndrome, pinta, occurs today in Central America and affects only the skin (Hackett 1967; Perine et al. 1984; Reeder and Palmer 1981; Steinbock 1976).

With the exception of pinta, each syndrome produces a similar pattern of bony involvement. Venereal syphilis presents the most extreme osseous changes in affected individuals. The spirochetes localize in the metaphyses of long bones, producing localized periostoses that spread to involve the entire cortex and medulla. Osteomyelitic necrosis and focal destruction that occur in venereal syphilis are rare in endemic syphilis and yaws, for which periosteal deposition is the main finding. Periosteal buildup on the anterior crest of the tibia leads to the so-called "sabre shin" deformity that is typical of treponematosis. Small erosive cranial lesions, known as "caries sicca," are common in the venereal disease but rare in the endemic syndromes, particularly yaws. Congenital syphilis can be identified by characteristic dental stigmata, along with systemic periostitis, osteomyelitis, and metaphysitis (Hackett 1951, 1976; Reeder and Palmer 1981; Rost 1942; Sengupta 1985; Steinbock 1976).

In tropical areas, such as the Maya Lowlands, two other causes of periosteal infection must also be considered in differential diagnosis of periostoses: tropical phagedenic ulcer and cutaneous leishmaniasis. Tropical ulcers are caused by infection with *Fusobacterium* together with *Treponema vincenti* following trauma (skin puncture or abrasion). The ulcers occur almost exclusively on the lower limb, are solitary, and often heal within six months. The initial lesion is small, but may proliferate to involve a large area and can penetrate to underlying tissues (Adriaans 1988; Meyers and Neafie 1991). Bone changes range from slight focal periostitis to large exostoses, with or without bone sequestration or osteolytic malignant change (Aufderheide and Rodríguez-Martín 1998; Brown and Middlemiss 1956; Ennis et al. 1972). Most reports document tropical ulcers in African or Southeast Asian populations, but they are also common in Jamaica (Ennis et al. 1972). Although Shattuck (1933) did not observe tropical ulcers in Yucatan, he suggests that they occur in wetter areas such as the Petén. Tropical ulcer is listed as cause of death for a 26-year-old Lacandon Maya male in 1888 (Baer and Merrifield 1971; Nations 1979a), although the diagnosis was not medically confirmed.

Similar, but less extensive, ulcers are characteristic of cutaneous leishmaniasis, with which tropical ulcer is sometimes confused (e.g., Steinbock 1976:151). American cutaneous leishmaniasis is endemic in the Petén, Yucatan, and Belize (Scrimshaw and Tejada 1970; Shattuck 1933). Both *Leishmania mexicana* and *L. brasiliensis* have been isolated from Petén sandflies, which transmit the infection with their bite (Rowton et al. 1992). Visceral leishmaniasis (kala-azar), transmitted by *L. donovani chagasi*, is also present in Guatemala but may have been introduced from the Old World (Lainson and Shaw 1987:74). Note that Resnick and Niwayama (1981) incorrectly attribute to leishmaniasis the rare bone changes in Donovanosis, or granuloma inguinale (Kirkpatrick 1970), a venereal disease with no relation to leishmaniasis. Mucocutaneous leishmaniasis is variously known in Central America as "chiclero ulcer," "bay sore," or "forest yaws" and typically affects the ear, face, or arms. This distribution is a consequence of modern clothing habits; where shorts are worn, lesions are common on the leg (Sanchez et al. 1992). Chiclero ulcers are small, discrete lesions characterized by dermal inflammation, epidermal necrosis, and granulomal development, but they normally heal within a year. Infection by *L. mexicana* typically produces a solitary lesion at the site of inoculation, but *L. brasiliensis* may be systemically disseminated to other mucocutaneous sites, such as the nose (espundia) (Costa et al. 1990; Manson-Bahr and Winslow 1975; Ridley 1987). Nasal destruction in "espundia" or "uta" (a localized Peruvian strain, *L. peruviana*) may be represented in pre-Columbian Moché ceramics from Peru (Urteaga-Ballon 1991). Where it is protected by little tissue, underlying bone can be affected following secondary bacterial infection (Marsden et al. 1977; Reeder and Palmer 1981).

Differentiation between possible causes of periostoses may be possible in some instances due to the distribution of bone deposition throughout the skeleton. On a populational level, age- and sex-specific patterns of periosteal deposition are important in diagnosing the presence of a specific pathogen in a sample. In many archaeological instances, diagnosis of the underlying cause of periostoses will not be possible due to the nonspecific nature of bone changes. In such cases, periostoses are often treated as a general index of the infectious disease load affecting a skeletal population.

Porotic Hyperostosis

Porotic lesions of the cranium are common in osteological collections and are widely considered to represent the bony response to anemia. Under anemic conditions, erythropoeitic tissues of the bone marrow and spleen expand to make up for blood deficit. In the skull, pressure on the external table from hyperplasia of the diplöe leads to porosity of the external table. In severe cases, the integrity of the external table is lost and new diplöic bone is deposited at right angles to the cortex, paralleling the direction of diplöic expansion. This new bone is visible as a characteristic "hair on end" pattern observed in radiographs. These bone changes are concentrated at the orbital roof, parietal boss, and the occipital squama (Burko et al. 1961; Caffey 1937; Stuart-Macadam 1987a, 1987b, 1989). Viewed in dry bone, they are referred to as "porotic hyperostosis."

In severe hemolytic anemias, such as Thalassemia and sickle cell anemia, cranial changes may be accompanied by analogous changes in short tubular bones of the hands and feet and in the vertebral bodies (Greenfield 1986). In iron deficiency anemia, bone changes are less pronounced, usually leading only to cranial lesions. Iron deficiency, at the hand of poor nutrition and parasitism, is the most common cause of anemia today (Ryan 1997). Iron deficiency anemia is widespread in Guatemala today, largely due to dietary insufficiency of iron (Wright and Chew 1998).

Bone changes occur in response to anemic episodes during childhood. The orbital roof appears to be the site of the initial bony response when children become anemic at very young ages. Orbital lesions have traditionally been termed "cribra orbitalia" but represent the same physiological process that causes the vault lesions referred to as porotic hyperostosis. Continued anemic stress in later childhood or a later onset of anemia affects the parietal bosses, occipital squama, and, rarely, frontal bosses. Recovery from anemic stress is indicated by sclerotic in-filling and remodeling of pores in the external table. Lesions observed in adult crania represent vestiges of childhood anemic experience that has not been completely remodeled. It is unlikely that anemia could result in porotic hyperostosis in robust adult bone because the gradual involution of hemopoeitic diplöe to fatty yellow marrow with age would leave sufficient space for diplöe expansion (Stuart-Macadam 1985, 1989).

Porotic lesions occurring on the ectocranial surface of the sphenoid bone and resembling porotic hyperostosis have recently been shown to be caused by scurvy (Ortner and Ericksen 1997). Given the similar appearance of the lesions, attention to the location and patterning of porosity is critical to accurate diagnosis.

In most skeletal samples, particularly those of the prehispanic Americas, it can be assumed that lesions of porotic hyperostosis located on the occipital bone and at the parietal bosses indicate iron deficiency anemia (Stuart-Macadam 1991). Early research on porotic hyperostosis in archaeological skeletal series attributed the apparently high prevalence of iron deficiency anemia to dietary insufficiency. In North America, the prevalence of porotic hyperostosis is often linked to maize consumption (El-Najjar 1977; Holland and O'Brien 1997; Lallo et al. 1977) and has been shown to increase with the adoption of maize agriculture (Cohen and Armelagos 1984). The contribution of parasitic infection to iron deficit also has been proposed as a significant factor in the expression of porotic hyperostosis (Carlson et al. 1974; Palkovich 1987), particularly in populations with high dietary iron intake (Walker 1986).

In subadults, the interaction of anemia and infection are indicated by the coocurrence of porotic hyperostosis and periosteal reactions (Mensforth et al. 1978). This pattern illustrates the synergistic relationship between nutrition and infection that is documented in modern populations (Scrimshaw et al. 1968; Sibrián and Elston 1990). Anemia at the hand of malnourishment has been thought to predispose children toward infection. In turn, chronic infection may contribute to the "anemia of infection." Recently it has been suggested that iron deficiency may be adaptive in combating infection (Strauss 1978; Weinberg 1992). The development of anemic skeletal lesions might then be interpreted as evidence of a "healthy" immune response to infection (Stuart-Macadam 1992). However, because the direction of causal arrows between anemia and infection continue to be hotly debated (Ryan 1997; Walter et al. 1997), at this time the lesions are best viewed as evidence of survived childhood anemic experience only.

Because of this synergistic relationship, periosteal reactions and porotic hyperostosis have been examined as indicators of health stress in archaeological skeletal series. Changes in the prevalence of both lesions have been noted in accord with changes in prehistoric settlement patterns and subsistence technologies in a number of world areas (Cohen and Armelagos 1984). High levels of porotic hyperostosis are found among prehistoric maize agriculturalists in North America (El-Najjar 1977; El-Najjar et al. 1976; Holland and O'Brien 1997; Lallo et al. 1977). Periosteal reactions increase dramatically with the adoption of sedentary lifeways in the American Midwest, a change that may reflect the development of endemic treponematoses with an aggregated settlement system (Cook 1976, 1984). In the Maya area, the high prevalence of anemia has been linked to the maize-reliant diet (Saul 1977; Wright and White 1996). Periosteal reactions are also common on Maya bones, but there is little consensus about their underlying etiology.

Here, I use periosteal reactions and porotic hyperostosis as general indicators of health status in the Pasión skeletal samples. Collapse models of environmental stress and agricultural failure have implications for both nutritional status and infectious disease that should be reflected in skeletal pathology. The proposed decline in childhood nutritional status whould have led to iron deficiency, diarrhea, and the synergistic interaction of anemia and infection. Increased population density could exacerbate endemic and epidemic infectious diseases, which would affect a greater proportion of the population. Hence, such models of collapse would be supported by an increase in the prevalence and severity of periosteal reactions and porotic hyperostosis in Pasión skeletons over the span of Maya occupation.

Methods

Periosteal Reactions

I examined all long bones and crania for evidence of subperiosteal new bone deposition. I scored each bone as observable or not observable for three units: proximal metaphysis, diaphysis, and distal metaphysis. The presence of at least two-thirds of each bone unit was required in order to score a unit as observable. Lesions were scored for each unit observable, as either active (presenting woven new periosteal bone) or healed (sclerotic bone). Additional notes were made describing the extent, nature, and severity of pathologic change for each affected bone. Unfortunately, systematic radiography was not feasible, so I could not evaluate endosteal involvement for many periostoses. Yet, postmortem fractures allowed assessment of cortical and medullary conditions for some bones.

In addition to long bones and crania that are used in statistical analysis, I inspected all other available skeletal elements for evidence of skeletal pathology. These data cannot be evaluated statistically due to the extreme inconsistency of preservation but are considered in the differential diagnosis of major disease patterns.

Porotic Hyperostosis

I scored cribra orbitalia after Nathan and Haas (1966) as follows:

absent: no apparent porosity
porotic: scattered fine openings in the roof of the orbit
cribrotic: numerous larger openings, tending to coalesce into larger apertures
trabecular: openings are coalesced into large irregular apertures, often arranged in radiating patterns from one or more centers in the orbital roof
healed: sclerotic in-filling of pores.

I scored porotic hyperostosis for each scorable frontal, parietal, and occipital bone as follows:

absent: no apparent porosity or cranial thickening
slight: active large pores in outer table, with diplöe expansion
extensive: spongy or coral-like outer table, with diplöe expansion
healed: sclerotic in-filling of pores, irregular sclerotic surface, obvious diplöic thickening
possibly healed: sclerotic surface with fine diffuse porosity but no diplöic thickening. This class was treated as "absent" in statistical analysis as the diagnosis was uncertain.

Because porotic hyperostosis is almost always bilaterally symmetrical (Stuart-Macadam 1989), I pooled the left and right sides to provide as large

Table 9.1. Occurrence of periosteal reactions in Pasión long bones

	Left side			Right side		
Bone	Proximal metaphysis	Diaphysis	Distal metaphysis	Proximal metaphysis	Diaphysis	Distal metaphysis
Woven Periostoses						
clavicle	0/17 (0)	0/51 (0)	0/28 (0)	0/15 (0)	0/48 (0)	0/31 (0)
humerus	0/18 (0)	0/85 (0)	1/37 (3)	0/12 (0)	1/94 (1)	0/42 (0)
radius	0/34 (0)	0/88 (0)	1/24 (4)	0/32 (0)	1/70 (2)	0/18 (0)
ulna	1/51 (2)	0/84 (0)	0/13 (0)	0/44 (0)	1/80 (0)	0/16 (0)
femur	1/36 (3)	0/95 (0)	3/19 (16)	2/39 (5)	3/91 (3)	2/22 (9)
tibia	1/18 (5)	1/83 (1)	0/21 (0)	1/19 (5)	1/91 (1)	1/22 (5)
fibula	0/9 (0)	0/61 (0)	0/18 (0)	1/9 (11)	3/66 (4)	0/15 (0)
Sclerotic Periostoses						
clavicle	1/17 (6)	4/51 (8)	3/28 (11)	0/15 (0)	3/48 (4)	3/31 (10)
humerus	1/18 (5)	2/85 (2)	3/37 (6)	0/12 (0)	2/94 (2)	0/42 (0)
radius	0/34 (0)	4/88 (4)	2/24 (8)	0/32 (0)	3/70 (5)	0/18 (0)
ulna	2/51 (4)	8/84 (10)	1/13 (8)	1/44 (2)	1/80 (1)	0/16 (0)
femur	0/36 (0)	27/95 (28)	4/19 (21)	0/39 (0)	26/91 (28)	3/22 (14)
tibia	2/18 (11)	53/83 (64)	5/21 (24)	3/19 (16)	56/91 (61)	9/22 (41)
fibula	0/9 (0)	30/61 (49)	5/18 (28)	0/9 (0)	26/66 (39)	4/15 (27)

Number of bones affected/number of bones observable (% affected).

a sample as possible. In addition to analysis at the level of each bone affected, I derived a composite index of vault involvement, in which occipital and parietal scores are considered, in order to raise the proportion of scorable individuals. I scored the vault as positive if a porotic reaction was observed on either bone; however, if only the occipital was scorable and showed no reaction, I considered the individual to be not scorable. As occipital reactions rarely occur in the absence of parietal change, this will not elevate anemia prevalence significantly. Statistical differences between subpopulations were considered to be significant at $p \leq 0.05$.

Results

Lesion Distribution and Differential Diagnosis

PERIOSTEAL REACTIONS

Periosteal reactions could be scored for some 144 postcranial skeletons from which one or more scorable bones were present, and for 154 crania. Many remains were excluded due to surface erosion of the bone or an absence of scorable units. Table 9.1 summarizes the distribution of woven and sclerotic periostoses by bone unit affected. Woven periostoses are rare, affecting only 26 bone units, with a peak prevalence of 16% for the distal metaphysis of the left femur. Woven periostoses also account for a larger proportion of periostoses located on metaphyses than on diaphyses, for all elements pooled ($X^2 = 16.35$, $p = 0.0001$). In contrast, sclerotic periosteal reactions occur mostly on diaphyses (Plate 9.1), with highest prevalence of 64% for the left tibial diaphysis (61% for the right). Sclerotic diaphyseal periostoses of the fibula are almost as common, at 49% (left) and 39% (right). Femoral diaphyseal periostosis prevalence is lower, at 28% (left and right). The distal metaphysis is more commonly affected than the proximal metaphysis for the tibia, fibula, and femur; and distal metaphysis of the lower limb bones are more

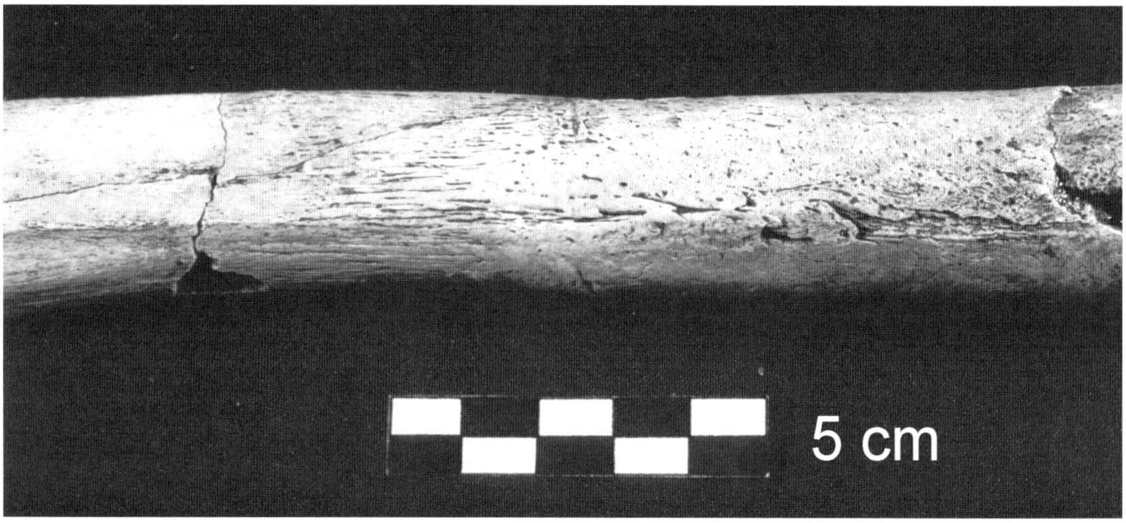

Plate 9.1. Sclerotic periostosis on the lateral aspect of the right tibial diaphysis of burial AG1.

commonly affected than any region of the upper limb.

Cranial periosteal reactions are rare (Table 9.2). Highest prevalences are recorded for the mandible and maxilla, in which infections are associated with periodontal disease, abscesses, and antemortem tooth loss. Excluding these, lesions are most common on the frontal bone but occur in only five skeletons (6%). The few remaining lesions are both woven and sclerotic. Most cranial periostoses are small focal patches of new bone. In AS54, a one-year-old with cranial deformation, a band of woven bone occurs along the coronal margin of the parietal, coinciding with the post-coronal sulcus, and may be a response to pressure in this area by the deforming apparatus. Only two skeletons showed active woven periostitis of the endocranial surface: the parietal of SE29 and the anterior squama of the left temporal of AS37; the remaining lesions are ectocranial.

The age and sex distributions of periostoses are presented in Tables 9.3 and 9.4 for cranial and diaphyseal periostoses in the series as a whole. A large proportion of subadult skeletons show periostoses, but the paucity of subadult skeletons hinders detailed analysis of this pattern. Woven lesions contribute differentially to the prevalence of subadult periostoses, with 9 subadults and only 12 adults contributing to the total distribution of woven periostitis. After adolescence, most bones show increasing prevalence of lesions into middle adulthood, implying that periostoses accumulate with age. Commonly, old adults show fewer periostoses, likely due to long-term remodeling. Table 9.3(b) lists differences in periostoses between adult age groups for lower limb bones; however, none of the differences among adults are statistically confirmed. Sex differences could not be substantiated for diaphyseal periostoses of any bones using Yates corrected X^2 or Fisher Exact tests (Table 9.4).

Table 9.5 is a matrix of phi (φ) coefficients calculated using pairwise deletion of missing data for 80 skeletons that exhibit two or more diaphyseal bones affected by periostitis. Periostoses are highly correlated in the two sides of the body for the femur, tibia, fibula, radius, and clavicle. In addition, periostoses of the left ulna are highly correlated with those of the left clavicle and left humerus. A significant co-occurrence is also noted between the right humerus and right radius. These results indicate that periostoses of the upper limb co-occur commonly in skeletons affected by systemic periostoses and are less common as isolated lesions.

Table 9.2. Distribution of cranial periostoses

Bone	Side	Woven N (%)	Sclerotic N (%)	Unaffected N	Scorable N
Frontal	L	0 (0)	5 (6)	73	78
	R	1 (2)	1 (1)	66	68
Parietal	L	1 (1)	1 (1)	85	87
	R	1 (1)	1 (1)	78	80
Occipital	L	1 (1)	1 (1)	70	72
	R	0 (0)	1 (1)	72	73
Temporal	L	1 (1)	0 (0)	71	72
	R	0 (0)	0 (0)	69	69
Zygomatic	L	0 (0)	1 (1)	28	29
	R	0 (0)	1 (1)	40	41
Maxilla	L	0 (0)	5 (18)	22	27
	R	0 (0)	5 (15)	28	33
Mandible	L	1 (1)	13 (14)	77	91
	R	0 (0)	14 (15)	81	95

Woven periostoses on adult skeletons tend to be slight and cover a restricted area. In contrast, sclerotic periostoses are often generalized, affecting a large area of bone, although discrete focal involvement also occurs. In some cases, sclerotic lesions incorporate discrete foci of thick subperiosteal deposition, often along the anterior crest of the tibia. Six skeletons show varying degrees of tibial bowing: AS112, AS135, DP1, DP38, SE3 and SE4-?. A number of other tibia may also be slightly bowed but cannot be definitely identified as such because only a 15 cm section of the diaphysis is present. Only two instances of pyogenic osteomyelitis are diagnosed by the presence of cloacae: the left clavicle of SE5 and the right ilium of AS63 (Saul 1972:Fig. 25).

One middle adult male skeleton, SE22, shows diffuse woven periostitis on the pleural surface of five rib fragments, as well as the inferiomedial aspect of the right clavicle, the supraspinous fossa of both scapulae, and the ventral surface of the left scapula. Few long bones were recovered, but the right humerus is unaffected. Although periosteal reactions of pleural rib surfaces have been attributed to tuberculosis (Kelley and Micozzi 1984), they are not pathognomic. No osteolytic lesions of Pott's disease have been described in Mayan remains to date, and I observed none in the Pasión skeletal series. This may partly be an artifact of poor vertebral preservation. Only five vertebral fragments were recovered from the aforecited skeleton with rib lesions (SE22). Salas Cuesta (1982) illustrates tuberculosis-like lesions in three vertebrae from a female skeleton of Tenochtitlan, which is the only published evidence for prehistoric tuberculosis in Central America to date. In the present case, a diagnosis of nonspecific periosteal inflammation, such as that of pulmonary hyperotrophic osteoarthropathy (Greenfield and Schorsch 1967), is more likely than tuberculosis.

The distribution of periostoses in Pasión skeletons conforms largely with the pattern shown by the treponematoses and encountered in other New World populations (Cook 1976; Powell 1988). Subadults are most often affected, and lesions in adults reflect healed conditions acquired in childhood. The intraskeletal distribution of lesions also parallels that affected by treponemes, with symmetrical involvement and an emphasis on the lower limbs. The sabre shin deformity of

Table 9.3. Age distribution of cranial and diaphyseal periostoses

(a) Number of bones affected/number of bones observable

Bone	Side	Infant	Child	Teen	Young Adult	Middle Adult	Old Adult	Adult
Frontal	L	1/2	0/2	0/7	2/27	1/32	1/8	-
Parietal	L	1/4	0/1	0/7	1/27	1/35	0/9	0/4
Occipital	R	0/4	0/2	0/6	1/24	0/25	0/7	0/4
Temporal	L	0/3	-	1/8	0/18	0/28	0/11	0/4
Zygomatic	R	0/3	-	0/4	0/12	0/14	1/8	-
Maxilla	R	0/1	-	0/3	0/8	4/14	1/6	0/1
Mandible	R	0/5	0/1	0/7	7/28	4/42	3/11	0/1
Clavicle	L	0/1	-	0/3	1/12	1/14	2/8	0/5
Humerus	R	0/4	1/1	0/7	0/22	1/31	1/13	0/9
Radius	L	0/2	0/2	0/6	0/19	3/33	0/10	0/7
Ulna	L	0/3	-	1/4	1/19	5/31	0/9	1/17
Femur	L	0/4	-	1/9	4/21	13/35	4/10	4/13
Tibia	R	1/2	-	3/10	14/25	22/28	4/8	4/9
Fibula	R	0/3	-	3/9	8/17	10/21	2/6	4/8

(b) Chi-square tests comparing the age distribution of periostoses among adults

Bone	Side	X^2	p
Femur	L	2.34	0.31
	R	0.84	0.66
Tibia	L	1.63	0.44
	R	3.97	0.14
Fibula	L	0.78	0.68
	R	0.41	0.81

tibiae and fibulae seen in a few Pasión skeletons is typical of treponematosis (Plate 9.2), but pathognomic caries sicca of the cranium are less evident. Isolated sclerotic depressions in the frontal of Burials AS86 and DP4 bear some resemblance to supposed healed caries sicca of yaws diagnosed by Stewart and Spoehr (1952) in Pacific crania but could equally well be the result of trauma. Tibiae of DP4 present bilateral generalized healed periostoses covering much of the diaphysis. The right tibia of AS86 is unaffected, but the left is absent. The Preclassic intersite burial TR3-1 shows a small osteolytic lesion of the right parietal that is depressed, with sclerotic in-filling at its margins (Plate 9.3). The same skeleton shows a second possible lesion, which is very well remodeled, along the left temporal line of the frontal. Marked periostoses occur on the humeri, ulnae, left radius, tibiae, fibulae, and left femur. Although they are not bowed, the tibiae show sclerotic and striate periostitis over the entire shaft, with several foci of superficial cavitation, diffuse cortical lysis, and endostosis (Plate 9.4). Although the cranial lesions are not unequivocally caries sicca, together with the postcranial changes, this skeleton provides a strong case for treponemal infection.

Few cranial lesions of treponematoses have been documented in Mesoamerica. Whittington (1989) did not observe caries sicca on any of 157 low-status skeletons from Copan. Goff (1953) diagnosed two crania from Postclassic Zaculeu as syphilitic on the basis of frontal caries sicca in one and an unhealed parietal defect in the second. In Mexico, crania from the Cueva de la Candelaria,

Table 9.4. Sex distribution of cranial and diaphyseal periostoses

Bone	Side	Males	Females	Unknown Sex	X^2	p
Frontal	L	3/45	1/25	1/8	0.21	0.64
Parietal	L	1/49	0/27	1/11	0.56	0.45
Occipital	L	0/39	2/24	0/9	3.36	0.07
Temporal	L	0/42	0/21	1/9	-	
Zygomatic	R	1/25	0/10	0/6	*	1.00
Maxilla	R	5/21	0/10	0/2	*	0.15
Mandible	R	8/59	6/25	0/11	1.38	0.24
Clavicle	L	4/25	0/15	0/11	*	0.28
Humerus	R	0/46	1/30	1/10	3.05	0.08
Radius	L	2/45	2/26	0/8	0.33	0.57
Ulna	L	4/39	3/29	1/7	0.00	0.99
Femur	R	14/49	11/32	1/12	0.31	0.58
Tibia	R	29/46	17/26	3/9	0.04	0.84
Fibula	R	15/32	8/21	4/11	0.40	0.53

Number of bones affected/number of bones observable.
* Fisher Exact probability was calculated for these elements, given the small sample size.

Coahuila, show apparent caries sicca (Goff 1967), and a Preclassic skull from Tehuacan exhibits similar destruction (Anderson 1965). Among Mexica skeletons encountered during subway construction in Mexico City (Tenochtitlan), Salas Cuesta (1982) identified one case each of venereal syphilis and yaws based on the extent of cranial lesions.

The pattern of periostoses in Pasión skeletons bears slightly greater resemblance to modern yaws than to endemic syphilis, in that lesions of the distal femur are common and cranial lesions rare. At Copan, Whittington (1989) also found a high prevalence of femoral involvement, yet the humerus was seldom affected. Periosteal involvement of short tubular bones—dactylitis—is typical of both syndromes. Two Pasión skeletons with severe sclerotic periosteal deposition of the tibiae also show irregular sclerotic periosteal reactions on metatarsals: SE20 is affected on the right fifth metatarsal and DP42 on the left fourth metatarsal. The tibiae of QCH10 are not scorable, but the skeleton shows marked fibular periostosis and dactylitis of three metacarpals. Burial 4 from nearby Los Quetzales/Pacayas also shows right first metatarsal dactylitis in conjunction with tibial and fibular periostitis (Wright, unpublished data), though the few burials from this site are not included here. A skeleton recently excavated at Piedras Negras also shows extensive periosteal changes that match the expectations for yaws (Wright and Witte 1998). I did not observe erosive arthropathy, described by Ortner et al. (1992) for yaws, but it might not be evident in these series given the generally poor preservation of metaphyseal bone.

Yaws is typically restricted to humid tropical climates like that of the Pasión region. Surprisingly, Shattuck (1933) found no evidence of yaws in the Yucatan earlier this century, yet Scrimshaw et al. (1970) report that it was endemic in Suchitepequez, Guatemala, and sporadic cases have been documented across lowland Guatemala. Although medically unconfirmed, Baer and Merrifield (1971) report yaws as the cause of death for a 39-year-old Lacandon Maya male in 1939. Endemic syphilis has not been reported from the Maya area and would not be expected, given the humid climate. Pinta is endemic to the Yucatan peninsula but does not produce bone changes.

Table 9.5. Matrix of phi coefficients (φ) for diaphyseal periostoses

	L. femur	R. femur	L. tibia	R. tibia	L. fibula	R. fibula	L. humerus	R. humerus	L. radius	R. radius	L. ulna	R. ulna	L. clavicle	R. clavicle
L. femur	1.000													
R. femur	**0.561**	1.000												
L. tibia	0.336	0.223	1.000											
R. tibia	0.302	0.122	**0.709**	1.000										
L. fibula	0.068	-0.023	0.013	0.108	1.000									
R. fibula	0.160	0.000	-0.058	-0.046	**0.689**	1.000								
L. humerus	0.266	0.250	0.098	0.110			1.000							
R. humerus	0.189	0.177	-0.349		-0.189	-0.189	-0.034	1.000						
L. radius	-0.031	0.019	0.121	0.117	0.239	0.236	-0.060	-0.035	1.000					
R. radius	-0.227	-0.222	0.105	0.131	-0.218	-0.254		**0.696**	0.471	1.000				
L. ulna	0.160	0.148	0.030	0.020	0.324	0.293	**0.501**	-0.066	0.342	0.208	1.000			
R. ulna	-0.124	0.006	0.127	-0.151	-0.17	-0.250	-0.038	-0.056	-0.053	-0.069	-0.073	1.000		
L. clavicle	0.150	-0.127	0.135	0.175	0.375	0.346			0.283	-0.149	**0.677**	-0.093	1.000	
R. clavicle	0.316		0.083	0.107	0.081	0.015		-0.069	0.553	-0.140	0.339	-0.079	**0.797**	1.000

Calculations used pairwise deletion, on 80 skeletons with two or more periostoses.
Values in **bold** are significant at $p \le 0.05$.

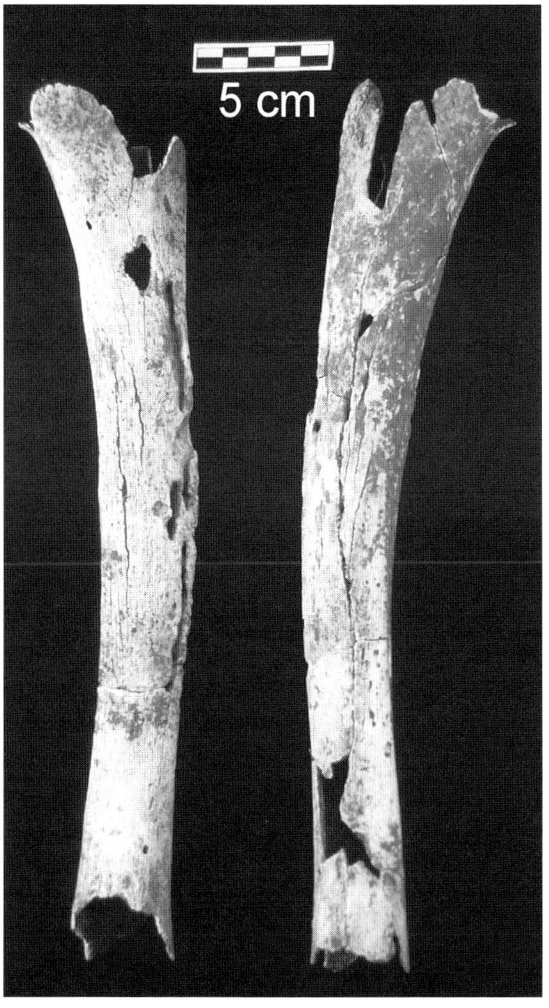

Plate 9.2. Sabre shin deformity in the tibiae of burial DP38, medial aspect.

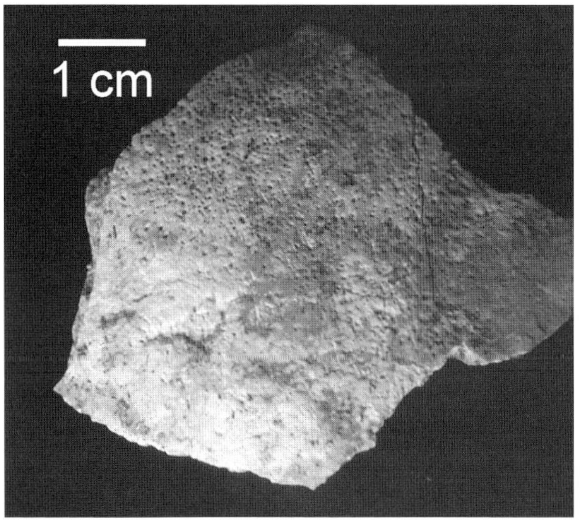

Plate 9.3. Possible caries sicca on the right parietal of burial TR3-1.

Studies of treponematoses in the Maya area have focused on venereal syphilis, which is rare in the indigenous population and when present seldom develops tertiary lesions even though (Western) medical treatment is rarely sought (Scrimshaw and Tejada 1970). Previous exposure to a prehispanic treponemal syndrome would likely provide some cross immunity and could account for the mild expression of syphilis documented in the indigenous population.

In addition to periostoses that involve the entire tibial shaft, discrete focal sclerotic reactions are also common, accounting for roughly 20% of Pasión skeletons with tibial periostoses. These lesions are small—from 2 to 7 cm in diameter—and involve only subperiosteal new bone. Some show multiple independent foci (e.g., Saul 1972:Fig. 37). These lesions may be the result of localized trauma but could also represent tropical phagedenic ulcer or leishmaniasis.

Like both endemic treponematoses, the prehistoric Pasión lesions show a predilection for involvement of the tibia, appear to be discrete inflammatory reactions to external pathogens (rather than hematogenous dissemination), and show healing. Given the rarity of modern reports of tropical ulcer in the Maya area and the slight extent of the lesions observed, leishmaniasis is a more probable diagnosis. In addition to cases affected only by focal periostoses, leishmanial infection might also contribute to more severe foci on bones that are otherwise affected by extensive periosteal reaction. Clearly, the observed pattern is not pathognomic of leishmaniasis, but given the modern distribution, it is likely that the disease did affect the inhabitants of the Pasión region and could well contribute to the high prevalence of tibial lesions.

In his description of pathology at Altar de Sacrificios, Saul (1972) described a number of lesions as ossified subperiosteal hemorrhages. He argued that this, together with the high rate of antemortem tooth loss, represented skeletal evidence

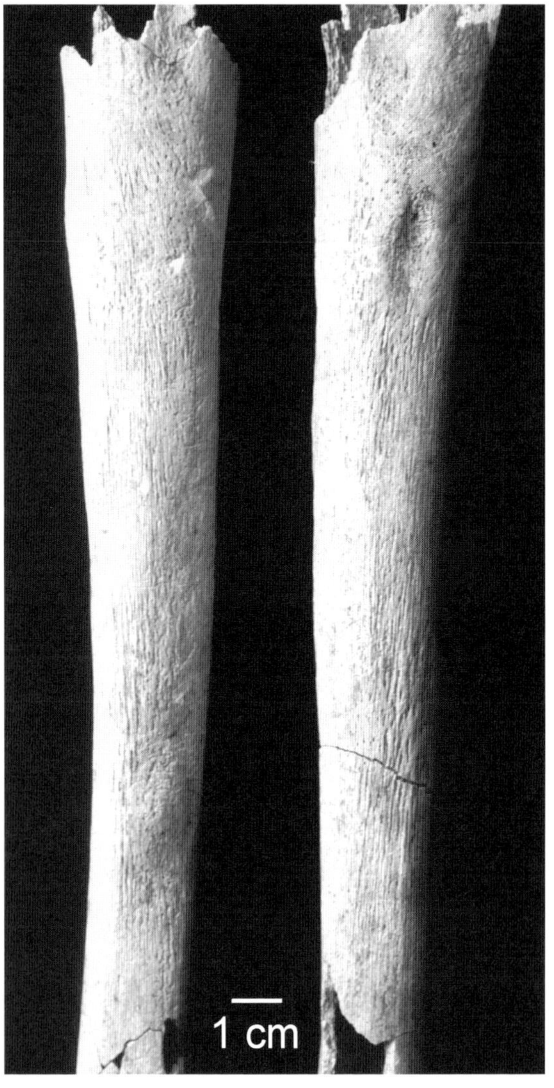

Plate 9.4. Bilateral periostoses with cavitation on the right proximal diaphysis of the tibiae of burial TR3-1, medial aspect.

for scurvy. As Ortner and Putschar (1985:273) note, the lesions are more characteristic of simple periostosis. In fact, lesions on the left tibia of AS62 are virtually identical to the "rugose" form of treponemal periostitis described by Hackett (1976). Antemortem loss of posterior teeth is common in Pasión skeletons and probably caused by abscess secondary to interproximal cervical caries that affect most skeletons. Whittington (1989) did not observe ossified subperiosteal hemorrhages in any skeletons from Copan. Similarly, lesions classified as hemorrhages by Saul (1972) were here considered to be periosteal reactions, a diagnosis that is more consistent with their morphology. Porous lesions of the sphenoid, recently identified as characteristic of scurvy, were not observed (Ortner 1997), but I was not specifically looking for them at the time these data were collected.

POROTIC HYPEROSTOSIS

Porotic hyperostosis commonly affects the crania of Pasión Maya skeletons. In total, 124 crania were examined for evidence of anemia. The age distributions of both active and healed lesions are presented in Table 9.6. The majority of subadults show active lesions, with remodeled lesions predominating among adults. Active cribra orbitalia occurs on 87.5% of children under age 12. Adolescents show more remodeled (37.5%) than active lesions (12.5%), while all orbital lesions in adults are remodeled. Most active lesions of cribra orbitalia are mild, consisting only of fine porosity. Only one infant (SE8) shows slight coalescence of foramina, and proliferative reactions were absent. Active vault lesions also predominate among subadults but persist in an unremodeled state into adulthood in a few individuals. All infants and children with hyperostotic lesions of the cranium also possess cribra orbitalia, but only two-thirds of those with cribra orbitalia show vault lesions. The paucity of subadult skeletons precludes detailed analysis of the age of anemic onset in subadults; however, the youngest scorable skeletons, aged at 12±4 months and 18±6 months, do show hyperostotic changes, suggesting an early onset of anemia.

Among adults, healed lesions are common, occurring in 63% of adult crania (Plate 9.5). The slight orbital porosity observed in subadult skeletons is not seen in adults, and few adults show any cribra orbitalia, indicating complete remodeling of orbital lesions. Healed vault lesions do not appear to decrease with adult age, suggesting that remodeling has not affected the visibility of the lesions dramatically, although the relationship between survival of childhood anemia and frailty remains uncertain. In the sample as a whole, no differences could be detected between the sexes in the prevalence of lesions on any bone (Table 9.7).

This pattern corresponds to that typically

Table 9.6. Age distribution of porotic hyperostosis by state, all sites

Bone	State	Infant	Child	Teen	Young Adult	Middle Adult	Old Adult	Adult
Orbit	Active	5/6	2/2	1/8	0/17	0/25	0/5	0/1
	Healed	0/6	0/2	3/8	3/17	4/25	0/5	0/1
Frontal	Active	0/2	1/2	0/10	0/28	0/34	0/9	0/1
	Healed	0/2	0/1	1/10	0/28	3/34	0/9	0/1
Parietal	Active	3/5	1/1	1/9	1/30	1/40	1/9	0/7
	Healed	0/5	0/1	4/9	16/30	21/40	5/9	5/7
Occipital	Active	4/5	2/3	1/6	2/26	0/30	1/7	0/5
	Healed	0/5	0/3	3/6	9/26	11/30	3/7	2/5
Vault	Affected	5/7	2/3	4/9	18/30	24/39	7/10	5/7

Number of bones affected/number of bones observable.

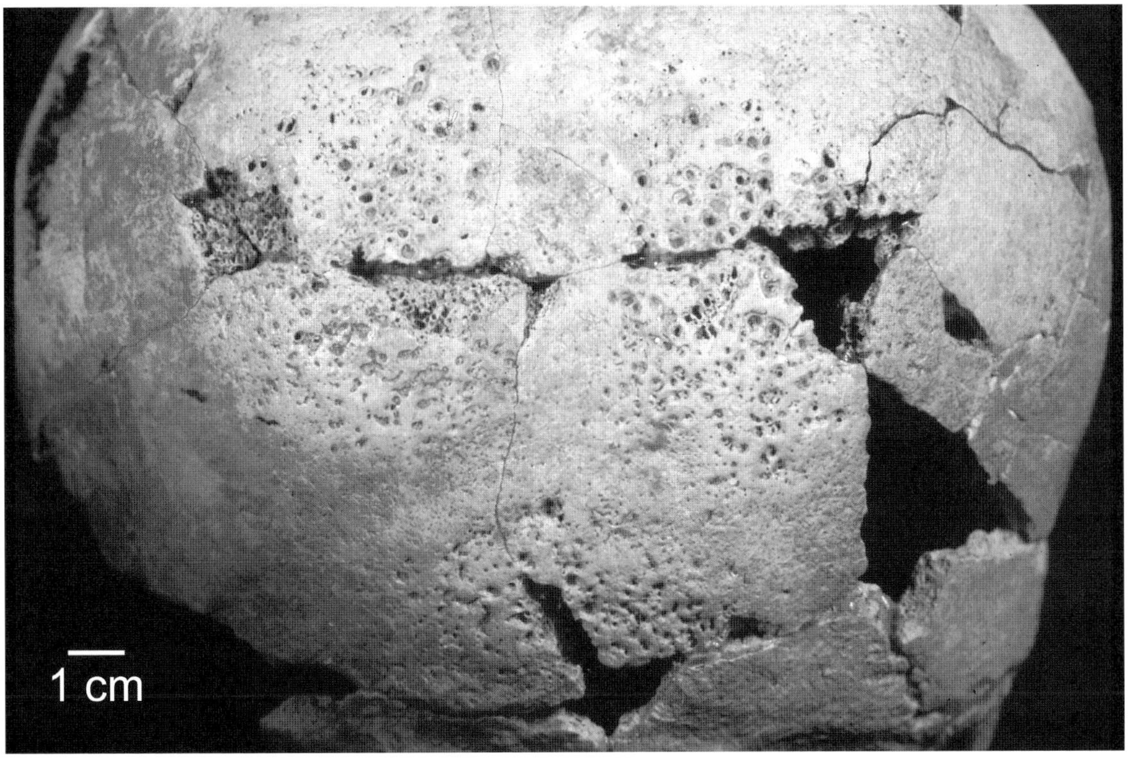

Plate 9.5. Healed porotic hyperostosis on the parietals and occipital of burial SE4-10, posterior aspect (Peabody number 986-38-20/N9876.4; Courtesy of the President and Fellows of Harvard College).

Table 9.7. Sex differences of porotic hyperostosis in adults, healed and active lesions considered together, all sites

Bone	Males	Females	Unknown Sex	X^2	p
Orbit	4/33	3/15	0/0	0.07	0.78
Frontal	3/46	0/25	0/1	1.70	0.19
Parietal	33/54	14/28	3/4	0.93	0.33
Occipital	19/42	7/23	2/3	0.36	0.24
Vault	34/54	17/28	3/4	0.04	0.84

Number of bones affected/number of bones observable.

seen in anemia. The locations where porous bone was observed is more consistent with a diagnosis of anemia than of scurvy. As the Maya do not suffer hereditary hemolytic anemias, the hyperostotic changes are best attributed to iron-deficiency anemia. Lesions in adults represent healed scars of childhood anemic experience from which the individuals recovered. The juvenile data is insufficient to evaluate whether the anemia is best explained as a response to a poor weanling diet or to endemic parasitism.

I calculated phi coefficients (φ) to examine the relationship between porotic hyperostosis (composite vault score) and diaphyseal periosteal reactions in adults (Table 9.8). A high correlation is not obtained for any bone, indicating that anemic expression in not closely linked to infectious disease in the rest of the skeleton. This pattern is contrary to that expected if synergistic interaction between nutrition and infection were responsible for the lesions (Mensforth et al. 1978). Because nutrition is not a major factor in resistance to treponemal infection (Hackett 1951), this finding may indirectly support the diagnosis of a yaws-like treponemal disease in this population.

TRAUMA AND MISCELLANEOUS CONDITIONS

Evidence of skeletal trauma is rare in the Pasión skeletal series. All fractures identified represent well-healed conditions. The high degree of bone fragmentation by root action and construction fill pressure precludes the identification of perimortem fractures for most burials. Partially reduced fractures of the clavicular shaft are visible on two skeletons—a left clavicle from AS135 and a right clavicle from SE4. A right femur from the latter feature also shows a compression fracture of the femoral neck and probably a second healed fracture of the proximal femoral shaft. Both are well healed and reduced, but they produce severe angulation of the femoral neck and twisting of the proximal shaft. AS115 exhibits a well-reduced parry fracture of the right ulna. A distal right ulna and radius labeled as AS86 show ankylosis, which Saul (1972:51) has suggested to be the result of amputation. Colles fracture of both bones is perhaps a more likely diagnosis. However, the fractured bones may not in fact belong with AS86 as they do not connect to proximal fragments or an ulnar capitus also present. The left fifth metacarpal of DP13 shows a healed and well-integrated diaphyseal fracture with slight angulation. Similarly, the right fourth metacarpal of TA6 shows a healed fracture that is well aligned. The left acetabulum of AS67 is rotated anteriorly and superiorly, the result of either dislocation or a healed iliac fracture. Unfortunately, only a fragment of the bone is preserved. The superior border of the acetabulum shows severe osteoarthritis with exposure of trabeculae. The femoral head is not fully preserved, but the left distal femur and proximal tibia present eburnation on the extreme medial edges, indicating a complication from the altered

Table 9.8. Phi coefficients (φ) for the correlation of porotic hyperostosis (composite vault score) with diaphyseal periosteal reactions in adults

Bone	Side	φ	N
Clavicle	L	0.325	19
Clavicle	R	-	22
Humerus	L	0.143	39
Humerus	R	-	39
Radius	L	0.133	41
Radius	R	-	31
Ulna	L	0.250	38
Ulna	R	0.146	34
Femur	L	0.092	42
Femur	R	-0.015	41
Tibia	L	0.104	34
Tibia	R	-0.036	34
Fibula	L	-0.086	24
Fibula	R	-0.116	27

gait that acetabular dislocation or iliac fracture would cause. Finally, AS118 exhibits spondylolysis of the fifth lumbar vertebra.

Most skeletons show some degenerative joint disease, but the degree of involvement is seldom severe. As might be expected, osteoarthritis is most common in elderly skeletons. Two skeletons, AS115 and DP30, show unilateral sacroiliac joint fusion, both of the right side. In both cases the ilium and sacrum are fused only along the superior margin from the auricular apex to the retroauricular area, but the joint surface itself is not involved. A third, but poorly preserved, right ilium, DP25, has a prominent exostosis along the superior margin of the auricular surface, suggesting incomplete fusion. Other vertebrae from these individuals do not show marked syndesmophyte development, so ankylosing spondylitis is an unlikely cause (cf. Saul 1972:50). Sacroiliac fusion in AS115 (Saul 1972:Fig. 27) is accompanied by isolated osteophytes along the iliac crest, the superior border of the pubis, and the linea aspera of the femora (Saul 1972:Fig. 36). A more probable diagnosis is diffuse idiopathic skeletal hyperostosis (DISH), a condition that affects males between 40 and 60 years of age (Resnick and Niwayama 1976) and is characterized by enthesophytes as well as vertebral fusion. The three Pasión skeletons are all male but were aged as young (DP25), middle (AS115), and old adults (DP30). One child, SE8, aged 2 to 4 years at death, shows scaphocephaly (premature closure of the sagittal suture) and is also affected by cranial periostoses and porotic hyperostosis.

Chronological Trends

PERIOSTEAL REACTIONS

Table 9.9 presents the temporal distribution of diaphyseal periostoses for all sites combined. Metaphyseal and cranial lesions are too scarce to permit temporal comparison. Series from the Preclassic and Early Classic periods have been pooled in order to increase the sample size for statistical comparison. Chi-square and Fisher Exact tests indicate few temporal differences in the prevalence

Table 9.9. Temporal comparisons of diaphyseal periostoses in adults, all sites

Bone	Side	Preclassic/ Early Classic	Late Classic	Terminal Classic	Preclassic/ Early–Late		Preclassic/ Early–Terminal		Late–Terminal	
					X^2	p	X^2	p	X^2	p
Clavicle	L	2/8	0/20	2/19	*	0.07	*	0.56	*	0.23
	R	2/10	1/13	0/20	*	0.56	*	0.10	*	0.39
Humerus	L	1/16	0/27	1/31	1.72	0.19	0.24	0.63	0.89	0.35
	R	0/17	2/31	0/34	1.14	0.28	-		2.26	0.13
Radius	L	2/15	1/28	1/34	1.43	0.23	1.96	0.16	0.02	0.89
	R	1/15	2/23	0/26	*	1.00	1.78	0.18	2.35	0.12
Ulna	L	3/15	1/28	3/33	3.12	0.08	1.12	0.29	0.75	0.38
	R	1/17	1/26	0/21	0.10	1.00	1.74	0.19	1.14	0.29
Femur	L	5/14	10/38	10/29	0.44	0.51	0.01	0.94	0.52	0.47
	R	7/16	9/36	11/28	1.83	0.18	0.08	0.77	1.50	0.22
Tibia	L	10/14	18/31	23/27	0.73	0.39	1.11	0.29	**5.12**	**0.02**
	R	10/16	16/33	27/30	0.85	0.36	**5.01**	**0.02**	**12.50**	**0.00**
Fibula	L	4/8	12/27	12/18	*	1.00	*	0.66	2.14	0.14
	R	4/10	11/25	11/19	*	1.00	*	0.45	0.83	0.36

Number of bones affected/number of bones observable.
* Fisher Exact probabilities were calculated for comparisons with $N < 40$.
A dash indicates that probability could not be calculated due to mutual absences.
Values in **bold** indicate a significant difference at the $p \leq 0.05$ level.

of lesions between either the early periods and Late Classic or Terminal Classic, or between the Late and Terminal Classic periods.

Statistical difference is obtained only for the tibia, with periostoses more prevalent in the Terminal Classic than the Late Classic period for both left and right diaphyses. For the right tibia, Terminal Classic periostoses are also more abundant than in the Preclassic/Early Classic sample. However, this difference is not significant for the left tibia. Few significant differences are detected in periostotic prevalence between Late and Terminal Classic periods at individual sites (Table 9.10). Only the right tibia shows a significant increase at Dos Pilas, where all four Terminal Classic skeletons were affected and contribute to the overall Terminal Classic distinction for this bone.

Given the large number of comparisons, one might expect that a few significant differences would be found due to Type I error, but, since the tibial pattern is bilateral, it is probably real. The question is whether or not this difference represents a true increase in the level of infectious disease experienced or whether it may be due to other factors. Certainly, sample size plays a substantial role in the detection of this difference. In a previous analysis of these data, which did not incorporate skeletons excavated at Tamarindito, Arroyo de Piedra, and Punta de Chimino, or the final few burials from Dos Pilas, only the right tibial periostoses were found to be significantly more common in the Terminal Classic period (Wright 1994, 1997a).

That only the tibia shows a significant change is interesting, as it might indicate that trauma or other conditions that led to direct infection of this bone may be at play. For instance, it may be an indication of a change in the proportion of focal

Table 9.10. Temporal comparisons of periostoses in adults

Bone	Side	Late Classic	Terminal Classic	Fisher Exact p
Altar de Sacrificios				
Femur	L	2/5	7/14	1.00
	R	1/5	7/13	0.31
Tibia	L	3/4	9/10	1.00
	R	3/4	8/10	1.00
Fibula	L	2/3	4/5	1.00
	R	1/3	5/8	0.54
Seibal				
Femur	L	4/8	2/11	0.32
	R	5/8	3/11	0.18
Tibia	L	5/6	10/13	1.00
	R	3/5	15/16	0.13
Fibula	L	4/5	6/10	0.60
	R	1/2	3/7	1.00
Dos Pilas				
Femur	L	1/9	1/4	1.00
	R	1/9	1/4	1.00
Tibia	L	5/9	4/4	0.23
	R	4/12	4/4	**0.04**
Fibula	L	2/11	2/3	0.18
	R	4/11	3/4	0.28

Number of bones affected/number of bones observable.
Values in **bold** indicate a significant difference at the $p \leq 0.05$ level.

versus systemic periostitis. Since periosteal reactions are often mixed and superimposed, I do not believe that is possible to discretely classify each skeleton as affected by systemic versus focal periostosis, but the skeletons on which periostoses were described as focal are predominantly from the Terminal Classic period. If these were caused by leishmaniasis, this change would suggest an increase in forest cover at this time when many sites were being abandoned. For intrasite comparisons, it is interesting to note that the Terminal Classic increase is significant only at Dos Pilas, where all four Terminal Classic skeletons are affected. At Dos Pilas we know that the final occupation was very small by Late Classic standards, so a local increase in systemic infection due to the combined effects of crowding and hygiene seems unlikely. Since there are some dietary differences between social groups, and nutritional adequacy may affect disease resistance, it also important to note that burials that can be identified as elite are rare from the Terminal Classic, and absent from both Dos Pilas and Altar de Sacrificios. If this is due to sampling bias, then the trend may be more simply an artifact of social status than an overall health change.

POROTIC HYPEROSTOSIS

Given the rarity of subadult skeletons, temporal comparisons are only feasible for healed anemic scars. Table 9.11 gives the prevalence of lesions and statistical comparisons for each bone in the total sample and for the composite vault score at each multicomponent site. Ideally, one would con-

Table 9.11. Temporal comparisons of porotic hyperostosis in adults

Bone	Preclassic/ Early Classic	Late Classic	Terminal Classic	Preclassic/ Early–Late		Preclassic/ Early–Terminal		Late–Terminal	
				X^2	p	X^2	p	X^2	p
All Sites									
Parietal	5/10	18/30	27/46	*	0.72	0.25	0.61	0.01	0.91
Occipital	2/9	9/20	17/39	*	0.41	1.40	0.24	0.01	0.92
Vault	5/10	19/30	30/46	0.56	0.46	0.81	0.37	0.03	0.87
Altar de Sacrificios									
Vault	3/6	6/7	8/13	*	0.27	*	1.00	*	0.35
Seibal									
Vault	2/3	5/6	13/19	*	1.00	*	1.00	*	0.64
Dos Pilas									
Vault	-	4/6	9/14	-		-		*	1.00

Number of bones affected/number of bones observable.
* Fisher Exact probability was calculated for these comparisons, given the small sample size.
A dash indicates that probability could not be calculated due to mutual absences.

trol for age in order to minimize remodeling bias in intersample comparison, but this is not feasible given the small samples. However, age-related bias is expected to be small, as the age-at-death distributions of the samples are comparable, with only slightly higher representation of middle adults in the Late Classic samples. No statistical differences are detected in the occurrence of porotic hyperostosis between chronological periods for the region as a whole or at individual sites.

Summary

The skeletal pathology data indicate that infection and malnutrition were common afflictions among the Pasión Maya. Porotic hyperostosis is very abundant in Maya skeletal remains, documenting persistent childhood anemia. However, this nutritional stress was felt equally during all periods of Pasión history. Undoubtedly, the synergistic interaction between nutritional stress and infection was responsible for the death of many children, a situation found in all preindustrial societies. It is possible that infectious disease increased slightly in the final phase of occupation of the region, after the collapse of political authority at some sites, but it is difficult to link this shift directly to changes in settlement density. Certainly, early occupants of the Pasión valley suffered a comparable burden of iron deficiency and infection to that experienced during the period of peak population density, yet this stress load did not hinder population growth into the Late Classic period.

CHAPTER 10

Human Biology and the Collapse of the Pasión Region

In this research I have attempted to use human burials—as repositories of both biological and cultural information—to examine the human biological implications of environmental and sociopolitical changes in Pasión Maya prehistory. In the preceding chapters, I treated each "database" in largely independent fashion. Here the results of diverse components of the work are integrated and discussed in the broader context of current perspectives on Pasión Maya history.

Environmental Models and Human Biology

Environmental models of collapse, in particular the model elaborated by Santley, Killion, and Lycett (1986), emphasize deleterious effects of heavy reliance on maize cultivation by the ancient Maya. In particular, nutritional deficiencies inherent in a maize-based diet are posited to provide a proximate biological cause for demographic instability. If this scenario were an accurate conception of the process of collapse that occurred in the Pasión region, the following patterns of diet and health would be predicted. In terms of dietary chemistry, (1) the isotopic composition of bone collagen should indicate heavy reliance on maize as a primary nutritional source. (2) Both isotopic and elemental bone chemistry data should indicate a trend to increasing maize consumption over the span of Pasión occupation, reflecting increasing emphasis on maize agriculture to the exclusion of other cultivated and wild plants and animals. (3) The chemical data should demonstrate a decline in consumption of animal protein over time, a consequence of increased predation pressure on wild fauna and of habitat reduction.

In turn, these dietary shifts are proposed to have brought about health changes. In response to declines in nutritional adequacy and increasing population density, (4) it is predicted that infectious disease increased in prevalence over time, becoming most severe in the Terminal Classic period, and this increasing disease load should be indicated by chronological trends in the abundance of periosteal reactions on long bones. Likewise, (5) severe malnutrition is expected to have increased over time, a consequence of increasing reliance on maize as a primary source of protein. One measure of malnutrition is anemia, which is responsible for lesions of porotic hyperostosis on crania, which are expected to increase in frequency over time. Food stress and malnutrition would have deleterious effects on young children, who are most susceptible to growth disruption. (6) Childhood morbidity should increase in the later periods of Pasión history and be measurable as increased prevalence of enamel hypoplasias in the teeth of adults, recording childhood stress history. Finally, it is important to note that these changes are argued to have come about very gradually as the population level rose. Therefore, changes in diet and health should occur in stepwise pattern across the major chronological divisions.

Diet in the Pasión Region

Pasión diets follow the pattern observed in other New World agricultural economies. Carbon isotopic composition of Pasión bone collagen ranges from −13.5‰ to −6.5‰, resembling the signal of

C4 plants that were important agricultural products. Similar values have been obtained for maize agriculturalists in central North America (Buikstra and Milner 1991; van der Merwe and Vogel 1978), the American Southwest (Ezzo 1992a; Spielmann et al. 1990), Mexico (Farnsworth et al. 1985), lower Central America (Norr 1991), and South America (Ericson et al. 1989). Thus, it seems likely that maize was an important dietary component for the Pasión Maya. Amaranth, vanilla, and CAM plants could also contribute to heavy $\delta^{13}C$, but it is safe to assume that these were less important, given the ubiquitous ethnohistoric and iconographic references to maize.

Although the observed $\delta^{13}C$ values resemble those of maize, recent work suggests that maize consumption is difficult to quantify from collagen $\delta^{13}C$ alone (Schoeninger et al. 1993). Experimental work demonstrates that estimates of C4-plant consumption may be refined using bone apatite $\delta^{13}C$ in conjunction with collagen $\delta^{13}C$, since apatite is constructed from a more representative mix of dietary macronutrients (Ambrose and Norr 1993). However, bone apatite $\delta^{13}C$ was found to be diagenetically contaminated at Dos Pilas (Wright and Schwarcz 1996), so apatite analyses are unlikely to constrain dietary signals with any greater precision in the Pasión region. Analyses of bone apatite from Altar and Seibal by Gerry and Krueger (1997) show a broad correlation with collagen data, as we would expect. Given the evidence for diagenesis at Dos Pilas, however, differences among burials in apatite-collagen $\delta^{13}C$ spacing should be interpreted very cautiously.

It is important to note, however, that the nitrogen isotopic composition of Pasión human collagen is heavier than that expected for a solely herbivorous diet. Indeed, consumption of plant foods alone should not produce a $\delta^{15}N$ in bone collagen higher than about 7‰ (as observed for Pasión herbivores), yet human collagen $\delta^{15}N$ ranges from 7‰ to 12‰. This result indicates that Pasión diets included a significant amount of animal protein. Furthermore, consumption of terrestrial herbivore meat should not raise human collagen $\delta^{15}N$ higher than about 11‰, so freshwater fish may also have been an important source of protein for some Pasión inhabitants. In view of the range of values obtained, it seems plausible that Pasión collagen $\delta^{15}N$ is largely from animal protein and that plant proteins contribute somewhat less to collagen synthesis.

The carbon isotopic composition of Pasión human collagen, spanning −13.5‰ to −6.5‰, must also incorporate this animal protein. The mean collagen $\delta^{13}C$ measured in a larger series of Pasión white-tailed deer was −20.55±1.0‰ (Emery et al. 2000), which would indicate an average meat value of −22.9‰. Thus, on average, meat consumption should produce human collagen values around −18‰. The further ^{13}C enrichment seen in the human collagen could be due to maize consumption both by humans and by some of the animals they consumed. For instance, the broad range in herbivore collagen values indicates that some animals did browse in maize fields. Similar ranges of $\delta^{13}C$ have been reported for archaeological herbivores from Belize (White et al. 1993; White et al. 2001), which White and colleagues discuss as evidence for "semi-domestication." Since one modern feral peccary from the Petexbatun had a C4-like signature, these values need not be taken as evidence for human intervention. With such heavy herbivore collagen $\delta^{13}C$, meat of the same animals could reach −15.4‰ (DeNiro and Epstein 1978), and a purely carnivorous diet of this enriched herbivore meat could produce human collagen as high as −11‰! The enriched $\delta^{13}C$ of −14.8‰ measured for one ancient puma, which approaches the human data, shows that it too consumed some C4-eating prey. However, enriched herbivores are quite rare among the prehistoric fauna sampled to date (Emery et al. 2000).

Animals that were purposely domesticated are more likely to have significantly enriched human diets. If, as one prehistoric sample indicates, domestic turkeys were fed maize, their consumption (meat $\delta^{13}C \approx -12.5$‰) would be significant. As at other sites in the Maya area (Tykot et al. 1996; White et al. 1993; White et al. 2001), the $\delta^{13}C$ data indicates that Pasión dogs were fed maize and would have had meat values as high as −10.5‰. Thus, dog consumption would also contribute to heavy human $\delta^{13}C$ and could explain the full range of human signals. However, archaeological, ethnohistoric, and ethnographic data indicate that

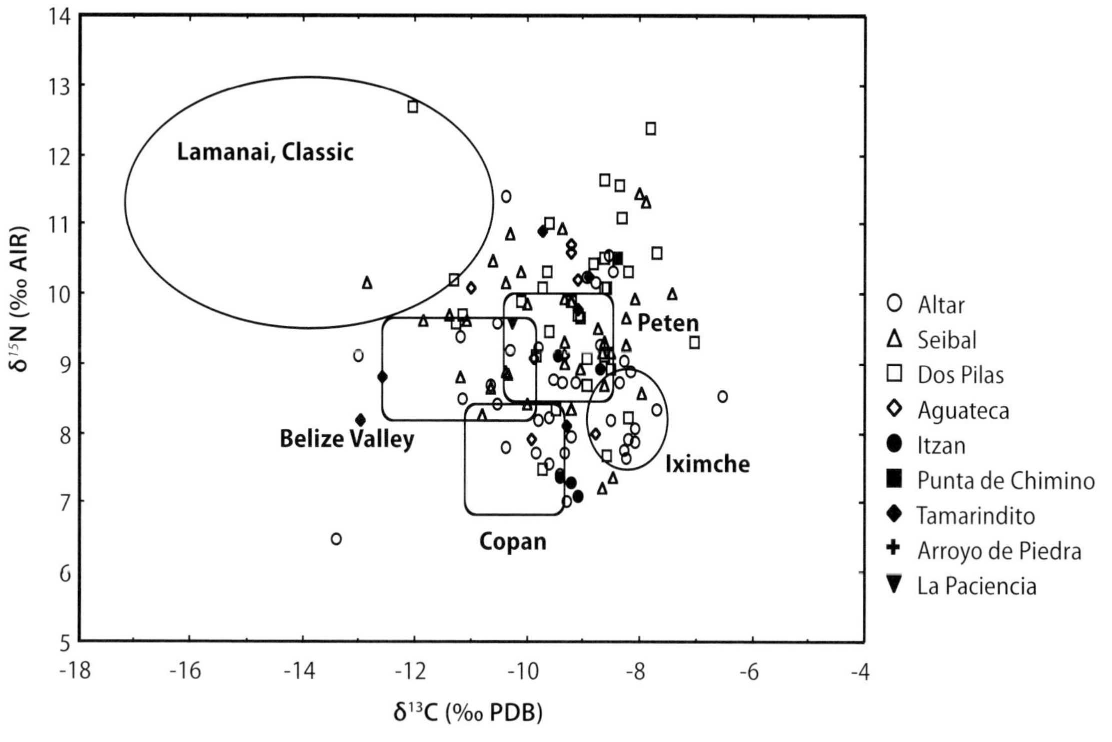

Figure 10.1. Isotopic composition of Pasion bone collagen in comparison with data from other Maya sites

maize consumption provided a significant amount of dietary proteins, so we must expect that maize consumption accounts for much of the observed human ^{13}C enrichment beyond ≈15‰.

The Pasión data can also be examined in relation to other Maya sites where isotopic analyses have been conducted (Figure 10.1). The rounded boxes in the graph illustrate the regional means plus or minus one standard deviation obtained by Gerry and Krueger (1997) for the Belize Valley region (Barton Ramie, Baking Pot), the Peten (Uaxactun, Holmul, Altar, Seibal), and Copan valley (the earlier Harvard excavations). The circle indicates the mean plus or minus one standard deviation for Whittington and Reed's (1998) data from Postclassic Iximche. The oval indicates the mean value for Classic period collagen from Lamanai (White and Schwarcz 1989). Postclassic burials from Lamanai are more enriched in $\delta^{13}C$ and overlap broadly with Peten values shown here. The Copan data reported by Reed (1998, 1999) are about one permil more enriched in $\delta^{13}C$ than the means shown here from Gerry and Krueger (1997), presumably due to social differences in sampling. Although not illustrated (to simplify the graph), isotopic data from Preclassic Cuello (Tykot et al. 1996) are similar to the Classic period Lamanai results, and diets at Pacbitun (White et al. 1993) give isotope values intermediate to Gerry and Krueger's Peten and Belize Valley groups.

Pasión diets reported here broadly overlap with the isotopic composition of Classic period sites in the central Peten, Belize Valley, and Postclassic/Colonial Lamanai. The Pasión and Lamanai regions share many ecological characteristics, particularly the availability of freshwater aquatic fauna; however, Lamanai's proximity to the coast availed it of estuarine and coral reef resources. In contrast, Pacbitun and the Belize Valley sites had local access to some freshwater foods and limited access to marine resources (by trade alone). Pacbitun in particular may have had greater access to terrestrial faunal reserves in the pine ridge ecozone of the nearby Maya Mountains. ^{13}C-enrichment from terrestrial faunal consumption like that proposed for the Pasión may contribute substantially to the δ^{13}C of Pacbitun collagen, given the comparable δ^{15}N observed (White et al. 1993).

Coastal diet from Mojo Cay in Belize falls at the upper range of Pasión data and is quite positive in δ^{13}C, owing to consumption of marine reef fauna that have δ^{13}C comparable to that of maize (Norr 1991). This marine faunal effect may also contribute to the Postclassic and Colonial signatures at Lamanai (White and Schwarcz 1989), in view of its location near the coast and its known participation in coastal trade (Pendergast 1986). Late Classic Lamanai diets are particularly distinctive for their low δ^{13}C, which suggested to White and Schwarcz (1989) very little maize or reef fauna consumption and greater reliance on C3 plants or terrestrial fauna. They state that freshwater fish were seldom consumed (White and Schwarcz 1989:467). Since freshwater fish had not been sampled from the Maya area prior to the Petexbatun data reported here, it seems likely that consumption of local lagoon fish would contribute to both the low δ^{13}C and high δ^{15}N—especially in the Early Classic tomb male—of Classic Lamanai diets. Marine foods are unlikely to contribute to the high δ^{15}N of Pasión diets due to the inland location. Although there is no direct evidence to support it, the possibility of salted and dried fish trade (Lange 1971) cannot be excluded. Such rare exotic foods would have been consumed by very few elite individuals and have a negligible effect on average collagen values.

Pasión human collagen is substantially more enriched in ^{15}N than is human collagen from Copan (Reed 1998, 1999; Gerry and Krueger 1997), indicating that meat consumption was more restricted at the latter site. While climatic conditions at Copan are very different than in the Pasión, an environmental distinction is unlikely to account for this discrepancy since greater aridity at Copan should be correlated with heavier δ^{15}N (Heaton et al. 1986), the opposite of the observed difference. Given this discrepancy in δ^{15}N, the comparable δ^{13}C cannot be taken to indicate equivalent levels of maize consumption at the two sites. Since greater meat consumption contributes to the δ^{13}C of Pasión samples, it is probable that maize was relatively more important to Copan diets than to Pasión diets. Whittington and Reed (1998) have suggested that the high δ^{13}C at Postclassic Iximche in the Guatemalan highlands is partly due to enrichment in maize δ^{13}C with high elevation. Like Copan, however, the Iximche collagen is also isotopically light in nitrogen, suggesting lower meat consumption than by most Peten individuals.

Maize was certainly an important component of ancient Pasión diets for both humans and fauna alike. Hence, the basic premise that maize constituted an important staple for the Pasión Maya is confirmed by the results of this work. Quantification of maize consumption is more difficult, however, considering the role of C4-meat enrichment, it is likely that maize was less important than has been suggested in previous isotopic studies of Maya skeletons. When the Pasión data are compared to data from other sites, regional variability in maize and meat consumption is clearly demonstrated, revealing considerable flexibility in dietary strategies and resources not so severely stressed as to enforce extreme reliance on maize as *the* primary source of sustenance.

The isotopic and elemental data from Altar partially support the hypothesis of increasing maize reliance, with an observed increase in maize consumption into the Late Classic period. Altar δ^{13}C rises from a Preclassic mean of –10.4‰ to a Late Classic mean of –8.3‰. Given the stability observed in δ^{15}N, the Late Classic ^{13}C-enrichment can be attributed with some confidence to maize consumption at the expense of C3 plants. Chronological trends in Ba/Ca mirror this pattern and can be taken as confirmation of increasing maize consumption over time at Altar. However, the lower δ^{13}C and Ba/Ca of the Terminal Classic samples at Altar contradicts the model. This decline in maize consumption indicates that a greater diversity of plant foods was exploited in the final occupation after the elite collapse of the site. If nutritional inadequacies of maize are to be blamed for health stress, then these more diverse Terminal Classic diets imply nutritional improvement in the final occupation, instead of the expected decline.

Chronological trends in maize consumption

at Seibal also violate the expectations of environmental models. Carbon isotopic ratios are stable over time at Seibal, indicating little increase in maize consumption from Preclassic through Terminal Classic times. Maize consumption did not increase in the Terminal Classic when the dramatic Bayal population increase ought to show the most rapid dietary change in the face of environmental catastrophe; however, maize consumption did not decline in the way seen at Altar either. If the high levels of maize consumption documented in Late Classic Altar had contributed to the early collapse of political authority there, it is difficult to see how coeval Seibal, where maize was consumed to an equivalent degree, could have escaped a simi-lar fate. Moreover, significant maize consumption in the Preclassic did not hinder the growth of large Late and Terminal Classic populations at Seibal.

At Dos Pilas, the mean Terminal Classic $\delta^{13}C$ is about one half permil lighter than in the Late Classic, but the difference is not significant, whether the decapitated crania—who are likely nonlocal—are included or not. Given the dramatic loss in population at Dos Pilas, this stability in maize consumption cannot be taken to indicate continued stress on dietary resources in the Terminal Classic occupation.

Chronological trends in maize consumption have been inferred from isotopic data for Lamanai and Pacbitun (White et al. 1993; White and Schwarcz 1989). As yet, the Copan data are restricted to the Coner phase (Reed 1998). At Lamanai, $\delta^{13}C$ declined over the course of the Classic period to a very low level during the Terminal Classic period (-15‰). While other nearby sites collapsed during the tenth century, Lamanai survived and flourished through the Postclassic, and was occupied into early Historic times. Postclassic Lamanai collagen shows a dramatic enrichment in ^{13}C over the Terminal Classic level, rising to –9.6‰ (White and Schwarcz 1989), a level comparable to the Pasión data. While it is tempting to speculate that Lamanai's populace weathered the collapse because of their minimal maize consumption, the high levels of Postclassic $\delta^{13}C$ cannot be so easily explained by maize reliance imposed by agricultural stress. White and Schwarcz (1989:469) suggest that the dietary change reflects cultural changes in "political and economic activities."

At Pacbitun, chronological trends in $\delta^{13}C$ closely resemble the pattern observed at Altar. As noted above, both the carbon and nitrogen isotopic data from Pacbitun are broadly comparable to the Pasión data, suggesting similar dietary strategies. Terminal Classic Pacbitun burials show a slight decrease in $\delta^{13}C$ (about 1.5‰) with respect to the Late Classic period. In contrast to my interpretation for Altar, White et al. (1993) infer that farmers were unable to produce sufficient maize to supply population demands and that the decline supports the role of environmental stress in the collapse. Yet, clearly, the Lamanai Maya were able to cope with a diet in which maize was substantially less important than at Pacbitun or in the Pasión. It is important to note that chemical data can only evaluate the relative contribution of different foods consumed and are unable to assess foodstuff availability or the prevalence of *under*nutrition (as opposed to malnutrition). For answers to those questions, we must look to paleopathology.

Trends in protein consumption do not strictly follow the predictions of environmental models either. Altar and Dos Pilas show no chronological trends in isotopic or elemental data that would confirm a decline in the quantity or quality of protein sources exploited. Human collagen is sufficiently enriched in ^{15}N at both sites (7.0–11.7‰) to indicate that animal protein was a significant component of the diet. Protein deficiency would seem to be an unlikely correlate of these data. If large Late Classic human occupations had decimated faunal populations in the environs of the sites, then a change in nitrogen isotopes would be expected. Despite the elite collapse, population density remained high at Terminal Classic Altar, so pressure on local fauna would not have diminished and a decline in $\delta^{15}N$ would be expected. It was not observed. Faunal populations might have recovered slightly near Dos Pilas, since the Terminal Classic population was so small there. Yet no change in protein procurement occurred—an indirect indication that Late Classic faunal populations were not unduly stressed.

At Seibal, $\delta^{15}N$ is quite high in Preclassic and

Late Classic collagen, indicating substantial animal protein consumption. When the isotopic and elemental data are considered together, Seibal's Late Classic inhabitants seem to have relied more heavily on freshwater protein consumption than did the Preclassic population. Terminal Classic (Bayal) diets do decrease in $\delta^{15}N$, providing *prima facie* support for the expectation of declining meat consumption. But this change probably signals a relative decrease in fish consumption, an interpretation that is supported by a coeval decline in Sr/Ca in bone mineral. Terminal Classic protein sources may have been based more terrestrially. Nonetheless, the mean $\delta^{15}N$ composition is still high overall (8.91‰), indicating that animal protein supplies were not compromised. The possible shift to aquatic protein sources in the Late Classic period might be taken to imply stressed faunal populations, but aquatic fauna are also very sensitive to overpredation.

These results are comparable to isotopic results obtained in previous studies of Maya diet. At both Lamanai and Pacbitun, nitrogen isotopic signals are remarkably steady over time, indicating little change in meat consumption. At Lamanai, $\delta^{15}N$ shows extreme stability in the face of dramatic changes in $\delta^{13}C$ over the site's history. At Pacbitun, a slight trend toward increasing $\delta^{15}N$ may be apparent, but it is statistically insignificant and compromised by the small Early Classic sample. If this trend were substantiated, it would imply an improvement in protein nutrition, directly conflicting with the expectations of environmental collapse models.

Both the absolute composition of prehistoric diets and the trends in dietary chemistry over the span of ancient Maya occupation in the Pasión region contradict the expectations of environmental models of the collapse. Furthermore, dietary differences among sites within the region also suggest that agricultural systems were not severely stressed. If environmental pressure were so great that all available land was dedicated to maize cultivation, thereby prohibiting further expansion, then we should expect all sites to show equivalent diets, with very narrow ranges overall. Preclassic diets differ markedly between Altar and Seibal in terms of both floral and faunal consumption. As these two sites had access to comparable ecozones, the dietary differences must be attributed to cultural factors rather than environmental variation (cf. White et al. 1993). The Late Classic sites are broadly comparable but show some important differences, particularly in the heavier $\delta^{15}N$ of Seibal and heavier $\delta^{13}C$ of Altar. Sampling biases that might account for these differences were discussed in Chapter 7; these patterns are unlikely to be artifacts of sampling bias. Instead, they indicate considerable heterogeneity in food preferences among sites.

This is sharply contrasted by the comparable diets among Terminal Classic sites. Yet, each Terminal Classic site shows a broad range of isotopic signatures, indicating that considerable diversity existed among members of these contemporary populations. Together with changes in social parameters symbolized in mortuary ritual, this dietary breadth may be a consequence of changing social privileges or population movement between sites within the region. The Pasión data contribute to the picture of dietary variability in the Maya Lowlands that is emerging as chemical data become available for more sites.

Health and Disease in the Pasión Region

Infectious disease loads can best be gauged through the occurrence of periosteal reactions, which are common on Pasión skeletons. The lower limb bones are most commonly affected, with sclerotic left-tibial diaphyseal reactions in 70% of adults. Chronological trends in periostitis abundance give a mixed answer to the question of disease load changes over time in the Pasión region. Trends are not apparent for most bones; however, a significant increase in Terminal Classic tibial periostitis is found for both left and right tibiae. These results might suggest an increase in infectious disease in the final occupation, especially at Seibal and Altar de Sacrificios, due perhaps to overcrowding as residents of the Petexbatun area abandoned sites and moved into the Pasión valley. As discussed in Chapter 9, this does not seem like a sufficient explanation because of the presence of bilateral tibial lesions on all four primary burials from Dos Pilas, where the Terminal Classic occupation cannot be described as crowded.

Although anecdotal data about periostitis is available for other Maya series, chronological trends in infectious disease have been examined at very few sites. An important exception is the large series from Copan, Honduras. Whittington (1989) found that the highest frequency of periosteal reactions occurred in Late Classic Copan skeletons (Early Coner) and that they declined in the Terminal Classic period (Late Coner), a statistically significant result. He attributes this decline to migration from the core to peripheral settlement following Copan's political collapse. Despite the apparent conflict with the expectation of deteriorating health, Whittington (1989:370) argues that "the low status population at Copan was highly stressed and unhealthy during the periods leading up to and following the political collapse" and implies that this illness contributed to the site's decline. He bases this conclusion on the interpretation that infection (and anemia) had a measurable impact on the longevity of Copanecos. Yet he found no significant relationships between the presence of periosteal reactions and age-at-death for any bone (Whittington 1989:336, 373).

In lower Central America, Norr (1991) found substantial variability in periosteal reactions among populations with differing subsistence strategies. However, she observed the greatest frequency of lesions in an early population with a mixed marine and terrestrial subsistence strategy, not in the later maize agriculturalists, so infection cannot be seen simply as a consequence of population density and maize reliance in lowland tropical environments.

The high frequency of periosteal reactions might be attributed to two tropical diseases: yaws and leishmaniasis. The prevalence and pattern of periostoses in Pasión skeletal material is very similar to that encountered in other prehistoric populations, such as the American Southeast and Midwest, where the pattern of periostoses has been interpreted as evidence for endemic infection by treponematosis (Cook 1976; Powell 1988). Lesion morphology is more consistent with yaws than endemic syphilis, as would be expected in this humid tropical climate. Leishmaniasis, a known prehispanic lowland parasite, could well account for many focal periostitic lesions, although its contribution to bone pathology has received little systematic attention to date. It is possible that an increase in leishmaniasis or other traumatically induced tibial infections contributes to the observed Terminal Classic trend, which might occur in an environment with increasing forest cover, as at Dos Pilas.

If a yaws-like treponematosis was endemic in the Pasión, this disease could account for a significant proportion of observed periostoses. In endemic regions, 60 to 100% of the population is seropositive for yaws, and bone lesions occur in up to 20% of individuals with clinical symptoms (Hackett 1951). Yet, yaws and endemic syphilis are chronic subacute conditions that seldom cause death and have a negligible effect on fertility. As Powell (1991) notes, the biological cost of treponemal infection is low despite its high visibility in a skeletal series. Similarly, leishmaniasis—particularly that due to *L. mexicana*, which was probably the only prehispanic species in the Petén—is a chronic condition with few repercussions for health status as a whole. Both conditions are unlikely culprits for population collapse. Neither is likely to hinder reproductive success or work capacity significantly. Moreover, there is little data to suggest that either condition is dramatically exacerbated by nutritional stress.

Hence, it is difficult to evaluate the implications of the observed trend in periostitis for the Pasión. The increase may indicate a rise in infectious disease levels in general, but might also indicate a rise in specific conditions for which crowding is not a contributing factor. In the absence of statistically significant results for other bones, I am hesitant to assert that the observed pattern is due to elevated disease load, although this cannot be excluded from consideration.

Porotic hyperostosis—a skeletal manifestation of iron-deficiency anemia—is very common in Pasión crania. About 65% of the population that lived to adulthood had survived a bout of chronic anemia during childhood. Most subadult skeletons also show anemic lesions, from which we can infer that childhood nutritional stress was severe and perhaps implicated in the early mortality of these individuals. Among adults in the Pasión, the prevalence of healed porotic hyperostosis is stable over time, indicating that equivalent proportions of the population had survived anemic episodes in later as in earlier times.

Lower levels of anemia are observed at Classic period Lamanai than in the Pasión, but increased levels are found in the Postclassic period skeletons, a time when maize consumption also increased dramatically (White 1986, 1988). Further increases in anemia at Colonial period Lamanai can be attributed to the effects of introduced Old World infection and parasitism (White et al. 1994).

The frequencies of porotic hyperostosis in "low status" Copan burials observed by Whittington (1989) are similar to those found in the Pasión. However, he found no difference between early and later anemic lesions, perhaps because of the paucity of early (Acbi) skeletons. Whittington (1989:306) argued that anemic stress had significant impact on Copan demographic stability because adult skeletons with anemic scars have a younger mean age-at-death (36.0 years, $n = 18$) than those without such lesions (45.1 years, $n = 12$). Although statistically confirmed, this trend is obtained from point estimates of age-at-death on a fairly small skeletal sample. If incorporated into the test, the broad error inherent in skeletal age might render the discrepancy nonsignificant. Remodeling of sclerotic lesions with age can also be expected to have obliterated lesions in older adults.

As noted in previous chapters, Pasión skeletons show no significant correlations between age-at-death and paleopathological indicators that demonstrate the impact of health stress on demographic processes in the region. The high frequency of healed anemic scars in adult remains indicates that this childhood experience did not prohibit survival. In view of the rarity of anemic lesions in modern highland Mayan skulls and the high levels of anemia their children experience, it is possible that the abundant lesions on Pasión crania are evidence that, despite anemia, significant numbers of Pasión children were able to survive to adulthood (Wright and Chew 1998). Regardless, stability of porotic hyperostotic prevalence over time in the Pasión indicates little deterioration of nutritional status over the span of occupation in the region.

Enamel hypoplasias are fairly common on Pasión teeth. Hypoplasias occur on 60% or more of canines and maxillary incisors in all time periods. Because these teeth are the most sensitive to growth disruption, they provide the best measures of total morbidity experience in childhood. For those teeth that are most susceptible to stress, no statistical difference in the proportion of teeth showing hypoplasias exists between chronological periods for the region as a whole, indicating a stable burden of childhood illness over Pasión history. As in the case of anemia, this result contradicts the expectation of deteriorating childhood health in the years preceding the collapse.

Significant chronological trends are documented for other teeth, however, that reveal a subtle change in the distribution of morbidity over the childhood years. Changes in the proportion of premolars showing hypoplasias in the Terminal Classic series point to a narrowing of the age of peak illness. This interpretation is bolstered by a decline in the mean age of formation of canine defects in this final occupation. These changes may be due to either of two possible explanations. First, they might occur because of a decline in social variability in child feeding practices. This hypothesis is supported by the apparent reduction in social correlates of dietary diversity in the Terminal Classic population of the Pasión region. Alternately, a shift to earlier weaning by some members of the Terminal Classic population, occasioned by reduced pressure on dietary resources, could lead to a decline in stress at older ages. This would occur if extended lactation during the Late Classic period had influenced the distribution of defects seen in adult teeth by improving the survivorship of frail children. For Dos Pilas and Altar de Sacrificios, reduced Terminal Classic maize consumption might hint at reduced pressure on food sources. However, at Seibal, increased population density might have the opposite effect. Thus, it is difficult to choose between these explanations of the trend. Indeed, it is possible that both contribute to the reduced peak age of childhood illness in the final years of Pasión history.

Although Bishop Landa's observation (Tozzer 1941:125) that the Maya weaned children at 4 years of age accords well with the peak age of hypoplasias, it probably refers to the end of breastfeeding rather than the initial supplementation of milk with solid foods. Oxygen isotope data from Kaminaljuyu suggest that the highland Maya may have weaned around 5 years of age (Wright and Schwarcz 1998), and this may also be true of the lowland Maya, for whom no direct data on weaning are yet available.

Danforth (1989:176) suggests that "weaning" (by which she means solid food supplementation) occurred around 2 years of age in both Late Classic Petén sites and Colonial Tipu. This is the same age that C_1 enamel microdefects peak. She contends that the later hypoplasia mode at 3.5–4.0 years of age is a consequence of continued post-weaning stress. Higher frequencies of hypoplasia occur around age 3.5 years in Late Classic skeletons than in Colonial Tipuans, though all defect profiles are similar for stress experienced at younger ages (Danforth 1989). This pattern complements the result obtained here. In the Pasión, the trend toward more concentrated childhood stress at younger ages, observed at Colonial Tipu, began in the Terminal Classic.

In a previous study of the Altar skeletal collection, Saul (1972) found hypoplasias affecting 92% of adult dentitions, with little change in prevalence over time. Because he reports the data by individual rather than by tooth, it is difficult to compare his results to mine. At Seibal, Saul (1973) also scored a higher prevalence of hypoplasias than I observed, with minimal change in occurrence over time. For Lamanai, White (1986) recorded a hypoplastic prevalence comparable to the Pasión data and, similarly, found no temporal trends despite the marked changes in diet and porotic hyperostosis in that series. Whittington (1989) observed that approximately 100% of low-status Copan skeletons are estimated to have been affected by hypoplasias on I_2, C_1, and P_3. He detected no statistical difference in hypoplastic occurrence between Acbi, Early, and Late Coner phase burials. As in the case of porotic hyperostosis, the effect of different scoring standards and reporting methods for hypoplasia used by different investigators hinder direct intersite comparisons of hypoplastic frequency. Although hypoplastic prevalence may be greater overall at Copan, the paucity of chronological trends in each of these studies corroborates the pattern of defect stability described here for the Pasión. Analysis of Late Coner subadult teeth (Storey 1992a) reveals that many elite Copanec children suffered growth disruptions in utero, suggesting that maternal health was compromised during pregnancy and lactation. Storey (1992b:166) argues that this high prevalence of subadult dental defects points to "problems . . . that may explain why the Copan area declined in population and was finally abandoned." Unfortunately, no data are yet available from earlier occupations at Copan with which to compare chronological trends in subadult teeth.

Summary

The results of paleodietary and paleopathological investigations in the Pasión provide little support for models that emphasize environmental pressures in the collapse of Classic Maya society. Bone chemical data indicate that Pasión diets included a substantial amount of animal protein and that dietary shifts did not follow the predicted maize increase and meat decrease. Instead, diets were socially and regionally heterogenous. Chronological trends in the total levels of anemia and childhood growth disruption were not observed, despite the widespread perception among archaeologists that Late Classic populations were much worse off than early Maya groups. However, evidence of infectious disease on the tibiae of Pasión skeletons is more common in the final occupation. This might indicate increased crowding at Seibal or perhaps increased interaction with a forested environment after the abandonment of many sites at the end of the Late Classic. Sampling bias is not a convincing explanation for the rarity of chronological trends in health indicators in the combined sample because the biases of individual sites (e.g., toward elites at Altar) are counter-balanced by opposing biases at other sites (e.g., toward nonelites at Dos Pilas and Seibal). Although paleopathology faces difficulty in determining whether changes in skeletal lesion abundances reflect a decline or improvement in overall frailty to disease (Wood et al. 1992), stability in most aspects of health experience is the most parsimonious explanation of these data. There is little reason to suppose that health stress was a significant factor in the collapse of the sites, since it apparently did not hinder the development of large Late Classic populations. This is not to say that the Pasión Maya were the picture of health. Levels of bone infection and anemia are high and illustrate that disease was a constant element of Maya life, as indeed it is to all human populations. Dietary choices surely played a role in the expression of these illnesses but cannot be held accountable for the trajectory of Maya society in the ninth- and tenth-century lowlands.

That natural resources were not under undue strain at the height of Maya occupation in the Pasión region is also supported by the results of recent paleoecological research, reported by Dunning and Beach (forthcoming). Sediment cores from the Lagunas Petexbatun and Tamarindito indicate a significant episode of erosion associated with the Preclassic colonization of the area but no exacerbation of the process during the Late Classic population peak. In fact, cores from the east part of Laguna Tamarindito show minimal silting despite dense Late Classic occupation on this side of the lake, and imply minimal landscape degradation. Although the pollen record is somewhat problematic, it seems to reveal the maintenance of substantial stands of primary forest throughout the occupation of the region. Relative to the Central Petén Lakes, the Petexbatun cores contain more primary forest pollen, demonstrating the maintenance of greater tree cover than in the former region (Dunning and Beach, n.d.; Dunning et al. 1997; Dunning et al. 1998; Dunning and Beach 1994). Faunal assemblages from Petexbatun excavations contain a significant component of primary forest species. Animals that require large areas of secluded forest—and are today facing habitat pressure—such as the tapir, large cats, and monkeys, are present in both the Petexbatun and Seibal faunal samples, indicating maintenance of these forest ecotypes (Emery 1997; Pohl 1985). Indeed, it has been suggested that the rarity of juvenile deer bones at Seibal implies that hunting pressure was low (Pohl 1985:138). These observations support the conclusion reached in the present work that Pasión agricultural systems were not stretched to the breaking point and that dietary patterns need not be attributed to strict environmental limitations.

For the Pasión, these results are not in keeping with White's (1997; White et al. 1993) argument that Terminal Classic maize consumption declined at Pacbitun due to inadequate maize supplies. If large areas of forest were maintained, then it should have been possible to intensify maize production by expanding agrosystems in step with demand. Biotic diversity of the Pasión was not dramatically reduced as would be expected if agricultural pressure had transformed the later Classic landscape to the extent required for an environmentally induced collapse. Although these results do not accord well with a model of progressively increasing nutritional and health stress over the span of occupation, they do not exclude the possibility of extremely rapid change in the nutritional environment, because the time spans considered are quite broad and thus homogenize chronological variability over time.

Problems with Environmental Models of Collapse

Even though it has not been rigorously evaluated, the hypothesis that inadequate diet and poor health directly contributed to the collapse of southern Lowland Maya cities has come to be accepted by many archaeologists (Culbert 1988; Rice 1993; Schele and Freidel 1990; Sharer 1994; Tainter 1988; Webster et al. 1992). In addition to a lack of concrete data, this tendency may be due to several long-standing assumptions regarding Maya subsistence and dubious interpretations of the biological cost of skeletal pathology.

Misconceptions about the nutritional value of maize diets founded in uncritical analogy with modern Mesoamerican diets and agricultural practices lie at the core of nutritional arguments about population collapse. The interpretation of maize as nutritionally poor is an omnipresent element in environmental collapse models. These arguments emphasize the low protein content of maize and imbalances among maize amino acids. For instance, Santley et al. (1986:137) focus on specific amino-acid deficiencies in maize. Although they mention that these are alleviated by alkaline processing, which removes the phytate-containing pericarp of the maize kernel (Bressani et al. 1958; Bressani and Scrimshaw 1958; Katz et al. 1974), nonetheless they conclude that "levels of tryptophan and methionine consumption were grossly inadequate. These deficiencies, together with the unfavorable leucine/isoleucine ratio and the intake of large quantities of phytate, produced niacin, zinc, and iron deficiencies" (Santley et al. 1986:138).

This conclusion is unwarranted because alkaline processing was almost certainly practiced by the ancient Maya just as it is by their modern descendants. In addition, preparation of maize for *pozole* improves the protein composition by partial fermentation (Cravioto et al. 1955). Together with consumption of beans, these two processing techniques make maize a rather good source of nutrition for most age groups.

Nutritional data collected in Mexico and Guatemala have been very important in modeling childhood health and nutrition in developing countries (Bongaarts and Delgado 1977; Chavez and Martinez 1982; Scrimshaw 1990; Sibrián and Elston 1990). Yet, many of these studies focus on ladino populations, on indigenous peoples in urban contexts, or on poor rural villages with minimal land holdings. These people have little control over food production. Although work in the 1960s identified protein as a limiting factor in maize diets and as the key deficiency of kwashiorkor, more recent research indicates that the relationship is ambiguous. For most children in Guatemala, maize diets do provide the recommended protein allowances; energy deficiency is the key problem. Growth is stunted because of inadequate total consumption (undernutrition), which, rather than being caused by the quality of available food, may be due to appetite loss at the hand of infection and social and behavioral factors (Behár 1977; Bogin 1988; Waterlow and Payne 1975:130–1). Childhood nutrition today is further complicated by the larger number of Old World infectious pathogens; when combating infections, a child's food intake declines dramatically.

In addition to radical changes in the pathogen load of native populations subsequent to contact between Old and New World populations, direct projection of this poor nutritional status into prehistory is not necessarily warranted. Undernutrition in Central America today is primarily a consequence of socioeconomic deprivation and reflects politically mediated inequality, not the inherent qualities of maize. Today, the low socioeconomic status of highland Maya peoples puts most animal protein beyond monetary reach, and wild faunal populations have been decimated by habitat destruction due to land appropriation for coffee, rice, and sugarcane *fincas* on a scale far exceeding that of ancient agriculture. With the arrival of new domestic fauna and cultigens from the Old World (Marcus 1982; Vargas 1990:153–4), indigenous foods came to be redefined as socially inferior, leading to abandonment of some advantageous prehispanic dietary practices, a trend that is ongoing today (e.g., Healy et al. 1990:178–80). Because Spanish diets emphasized cereals, the early colonists were particularly impressed with *Zea mays* and encouraged cultivation of maize over other crops. In order to keep up with Spanish maize demands, complex indigenous agricultural systems that exploited a variety of crops shifted toward maize monocropping (Atran 1993). Although this cereal demand did not greatly modify agricultural systems of some indigenous Maya in lowland frontier areas (such as the Lacandon Forest and parts of Petén), diets of the emerging Yucatec and highland mestizos and ladinos may have shifted toward the Spanish cereal emphasis in which maize may have provided most of the protein and calories consumed.

The conquest may also have precipitated a change in Maya culinary uses of maize. Throughout Mesoamerica today the bulk of maize is consumed as tortillas, but ceramic and iconographic evidence points to the tamale as the primary maize product consumed during the Classic and, perhaps, Postclassic periods (Taube 1989). While comales that could have been used for cooking tortillas have been found in the lowlands, they are quite rare and other functions have been proposed, such as cacao toasting (Smith 1971:84). The comal is often thought to have been introduced to the Maya area during the Postclassic when interaction with Central Mexico intensified; however, a few have been found in Classic period contexts in the Petexbatun region (Inomata, personal communication 1999). Because of the rarity of comales even in Postclassic ceramic assemblages, it is fairly certain that the heavy emphasis on tortilla consumption is a recent phenomenon (Taube 1989:33–34; Marcus 1982:248). Tortillas require less complex preparation than do tamales, so can be produced more efficiently, but they are of lower nutritional value than tamales. Moreover, tamales are usually stuffed with meat. In conjunction with Spanish starch preferences, this technological shift has implications for consumption of both maize and meats in modern Mesoamerican diets, especially those in easily accessible and urban areas, where most nutrition research has been done.

Such colonial changes in diet are clearly relevant to the idea that prehispanic diets may have been deficient in vitamin C. Saul's diagnosis of scurvy (vitamin C deficiency) in Maya skeletons (Saul 1972, 1973) was bolstered by the observation that 20th-century Yucatec consume little fruit, despite the abundance of both cultivated and wild fruit trees (Benedict and Steggerda 1937; Shattuck 1938). This diagnosis is problematic on pathological grounds (Chapter 9), but neither is the Yucatec analogy directly applicable to a prehispanic context. Danforth (1989:20–21) cogently argues that fruit provided an important source of sugar in the prehispanic diet. The low fruit consumption of modern Yucatecans is directly related to the mass production of processed sugar from sugarcane—an Old World import—which has replaced fruit as the primary sugar source (Benedict and Steggerda 1937). Danforth also notes that the Maya consume greens, such as chaya, that are high in vitamin C. Perhaps more significant is the contribution of chili peppers, which are eaten in large quantities with virtually every Maya meal and have much higher levels of vitamin C than fruits (I.N.C.A.P. 1961:34–36).

Students of native farming systems are now beginning to appreciate the complexity of agricultural strategies employed by Maya peoples in tropical forest environments. Surprisingly resistant to Spanish influence over the last 500 years, Lacandon and Itza Maya practice complex agroforestry, which exploits a diversity of wild and cultivated species and incorporates sophisticated forest management into the agricultural cycle (Atran 1993; Barrera et al. 1977; Nations and Nigh 1980). Continuing research into ancient agronomic technology is beginning to reveal the complexity of Maya microenvironmental adaptation (Dunning et al. 1997; Dunning and Beach 1994; Fedick and Ford 1990), but the preconception that Late Classic agriculture emphasized maize monocropping is particularly tenacious (Atran 1993; c.f. commentary by Chase, Webb, and Fedick). The existence of land-form modification, such as terracing and raised fields, does not thereby imply use of a monocropping system.

Skeletal pathology of ancient Maya burials has played an enormous role in bolstering the ecological model, but interpretations about the biological cost of bone disease and the implications of changing lesion abundance have seldom been firmly grounded. To this day, we have a poor understanding of the correspondence between levels of bone disease in mortality samples and the actual health status of the living population from which it was derived, a factor that hinders comparison of ancient health to modern standards (Wood et al. 1992; Wright and Chew 1998). Today the proliferation of skeletal research provides a framework against which to judge the distinctiveness of health patterns in a sample, but Frank Saul's (1972) documentation of skeletal pathology at Altar was published at a time when few other paleopathology studies were available. Saul was surprised by the apparent severity of disease shown in Altar bone, commenting, "In fact, one might wonder, not *why* they declined, but rather, *how* they managed to survive for so long" (Saul 1972:73, emphasis in original).

Likewise, archaeologists have been impressed by Saul's "gruesome" photos and further misinterpret the impact of disease on Maya peoples by exaggeration. For instance, Lowe (1985:92, emphasis added) discusses the Altar osteological data as "evidence from some burials of severe malnutrition and *starvation*." More recent work at Copan is similarly miscited or is cited secondhand (Rice 1993:43; Tainter 1988:174).

This "shock effect" of skeletal pathology is exacerbated by the relative lack of good comparative data on ancient Maya health. Indeed, Saul (1972) cautiously hesitated to describe chronological trends in skeletal pathology at Altar de Sacrificios because of the small sample sizes. Although some characteristic bone diseases can be diagnosed on an individual basis, paleopathology is by its very nature a comparative exercise. Often, Maya osteological data is derived from skeletal samples that are too small to estimate population health parameters confidently. Unfortunately, reservations about sampling are generally lost in subsequent citation, and hypothesized trends become reified as demonstrated facts.

The effects of small sample size are particularly apparent in studies of skeletal stature (Danforth 1994). Haviland's (1967) classic study at Tikal illustrated a decline in male stature between Early and Late Classic times, accompanied by increasing difference between elite stature of tomb burials and low-status stature. However, the ranges overlap substantially (see Haviland and Moholy-Nagy 1992), and it is unlikely that the trends would be confirmed statistically. Saul (1972) described a similar trend at Altar, but it was based on only 12 individuals from the entire sequence. Márquez Morfín's survey of Maya stature data demonstrates the paucity of samples with sizeable numbers of measurable bones (Márquez Morfín 1984; Márquez Morfín and del Angel 1997). Although Márquez and del Angel (1997) attempt to synthesize a pan-lowland trend from these data, Danforth (1994) cogently points out the perils of such an approach.

It is possible, but unlikely, that the paucity of chronological health trends detected for the Pasión region is likewise due to small sample size. Yet, a number of statistical trends exist, specifically in the prevalence of hypoplasias on posterior teeth and in the timing of hypoplasias, indicating that sample sizes are adequate. Moreover, chronological trends in pathology are absent at Copan over the Classic period (Whittington 1989) but do occur for small sample comparisons between Postclassic and Historic periods at Lamanai (White et al. 1994). It seems, instead, that health changed little over time in the Pasión region and was relatively immune to changes in settlement density and the political fortunes of competing dynasties. All available evidence suggests that Pasión peoples had access to an adequate variety of foodstuffs throughout their history and that the health implications of these dietary choices were not directly implicated in the decline of complex society and loss of population in this region.

Dietary Privilege in Changing Pasión Society

Although bioarchaeological data do not support a model of environmental deterioration for the Pasión region, the results obtained here do suggest some changes in Pasión bioarchaeology that shed light on the collapse. In particular, the results highlight changes over time in the nature of social inequality between segments of Pasión society that are correlated with political processes which may be implicated in the collapse. These changes were detected by mortuary analysis and by comparison of dietary chemistry with social distinctions among burials.

Mortuary data document the development of a superordinate-status dimension (*sensu* Peebles and Kus 1977) during the Classic period that is reinforced by redundant mortuary symbolism. The Late Classic burial samples demonstrate a clear distinction between superordinate and subordinate mortuary groups by the presence of a highly redundant set of symbols employed to distinguish elite (or possibly royal) from nonelite burials. In the northeast Petén, this elite mortuary program appears to have emerged during the Early Classic period (Hall 1989), and it is possible that the less redundant distribution of these traits in the Early Classic sample from Altar—the only Early Classic data for the Pasión—reflects a fundamental bias toward elite burials in Group B at Altar. Certainly, the clearly "royal" tombs like those from Tikal and Rio Azul are missing from the Early Classic Pasión sample. That this superordinate dimension was associated with dietary privileges during the Late Classic period is indicated by patterning of isotopic and elemental signatures at both Altar and Dos Pilas, as well as in the Petexbatun subregion as a whole. The emergence of this superordinate dimension corresponds well with the view that Late Classic elites obtained power through charismatic display of symbols of authority (Demarest 1992; Fash 1988; McAnany 1993).

Lesser distinctions are evident among burials in the Late Classic samples and represent further differentiation within the subordinate-status group. These mortuary distinctions also demonstrate subtle dietary discrepancies, indicating that the structure of Late Classic society was indeed more complex than a simple two-class structure. Moreover, this finding confirms that mortuary patterning among the subordinate burials is in some measure congruent with economic or social inequality. Due to the small sample sizes, however, these differences should be interpreted with some caution.

Organizing these subordinate mortuary groups and diets into a discrete ranked order or hierarchy is problematic. Unlike the superordinate dimension, which is characterized by a similar symbolic vocabulary across the region, distinctions among the subordinate statuses seem to be heralded with different symbols at each site, in accord with the local audience for whom funeral rituals were performed. Many of these differences involve emphasis on body position and orientation rather than grave accompaniments. In turn, subordinate dietary distinctions are not identical at all sites. Thus, we cannot simply assume that similar burials at different sites indicate identical social roles or economic benefits in life. In part, these differences may be due to sampling error between sites, but extreme variability in expression of mortuary traits at sites within any region has been observed in other surveys of Maya burial patterns and argues for more fundamental differences than merely sampling error (Ruz Lhuillier 1968; Welsh 1988). Cross-cultural surveys (Carr 1995) suggest that ethnic or kinship distinctions are symbolized in burial body position and orientation in many cultures. If this were the case among the Maya, then some of these status distinctions may be horizontal rather than vertical, and dietary discrepancies may reflect familial menu choices rather than a simple ranking of dietary quality.

These Late Classic patterns contrast with the picture observed in the Terminal Classic burials from both Altar de Sacrificios and Seibal. Evidence for a superordinate dimension that manifests the redundant symbolism of the Late Classic royalty is absent from both sites. At Seibal, one burial may demonstrate some arguable elite ties (with redundant variables, albeit different ones than in the Late Classic PC1s), and excavation did not uncover any graves of the site's documented Bayal rulers. At Altar, excavation was biased toward monumental architecture, so evidence of a Terminal Classic superordinate status should have been found if it was present in a form analogous to that of the Late Classic. Other aspects of Altar's archaeology also point to an absence of strong political authority, specifically the absence of architectural, sculptural, and, most importantly, hieroglyphic traditions (Mathews and Willey 1991; Willey 1973). The production of Fine Orange ceramics was a vigorous industry at Altar, and the dissemination of these ceramics throughout the Pasión drainage attests to continued community vitality, albeit subject to a modified form of governance.

Sampling issues aside, the Terminal Classic Pasión burials that were recovered do not show the same formal structure as those found in the Late Classic assemblages, indicating a fundamental change in the correspondence between funerary ritual and social status. The most representative sample, that from Seibal, is derived primarily from domestic contexts and is roughly comparable to that of Late Classic burials at Dos Pilas. Unlike the latter case, however, the Bayal mortuary program at Seibal shows little formal structure, and mortuary clusters obtained are not congruent with dietary chemical distinctions as seen at Dos Pilas. Perhaps some formal principles govern the expression of Bayal mortuary traits that the clustering method did not identify, but in itself this is a significant finding since the method successfully identified meaningful groups at Late Classic Dos Pilas and Altar. Instead of mortuary distinctions in diet, the Seibal data indicate broad variability in chemical signatures among individuals who were afforded similar funerary treatment. Sexual differences in carbon isotopes crosscut these loose mortuary divisions, indicating a more basic dietary pattern. Since a sexual difference in $\delta^{13}C$ was also observed at Late Classic Dos Pilas, it is unlikely that this sexual partitioning represents new dietary rules for males and females in the Bayal population, but it is more likely a simple consequence of sex-specific activity roles. For instance, males working in agriculture might consume proportionately more portable maize products like *pozole* or tamales than women at the home did.

Likewise, at Altar de Sacrificios mortuary traits show little formal organization in the Terminal Classic sample. Since Late Boca, Boca/Jimba, and Jimba graves are considered together, the sample is not simply biased toward a narrow social group by artificial separation of these two ceramic complexes, as would be the case if only Jimba features were considered. Instead, the Terminal Classic Altar burials show a very different set of mortuary practices than those adhered to at Altar during the Late Classic. Terminal Classic burials are common in monumental architecture at Altar but differ fundamentally from those of the Late Classic. They are virtually all intrusive shallow graves that were dug into existing architecture and are not associated with episodes of construction, either as "dedicatory" interments or elite deaths that might precipitate construction. Other Terminal Classic burials at Altar were recovered from small domestic architecture or the low burial mound #2, indicating some continuity with earlier locational choices. Given this partial shift in interment location, the lack of formal structure in the Altar Boca/Jimba burial sample cannot be dismissed as due to excavation bias alone.

As at Seibal, the Terminal Classic Altar clusters do not correlate with dietary distinctions, suggesting a comparable loss of correspondence between the social identities expressed in funerals and economic or dietary inequality among members of the community. Although the sexual distinction noted for Seibal is not statistically confirmed in the Altar sample alone, the isotopic difference remains if the two sites are lumped together, hinting that the dietary sex difference may have been a trend at Altar as well.

The first possibility that may account for this shift in the interdigitation of mortuary and dietary patterns is a corresponding loss of structure in the population from which the sample is drawn. A breakdown of formal rules defining status and, concurrently, socially mediated inequality might result in the unstructured pattern observed. If rules defining hierarchical groups came to be redefined along new lines or forsaken altogether, then dietary distinctions among mortuary groups would be less evident than in the Late Classic samples.

Two other possibilities must be considered before elaborating further on this idea. First, rapid chronological change in mortuary behavior might blur formal distinctions between groups (Bradley 1988). The Bayal occupation at Seibal is thought to span a short period, A.D. 830 to 950, especially in comparison with earlier periods. Chronological leveling is more likely to obscure patterning in the Late Classic, which spans twice this time depth, A.D. 600 to 830. It is probable that chronological change is a factor contributing to inconsistencies among, and indeed definition of, the observed Late Classic clusters. If, however, the rate of social change increased dramatically in the Terminal Classic—as might be suspected with the apparent political upheaval and imminent collapse—then rapid chronological change of funerary symbols must be kept in mind as a contributing factor.

The second issue is that of population movement in Terminal Classic times. An incursion of new peoples bringing with them new mortuary practices and dietary preferences might introduce sufficient "noise" into the data to obscure any patterning present within any subpopulation, whether local or immigrant. For Seibal, the Bayal king "Wat'ul-Chatel" presumably brought his own retinue from Ucanal (Schele and Mathews 1998), who may have contributed to this funerary noise. However, it is likely that population influx to Terminal Classic Seibal, and perhaps Altar, was largely of local Pasión Maya peoples from other sites that collapsed before Seibal, especially from the Petexbatun sites (Demarest and Escobedo 1998, Demarest 2006). Following the demise of one's own home dynasty, such intraregional migration was presumably undertaken in search of some form of political authority and the social, economic, and religious advantages that city life had previously afforded. If this migration can be viewed as an attempt to cling to the last vestiges of the traditional social order, then we might expect the carryover of local mortuary distinctions to be brief, with migrants eager to adopt the mortuary traditions and site-specific identities of their new communities. Hence, the lack of redundancy in Terminal Classic mortuary programs and dietary distinctions may well indicate a diminished social hierarchy among these populations.

During the Late Classic, dietary differences among redundantly defined burial clusters indicate that social divisions were, in part, economically based. Reconstructions of Late Classic social composition argue for increasing complexity of status levels, both in terms of economic wealth and social power through genealogical descent. The proliferation of elite-status identities is suggested by new hieroglyphic titles and increasing diversity of personages illustrated in iconography. If polity leadership was grounded in the ability to manipulate material symbols of social power, these social changes would have put pressure on rulers toward further elaboration of ritual display. Maintenance of royal prerogatives in the face of this growing subordinate body is often seen as a primary factor contributing to the intensification of interpolity aggression and escalating warfare of the eighth century (Demarest 1992, 1996; Houston 1993; McAnany 1993).

Hodder (1979) has argued that a social group will react to increasing stress or pressure on the definition and isolation of that group by projecting a louder ritual statement visible in the patterning of material remains. This argument is particularly appropriate to analysis of funerary remains. In Pasión burials, this is seen in the elaboration of redundant symbol sets that serve to distinguish Late Classic status groups. Some of the subordinate burial clusters contain elements that are also common in the superordinate dimension, such as jade and cylinder vases. In societies in which access to status symbols is regulated by economic means, elite groups may react to such emulation and counteract the pressure of subordinate-status groups by shifting to a more conservative, simplistic expression of group solidarity, a behavior that produces cyclical trends in expressive redundancy and restraint of funerary symbols (Cannon 1989). This strategy was not available to Late Classic rulers because the display and manipulation of material symbols was a primary means to obtain social power. Thus, polity leadership was locked into a cycle of escalating competition.

Rising militarism was not conducive to the smooth conduct of extraregional trade, which provided the raw materials from which power was drawn. Terminal Classic burials lack these power symbols, with jade and shell much rarer than in the Classic period, suggesting the disruption of trade routes along the Pasión. In addition to local power struggles, the realignment of long-distance exchange networks in Mesoamerica at large may also have contributed to this disruption (Freidel 1986; Webb 1973). Terminal Classic sculptures from Seibal portray a diverse set of characters, among whom the elaborately decked-out ruler of Late Classic art is less conspicuous. Whether these new characters depict foreign features (Graham 1973) that imply a local attempt to achieve power by drawing on foreign connections (*sensu* Helms 1979, 1991) in lieu of genealogical purity or illustrate members of lesser elite groups (Stuart 1993:337) and thereby new public roles for these individuals, they would seem to herald a weakening of the charismatic power of the ruler in his own right. If peer polities are legitimized by the existence and success of neighboring polities (Renfrew 1982:289), then the faltering of dynasties in the Petexbatun area would have cast doubt on the value of elite display and the very foundations of Pasión Maya ideology, weakening the fabric of the society as a whole. The lack of social distinctions in both mortuary ritual and dietary choices in the final occupations points to a fundamental change in the structure of Pasión society. Despite desperate attempts, the Terminal Classic Maya had lost the "capacity to make inequality enchant" (Geertz 1980:123). Instead of environmental degradation, these social transformations may hold the key to unraveling the process of collapse.

Directions for Future Research

The results of this work demonstrate that the bioarchaeological approach can provide insight into the changing nature of Maya interactions with the lowland ecosystem over time and space. In particular, three research areas can be highlighted that will be productive in future work: ecosystem sampling for dietary chemistry, skeletal pathology, and the intercorrelation of mortuary programs with bone chemistry.

Here, chemical analysis of wild and cultivated plants and animals provide a more complete picture of chemical dynamics in this tropical rain forest. Several food sources proved to have unexpected isotopic and elemental signatures. For instance, the freshwater ecosystem has distinctive low Ba/Sr due to Sr leaching. Likewise, isotopic analysis of foods revealed the unusually light $\delta^{13}C$ of freshwater fish in the study region. These are the first substantial isotopic and elemental analyses that have been conducted on freshwater fauna from the Maya area. However, sample sizes for each species are very small. Future studies of Maya diet would benefit from analysis of larger numbers of samples to better define the variation within a given species, such as that carried out for Petexbatun deer by Emery et al. (2000). Indeed, a broader range of species would be of further utility. For $\delta^{13}C$, a better understanding of the relative exploitation of hunted versus domesticated animals is critical for evaluating the contribution of meat to collagen synthesis.

If herbivore meat contributes to collagen $\delta^{13}C$, as is suggested by the data reported here, then the collagen $\delta^{13}C$ data may not provide a sufficiently precise measure of maize consumption. While apatite $\delta^{13}C$ more faithfully measures whole diet $\delta^{13}C$ (Ambrose and Norr 1993; Tieszen and Fagre 1993b) and thus maize consumption, bone mineral is likely to be contaminated at Maya sites (Wright and Schwarcz 1996). Therefore, future studies should focus on tooth enamel, which is less likely to be affected by diagenesis. Such studies must take care to sample the same tooth and portion of the tooth, however, in order to control for age differences in maize consumption during childhood. Such studies would of course measure childhood rather than adult diets.

This work has demonstrated that mortuary behavior is congruent with social distinctions in life that afforded differential access to foods. I applied a simplistic classification to all burial assemblages for the sake of consistency. It is possible that more refined distinctions would be detectable upon more detailed analysis, employing several different classificatory methods. Clearly, the samples analyzed here are small and more detailed analysis of larger burial series would be useful to better understand the nature of Classic Maya burial ritual, and, in conjunction with dietary chemistry, may reveal subtle changes in Maya social interaction over time. Such work would allow a fine-grained glimpse of social changes leading up to the collapse and of Maya social evolution in general.

Once the nature of social partitioning of resources is better understood, we will be in a better position to evaluate the impact of social complexity on the health of subpopulations within ancient Maya society. Given the limitations of skeletal preservation and the size of existing skeletal collections, paleopathology may be most productive if it focuses on select conditions that are frequently preserved, such as enamel developmental defects. Hypoplasia data obtained here hints at changes in child-care practices over time in the Pasión. Since enamel microdefects (Wilson bands and striae of Retzius) are typically more abundant than macroscopic defects, they may permit more sensitive indications of health change and be useful for examining intrapopulational distinctions in small samples. If sampling difficulties can be overcome, paleopathological analysis has the potential to evaluate the impact of social inequality on Maya society in greater depth than was possible here.

Summary

I undertook analysis of skeletal remains and mortuary practices in the Pasión region of the Maya Lowlands in order to evaluate the hypothesis that ancient Maya cities in the southern lowlands were abandoned because of environmental mismanagement and agricultural failure. This argument emphasizes the role of maize monocropping in the deterioration of the agricultural landscape and in the etiology of hypothesized nutritional and health problems that were directly implicated in population decline. Isotopic and elemental analyses of diet and paleopathological analysis of human skeletons from sites in the Pasión region do not reveal the chronological trends in diet and health that would be expected if the posited environmental scenario had taken place. Chemical analysis reveals substantial regional variability in diet and indicates that ancient Pasión diets contained substantial quantities of protein, implying that protein-calorie malnutrition was not sufficiently widespread to account for the collapse. Chronological trends in diet do not follow the expectations of increasing maize reliance and decreasing animal protein consumption over time. Paleopathological analysis reveals that Pasión peoples suffered a significant health burden, but disease is not a likely cause of the population collapse because few health indicators show chronological trends. Statistical analysis of mortuary features reveals changes in the definition and composition of social groups within Maya society toward the end of the Classic period. The Terminal Classic samples lack the discrete patterning of mortuary features that had been correlated with dietary distinctions in the Late Classic samples. Terminal Classic diets varied widely among members of a single population but suggest some sexual trends.

For the Pasión region, there is little reason to suppose that environmental degradation played a significant role in the collapse of political authority or the subsequent abandonment of sites. Instead, political and social conflict within the region is key to resolving the issue. Continued work on skeletal biology has a vital role to play in elucidating the process of collapse as changes in the social distribution of resources may have been an important element in the transition.

APPENDIX A

Definitions of Skeletal Measurements Considered for Use in Discriminant Functions

Acronym	Definition	Reference
mastoid*	mastoid height	Whittington 1989
mandboht*	mandibular body height, measured between M1 and M2	Giles 1970
clavcirc*	midshaft circumference of the clavicle	Bass 1987
scapglht	height of the glenoid cavity of the scapula	Giles 1970
hubiepic	maximum epicondylar width of the humerus	Giles 1970
huartic	width of the trochlea and capitulum of the humerus	Bass 1987
hutrhead	transverse diameter of head of the humerus	France 1983, cited in Bass 1987
huvehead	vertical diameter of the head of the humerus	France 1983
huminsh*	minimum diameter of the humerus shaft	France 1983
humaxsh	maximum diameter of the humerus shaft, taken at right angle to huminsh	France 1983
humincir*	minimum circumference of humerus shaft	Giles 1970
ulmaxcr*	transverse diameter of the ulna at point of greatest crest	Giles 1970
ulprmet	transverse diameter of the ulna below radial notch	Storey, personal communication 1990
ulmaxcap	maximum diameter of the capitulum of the ulna	Giles 1970
radcirc*	midshaft circumference of the radius	Giles 1970
femaxhead*	maximum diameter of the femoral head	Giles 1970
feverhead	vertical diameter of the femoral head	Bass 1987
femidcir*	midshaft circumference of the femur	Bass 1987
femidapw*	midshaft antero-posterior diameter of the femur	Bass 1987
tinfcirc*	circumference of the tibia at the nutrient foramen	Bass 1987
timaxap*	maximum midshaft antero-posterior diameter of the tibia	Giles 1970
timincir*	minimum circumference of the tibia	Giles (1970)

An asterisk indicates measurements ultimately used.

Key to Appendix B

For sex estimations

M = male
F = female
? = uncertainty
c = cranial morphology
p = pelvic morphology
K = considered to be of known sex in calculation of discriminant functions.

For age estimations

I = infant (0–5)
C = child (6–11)
T = adolescent (12–19)
Y = young adult (20–34)
M = middle adult (35–49)
O = old adult (50+)
A = adult
e = dental eruption
f = epiphysial fusion
c = cemental annulation
s = cranial sutures
p = pubic symphysis
a = auricular surface

An asterisk indicates sex and age identified by Saul (1972; Tourtellot 1990) as no field estimates are published.

APPENDIX B

Summary of Age and Sex Identification of Skeletons, with Chronological Placement

	Sex Identification					Age Identification				
Burial	Field	Lab	Skeletal D.F.	Dental D.F.	Final Sex	Field	Lab	Attrition	Final Age	Date
Altar de Sacrificios										
AS1a	?				?	A			A	Late
AS1b	?				?	C			C	Late
AS2	?				?	A			A	Terminal
AS3	?				?	A			A	Late
AS4	F*	M?	F?		?	Y	Ae	T	Y	Late
AS5	?*	?			?	I	9m±3e		I	Late
AS6	M	F?	M?		?	Y	<35s		Y	Early
AS7	?				?	A			A	Early
AS8	M	Mcp	K	K	M	A			A	Preclassic
AS9	?				?	A			A	Terminal
AS10	F*	M?c		M	M	M	>35s	M	M	Terminal
AS11a	F*	?c	F?		F	Y	Ae	Y	Y	Terminal
AS11b	?*	?			?	I	6±2		C	Terminal
AS12	?				?	C			C	Early
AS13	M*	Mcp	K	K	M	O	45.2±12.6s	O	M	Preclassic
AS14	F				F	A			A	Preclassic
AS15	?*	?			?	Y	Ae	M	M	Terminal
AS16	?				?	A			A	Late
AS17	?				?	I			I	Late
AS18	?				?	A			A	Late
AS19	F				F	A			A	Terminal
AS20	?				?	A			A	Terminal
AS21	M				M	A			A	Terminal
AS22	M				M	A			A	Late
AS23	M*	?	M		M	M	Af		A	Terminal
AS24	?				?	A			A	Early

Burial	Sex Identification: Field	Lab	Skeletal D.F.	Dental D.F.	Final Sex	Age Identification: Field	Lab	Attrition	Final Age	Date
AS25	?				?	A			A	Early
AS26	?	?	M		M	A	A?		A	?
AS27	F				F	A			A	Early
AS28	?				?	A			A	Early
AS29	?				?	C			C	Early
AS30	F	?	M		M	A	Ae	M	M	Late
AS31	F	Mcp	K	K	M	A	35-39a	O	M	Preclassic
AS32	?				?	A			A	Late
AS33	?				?	A			A	?
AS34	?				?	A			A	Terminal
AS35	?				?	A			A	?
AS36a	F				F	A			A	Late
AS36b	?*	?		F	?	C	8±2e		C	Late
AS37	?*	?		F	?	T	10±3e		T	Terminal
AS38	?				?	A			A	Late
AS39	F*	Fcp	K		F	M	32.0±8.3s >50a	O	M	?
AS40	M*	M?cp	M?	K	M	M	50-60a	O	O	Terminal
AS41	M*	?	M		M	M	Ae	M	M	Preclassic
AS42	F				F	A			A	Early
AS43	F*	Fcp	K	K	F	Y	>60a	O	O	Terminal
AS44	?				?	C			C	Early
AS45	?*				?	I			I	?
AS46	?*	?			?	I	18m±6e		I	?
AS47	F*	Fcp	K	K	F	M	>60a 34.7±7.8s	M	M	Late
AS48	M*	M?c	M?	M	M	Y	Ae	O	O	Late
AS49	M				M	A			A	Late
AS50	?				?	C			C	?
AS51	?*	?			?	I	3±1e		I	Early
AS52	M*	F?cp	F?	F	F	M	<43s 45-49a	O	M	Terminal
AS53	F				F	A			A	Preclassic
AS54	?*	?			?	I	12m±4e		I	Early
AS55	M*	M?c	M		M	Y	Af		A	Early
AS56	M*	M?c	M		M	Y	Ae		A	?
AS57	F*	Fc	K	K	F	M	39.4±9.1s	M	M	Terminal

	Sex Identification					Age Identification				
Burial	Field	Lab	Skeletal D.F.	Dental D.F.	Final Sex	Field	Lab	Attrition	Final Age	Date
AS58	M*	M?c	M	K	M	M	Ae	M	M	Terminal
AS59	F*	?		F	F	Y	Ae	Y	Y	Terminal
AS60	F*	Fcp	K		F	Y	43.4±10.7s 40-44a	O	M	Terminal
AS61	F*				F	O			A	Terminal
AS62	M*	Mc	K	K	M	O	41.1±10.0s	O	M	Terminal
AS63	F*	Fc	K	K	F	M	45.2±12.6s	M	M	Terminal
AS64	M*	Mc	K	K	M	M	34.7±7.8s	Y	Y	Terminal
AS65	M*	Mcp	K	K	M	Y	18.5±2.1p	Y	Y	Preclassic
AS66	F*	Fp	K		F	M	40-44a		M	Terminal
AS67	F*	Fcp	K		F	Y	30-34a 41.1±10.0s		Y	Terminal
AS68	F*	F?c	F	K	F	O	34.7±7.8s	O	Y	Terminal
AS69	?*	?		M	?	C	7±2		C	Terminal
AS70	M*	Mc	K	K	M	Y	41.1±10.0s	O	M	Terminal
AS71a	?				?	C	10±2e		C	Terminal
AS71b	M*	M?c	M	K	M	Y	Ae	Y	Y	Terminal
AS72	?*	?	F?	M	F	T	Ae	Y	Y	Terminal
AS73	?*	?			?	T	9±2e		C	Terminal
AS74	M*	M?cp	M	K	M	M	41.1±10.0s 50-60a	O	O	Terminal
AS75	M*	Mc	K	K	M	M	Ae	O	O	Terminal
AS76	F*	?			?	M	Ae	M	M	Terminal
AS77	?				?	I			I	Terminal
AS78	?*	?		F	F	Y	Ae	T	Y	Late
AS79	?*	?			?	T	12-17f		T	Late
AS80	?*	?	M?	M	M	Y	Ae	M	M	Late
AS81	?				?	A			A	Terminal
AS82	?*	?		M	?	T	12±2.5e		T	Terminal
AS83	M				M	A			A	Terminal
AS84	?*	?		F	?	T	12±2.5e	T	T	Terminal
AS85	M	M?c			M	O	45.2±12.6s	M	M	Late
AS86	M	Mcp	M	K	M	M	>60a	O	O	Terminal
AS87	?				?	I			I	Late
AS88	M*	Mc	M		M	M	43.4±10.7s		M	Late
AS89	M*	M?	M		M	Y	23.4±3.6p		Y	Late
AS90	M*	M?c	M	K	M	Y	Ae	M	M	Terminal

	Sex Identification					Age Identification				
Burial	Field	Lab	Skeletal D.F.	Dental D.F.	Final Sex	Field	Lab	Attrition	Final Age	Date
AS91	?				?	A			A	Late
AS92	M*	?	M	M	M	O	Ae	O	O	Terminal
AS93	M				M	A			A	Late
AS94	?*	?			?	I	5±1.3e		I	Terminal
AS95	F*	Mc	K	K	M	Y	Ae	M	M	Terminal
AS96	F*	Fp	K		F	Y	18.5±2.1p 25-29a		Y	Late
AS97a	F				F	A			A	Preclassic
AS97b	?				?	I			I	Preclassic
AS98	M*	?			?	Y	A?		A	Early
AS99	M				M	A			A	Early
AS100	?				?	I			I	Early
AS101	?*	?			?	I	6m±3e		I	Early
AS102	?				?	A			A	Late
AS103	?	?		F	?	A	12±2.5e		T	Early
AS104	?	?			?	Y	Ae	O	O	Preclassic
AS105	M*	M?c	M	K	M	Y	Ae	Y	Y	Preclassic
AS106	?*	?	M		M	Y	Ae	M	M	Early
AS107	F*	Fcp	K	K	F	M	40-44a	O	M	Preclassic
AS108	?*	?		F	F	Y	17-21e	T	T	Preclassic
AS109	?*	?			?	M	Ae	Y	Y	Terminal
AS110	?*	?			?	M	A?	O	O	Preclassic
AS111	?*	?			?	I	18m±6e		I	Late
AS112	M*	?	F?		F	M	Af		A	Early
AS113	?				?	A			A	Early
AS114	?*	?			?	M	Ae	O	O	Early
AS115	M*	Mcp	K	K	M	O	35-39a	O	M	Early
AS116	F*	Fcp	K		F	O	35-39a	O	M	Early
AS117	M*	Mcp	K	K	M	Y	25-29a	M	Y	Early
AS118	M*	Mcp	K	K	M	Y	35.2±9.4p 30-34a 32.0±8.3s	M	Y	Early
AS119	M*	?		M	M	M	Ae	O	O	Preclassic
AS120	?*	?		M	M	M	Ae	O	O	Late
AS121	?				?	A			A	Late
AS122	?*	?			?	Y	Ae	M	M	Early
AS123	?*	?			?	I	18m±3e		I	Late

	Sex Identification					Age Identification				
Burial	**Field**	**Lab**	**Skeletal D.F.**	**Dental D.F.**	**Final Sex**	**Field**	**Lab**	**Attrition**	**Final Age**	**Date**
AS124	F*	Fcp	F?	K	F	Y	20-24a <35s	Y	Y	Preclassic
AS125	?*	?			?	I	9m±3e		I	Preclassic
AS126	?				?	A			A	Terminal
AS127a	?*	?			?	I	2.5±1e		I	Preclassic
AS127b	?*	?			?	I	18m±6e		I	Preclassic
AS127c	?*	?			?	I	6m±3e		I	Preclassic
AS128	F*	F?p	K		F	M	Af		A	Late
AS129	M*	M?cp	M	K	M	Y	35.2±9.4p 40-44a	O	M	Preclassic
AS130	?*	F?c			?	T	12±2.5e	T	T	Preclassic
AS131	M*	M?c	M	K	M	O	Af	O	O	Preclassic
AS132	?				?	A			A	Late
AS133a	?*	?			?	C	6±2e		C	Late
AS133b	?*	?			?	I	6m±3e		I	Late
AS134	?*	?		M	?	C	8±2e		C	Early
AS135	M*	Mp	K		M	Y	28.7±6.5p 30-34a		Y	Preclassic
AS136	?*	?			?	I	9m±3e		I	Preclassic
Seibal										
SE1	F*	Fcp	K	K	F	Y	Ae	O	O	Terminal
SE2	M*	Mcp	M	K	M	Y	34.7±7.8s 35-39a	M	M	Terminal
SE3	?*	?			?	C	1-6ef		I	Terminal
SE4-2	M*	M			M	A	30.5±9.6s	Y	Y	Terminal
SE4-3	M*	M			M	A	Ae	M	M	Terminal
SE4-4	M*	M			M	A	34.7±7.8s	M	M	Terminal
SE4-5a	M*	M			M	A	Ae	Y	Y	Terminal
SE4-5b	M*	M			M	A	39.4±9.1s	Y	M	Terminal
SE4-6	M*	M			M	A	Ae	M	M	Terminal
SE4-8	M*	M			M	A	<35s	Y	Y	Terminal
SE4-9	M*	F			F	A	<35s	Y	Y	Terminal
SE4-10	M*	M			M	A	45.2±12.6s	O	O	Terminal
SE4-11	M*	F			F	A	<35s	M	M	Terminal
SE4-J		?			?		15-18f	T	T	Terminal
SE5	M*	Mcp	K	K	M	M	>60a	O	O	Preclassic

Burial	Sex Identification: Field	Lab	Skeletal D.F.	Dental D.F.	Final Sex	Age Identification: Field	Lab	Attrition	Final Age	Date
SE6	M*	M?c	M	K	M	A	45.2±12.6s		M	Late
SE7	F*	M?c	M	K	M	M	A?		A	Late
SE8	?*	?			?	C	3±1e		I	Terminal
SE9	F*	Fc	K	K	F	A	Ae		A	Late
SE10a	F*	F?	F?		F	T	12±2.5e <15f	T	T	Terminal
SE10b	?*	?			?	C	0-3 size		I	Terminal
SE11	M*	Mc	K	K	M	M	39.4±9.1s 50-60a	O	O	Preclassic
SE12	?*				?	A?			A	Late
SE13	?*				?	C			C	Terminal
SE14	M*	M?cp	M	K	M	A	25-35a		Y	Terminal
SE15	F*	Fcp	K	K	F	Y	35-39a 30.5±9.6s	M	M	Terminal
SE16	F*	?	F		F	Y	34.7±7.8s		Y	Preclassic
SE17	M*	Mc	K	K	M	M	Ae	M	M	Late
SE18	F*	F?c	F		F	A	Af		A	Preclassic
SE19	?*				?	C			C	Late
SE20	M*	?	M		M	M	30-34a	M	Y	Terminal
SE21	?*	M?c			M	A	Ae	Y	Y	Terminal
SE22	F*	M?c	F?	M	M	A	Ae	M	M	Preclassic
SE23	M*	?	M?		M	A	Af		A	Late
SE24	M*	?	M		M	A	A?		A	Late
SE25	M*	M?c	M		M	M	Ae	O	O	Late
SE26	M*	M?c	F	F	F	Y	25-29a 34.7±7.8s	M	Y	Terminal
SE27	?*	?			?	C	2±0.6e		I	Late
SE28	F*	Fcp	K	K	F	Y	17-21ef 25-29a	T	T	Terminal
SE29	M*	Mcp	K	K	M	Y	30-34a	M	Y	Late
SE30	M*	M?cp	M?	K	M	A	35-39a <35s	M	M	Preclassic
SE31	M*	?	M?	M	M	A	Af	Y	Y	Terminal
SE32	M*	?	F?		F	A	A?		A	Terminal
SE33	?*				?	C			C	Preclassic
SE34	M*	Mcp	K	K	M	Y	45-49a 34.7±7.8s	Y	M	Terminal
SE35	?*	F?c	M	M	M	A	Ae	Y	Y	Terminal

	Sex Identification					Age Identification				
Burial	Field	Lab	Skeletal D.F.	Dental D.F.	Final Sex	Field	Lab	Attrition	Final Age	Date
SE36	M*	M?c	M	K	M	Y	Ae	M	M	Late
SE37	M*	M?c	M	K	M	M	Ae	M	M	Late
SE38	M*	M?c	M	K	M	A	Ae	M	M	Terminal
SE39	M*	M?c	M?	K	M	M	20-24a 34.7±7.8s	T	Y	Terminal
SE40	M*	?	M		M	A	As		A	Late
SE41	M*	?	M		M	A	35-39a	Y	M	Late
SE42	M*	?	M	M	M	A	Ae	M	M	Preclassic
SE43	M*	M?c	M	K	M	A	Ae	Y	Y	Late
SE44	?*	?			?	A	?		A	Late
SE45	M*				M	A			A	Late
Dos Pilas										
DP1	?	M?c	K	K	M	A	Ae	M	M	Late
DP2	?	M?c	M?	M	M	A	Ae	Y	Y	Terminal
DP3	?	Mc	K	K	M	A	43.0c	O	O	Terminal
DP4	?	M?c	F	M	F	?	20.1c	O	Y	Late
DP5	?	Fc	K	K	F	?	Ae 16.7c	M	M	Late
DP9	?	Mc	M		M	A	39.4±9.1s	M	M	Terminal
DP10a	M	Mc	M?	K	M	A	Ae	Y	Y	Terminal
DP10b	M	Mc	M?	K	M	A	18-25e	T	T	Terminal
DP10c	?	?		F	F	A	Ae	M	M	Terminal
DP11	?	?			?	?	Ae		A	Terminal
DP12	M?	Mc	K	K	M	A	Ae	M	M	Terminal
DP13	F?	Fc	K	K	F	A	34.7±7.8s 35-39a 25.2c	M	M	Terminal
DP14	?	?			?	C	5±2.3e		I	Terminal
DP16	F	Fc	K	K	F	A	Ae	Y	Y	Terminal
DP17	M?	Mc	K	K	M	O	39.4±9.1s	O	M	Terminal
DP18	?	?	F?	F	F	A	Ae	M	M	Late
DP19	?	?			?	?	?		?	Late
DP20	F?	F?c	F	K	F	A	Ae	O	O	Late
DP21	?	?			?	A?	Ae		A	Late
DP22	?	M?c	K	K	M	?	24.2c	Y	Y	Late
DP23	?				?	?			?	Late
DP24	?	?		F	?	C	7±2e		C	Late

	Sex Identification					Age Identification				
Burial	**Field**	**Lab**	**Skeletal D.F.**	**Dental D.F.**	**Final Sex**	**Field**	**Lab**	**Attrition**	**Final Age**	**Date**
DP25	M?	Mcp	K	K	M	A	Ae	Y	Y	Late
DP26	?	?	M	M	M	A	Ae	Y	Y	Late
DP27	?	?			?	A	Ae	M	M	Late
DP28	?	?		F	F	A	A?	Y	Y	Late
DP29	?	?	F?	M	F	A	Ae	M	M	Late
DP30	M	Mcp	K	K	M	M	45.6±10.4p 50-60a 51.9±12.5s	Y	O	Late
DP31	?	?		M	M	A	>39.4±9.1s 20.4c	Y	Y	Late
DP33	?	?	F	F	F	A	17-19f 16.4c	T	T	Late
DP34	M?	F?	F	M	F	A	Ae	Y	Y	Late
DP35	M	Mcp	K	K	M	A	34.7±7.8s	Y	Y	Late
DP36	?	?	M		M	A	A?	M	M	Late
DP37	?	?		M	M	A	Ae	O	O	Late
DP38	M?	Mc	K	K	M	A	Ae	M	M	Late
DP39	?				?	?			?	Late
DP40	?	?		F	F	?	21.4c	M	Y	Late
DP41	?	?			?	?	A?f		A	Late
DP42	?	?	F	M	?	T	15±3e 14-21f	Y	T	Late
DP43	F	Fcp	K	K	F	M	48.1±14.6p >56.2±8.5s	M	M	Late
DP44	?	?	F		F	A?	Ae		A	Late
DP45	M?	M?c	M	K	M	A	Ae		A	Late
DP46	?	?	F		F	A	A?f		A	Late
DP47	M	Mc	K	K	M	A	Ae	Y	Y	Late
DP48	?	?		M	M	A	Ae		A	Late
DP49	?	?	M		M	A	Ae	Y	Y	Late
DP50	M	Mp	K		M	O	45.6±10.4p 45-49a		M	Late
DP51	M	Mcp	K	K	M	A	>60a	O	O	Late
DP52					F				A	Late
DP53					?				A	Late
DP54					?				A	Late
DP55					?				A	Late
DP-PD1A	?	Mc	K	K	M	A	>39.4±9.1s 15.7c	O	M	Terminal

	Sex Identification					Age Identification				
Burial	Field	Lab	Skeletal D.F.	Dental D.F.	Final Sex	Field	Lab	Attrition	Final Age	Date
DP-PD1B	?	Mc	K	K	M	A	39.4±9.1s	M	M	Terminal
DP-PD1C	?	?		M	M	A	Ae	Y	Y	Terminal
DP-PD1D	?	?			?	A	Ae	Y	Y	Terminal
DP-PD1E	?	M?c	F		F	A	>30.5±9.5s	Y	Y	Terminal
DP-PD1G	?	M?c		M	M	A	>39.4±9.1s	M	M	Terminal
DP-PD1H	?	M?c	F	F	F	A	30.5±9.6s	Y	Y	Terminal
DP-PD1I	?	Mc	K	K	M	A	34.7±6.8s	M	Y	Terminal
DP-PD1J	?	Mc	K	K	M	A	15±3e	T	T	Terminal
DP-PD1K	?	?			?	A	30.5±9.6s	Y	Y	Terminal
Aguateca										
AG1	F?	F?c	F		F	O	Ae	O	O	Late
AG2	M	Mc	K	K	M	A	Ae	Y	Y	Late
AG3	M?	?	M		M	A	Ae		A	Late
AG4	?	?			?	?	?		A	Late
AG5a	?	Fcp	K	K	F	A	19.4±2.6p 20-24a <35s	T	T	Late
AG5b	?	Fcp	K	K	F	A	>60a 34.7±7.8s	M	M	Late
AG6	?	?	?		?	A?	Ae	O	O	Late
AG7	?	?			?	A?	Ae	M	M	Late
AG8	?	?	M		M	A	Ae	M	M	Late
QCH1a	?	M?c	M		M	?	39.4±9.1s >40a	M	M	Late
QCH1b	?	?	M	F	M	?	Ae	M	M	Late
QCH2	?	?			?	A	Ae	M	M	Late
QCH3	?	M?c	F?		?	A	Aef	Y	Y	Late
QCH4	?	?	F?		F	A	A?	T	T	Late
QCH5	?	M?c	M	M	M	A	Ae	M	M	Late
QCH6	F?	Mc	K	K	M	A	>41±10s	M	M	Late
QCH7	?	F?c	F		F	C?	Af		A	Late

	Sex Identification					Age Identification				
Burial	Field	Lab	Skeletal D.F.	Dental D.F.	Final Sex	Field	Lab	Attrition	Final Age	Date
QCH8	?	?			?	A?	Ae	M	M	Late
QCH9	?	?	F		F	?	A?		A	Late
QCH10	?	?	F	F	F	?	Ae		A	Late
CCH1	?	?	F	F	?	A	14-18		T	Late
Itzan										
IT1	?	Fc	K	K	F	?	34.7±7.8s	M	Y	Late
IT2	?	M?c	M?		M	?	Ae	M	M	Late
IT3	?	F?c			F	?	>39.4±9.1s		M	Late
IT4	?	?	M		M	?	A?		A	Late
IT5	?	?	M		M	?	A?		A	Late
IT6	?	?	F	F	F	?	A?		A	Late
IT7	?	F?c	F		F	?	15-25e	T	T	Late
IT8	?	?	M		M	?	A?		A	Late
IT9	?	?			?	A?	A?	Y	Y	Late
IT10	?	?			?	A	Ae	O	O	Late
IT11	?	?		F	F	A	Ae	Y	Y	Late
IT12	?	M?c			M	A	>39.4±9.1s	Y	M	Late
IT13	?	?			?	I	9m±3e		I	Late
ITDE3	?	?			?	?	Ae	M	M	Late
Tamarindito										
T1a	M?	Mc	K	K	M	A	39.4±9.1s	Y	M	Late
T1b	?	Fc	F		F	?	A?		A	Late
TA2	?	Fp	K	K	F	OA?	20-29a	M	Y	Late
TA3	?	?			?	?	Aef		A	Late
TA4					M	A			Y	Late
TA5					?				C	Late
TA6					M				Y	Late
TA7					?				A	Late
TA8					?				Y	Late
TA9					F				Y	Late
TA10					?				A	Late
TA11					M				M	Late
TA12					?				A	Late
TR3-1					M?				M	Preclassic

Burial	Sex Identification: Field	Lab	Skeletal D.F.	Dental D.F.	Final Sex	Age Identification: Field	Lab	Attrition	Final Age	Date
TR3-2					?				A	Late
Punta de Chimino										
PC1	?	M?c	F		?	T	15±3e <20f 30.5±9.6s	Y	T	Late/ Terminal
PC2	?	?			?	A	Af		A	?
PC3a					M	A			A	
PC3b					F?				A	
La Paciencia										
LP1	?				M?	A			M	Late
Arroyo de Piedra										
AP1	?	?		M	?	?	9±2e		C	Late
AP2	?	?			?	?	I?		I	Late
AP3	?	M?c	M?		M	?	Ae	M	M	Late
AP4					M?				Y	Late
AP5					M?				T	Late

References

Abbreviations

AA	*American Anthropologist*
AAnt	*American Antiquity*
AJPA	*American Journal of Physical Anthropology*
AM	*Ancient Mesoamerica*
JAS	*Journal of Archaeological Science*
LAA	*Latin American Antiquity*
PMAE	Peabody Museum of Archaeology and Ethnology, Harvard University, Cambridge, Massachusetts
VIMA	Vanderbilt Institute of Mesoamerican Archaeology

Abrams, Elliot M., and David J. Rue

1988 The Causes and Consequences of Deforestation among the Prehistoric Maya. *Human Ecology* 16(4):377–96.

Acsadi, G., and J. Nemeskeri

1970 *History of Human Life Span and Mortality*. Budapest: Akedemiai Kiado.

Adams, Richard E. W.

1971 *The Ceramics of Altar de Sacrificios*. Papers of the PMAE vol. 63, no. 1.

1973a The Collapse of Maya Civilization: A Review of Previous Theories. In *The Classic Maya Collapse*, edited by T. Patrick Culbert, pp. 21–34. Albuquerque: University of New Mexico Press.

1973b Maya Collapse: Transformation and Termination in the Ceramic Sequence at Altar de Sacrificios. In *The Classic Maya Collapse*, edited by T. Patrick Culbert, pp. 133–64. Albuquerque: University of New Mexico Press.

1983 Ancient Land Use and Culture History in the Pasión River Region. In *Prehistoric Settlement Patterns*, edited by Evon Z. Vogt and Richard M. Leventhal, pp. 319–35. Albuquerque: University of New Mexico Press.

Adriaans, B.

1988 Tropical Ulcer: A Reappraisal based on Recent Work. *Transactions of the Royal Society of Tropical Medicine and Hygiene* 82:185–89.

Alcocer, Ignacio

1938 Las Comidas de los Antiguos Mexicanos. In *Historia General de las cosas de Nueva España*, supplement to vol. 3, by B. de Sahagun, pp. 367–74. Mexico City: Editorial Pedro Robredo.

Altschuler, Milton

1958 On the Environmental Limitations of Maya Cultural Development. *Southwestern Journal of Anthropology* 14(2):189–98.

Ambrose, Stanley H.

1990 Preparation and Characterization of Bone and Tooth Collagen for Isotopic Analysis. *JAS* 17:431–51.

1991 Effects of Diet, Climate, and Physiology on Nitrogen Isotope Abundances in Terrestrial Foodwebs. *JAS* 18:293–317.

1993 Isotopic Analysis of Paleodiets: Methodological and Interpretive Considerations. In *Investigations of Ancient Human Tissue: Chemical Analyses in Anthropology*, edited by M. K. Sandford, pp. 59–130. Amsterdam: Gordon and Breach Science Publishers.

Ambrose, Stanley H., and Lynette Norr

1993 Experimental Evidence for the Relationship of the Carbon Isotope Ratios of Whole

Diet and Dietary Protein to Those of Bone Collagen and Carbonate. In *Prehistoric Human Bone: Archaeology at the Molecular Level*, edited by J. Lambert and G. Grupe, pp. 1–37. Berlin: Springer-Verlag.

Anderson, D. L., G. W. Thompson, and F. Popovich
1976 Age of Attainment of Mineralization Stages of the Permanent Dentition. *Journal of Forensic Science* 21:191–200.

Anderson, J. E.
1965 Human Skeletons of Tehuacan. *Science* 148:496–97.

Angel, J. Lawrence
1969 The Bases of Paleodemography. *AJPA* 30:427–37.

Arriaga, Eduardo E.
1968 *New Life Tables for Latin American Populations in the Nineteenth and Twentieth Centuries*. Population Monograph Series, no. 3. Berkeley: Institute of International Studies, University of California.

Atran, Scott
1993 Itza Maya Tropical Agro-forestry. *Current Anthropology* 34(5):633–700.

Aufderheide, Arthur C., and Conrado Rodríguez-Martín
1998 *The Cambridge Encyclopedia of Paleopathology*. Cambridge, England: Cambridge University Press.

Bada, J. L., M. J. Schoeninger, and A. Schimmelmann
1989 Isotopic Fractionation during Peptide Bone Hydrolysis. *Geochimica et Cosmochimica Acta* 53:3337–41.

Baer, P., and W. R. Merrifield
1971 *Two Studies on the Lacandones of Mexico*. Norman: Summer Institute of Linguistics, University of Oklahoma.

Ball, Joseph W., and Jennifer T. Taschek
1989 Teotihuacan's Fall and the Rise of the Itza: Realignments and Role Changes in the Terminal Classic Maya Lowlands. In *Mesoamerica after the Decline of Teotihuacan A.D. 700–900*, edited by R. A. Diehl and J. C. Berlo, pp. 187–200. Washington: Dumbarton Oaks.

Baraybar, José Pablo
1999 Diet and Death in a Fog Oasis Site in Central Coastal Peru: A Trace Element Study of Tomb 1 Malanche 22. *JAS* 26(5):471–82.

Barrera, A., A. Gómez-Pompa, and C. Vázquez-Yanes
1977 El Manejo de las Selvas por los Mayas: Sus Implicaciones Silvícolas y Agrícolas. *Biótica* (Xalapa, Mexico) 2(2):47–61.

Barrett, John C.
1990 The Monumentality of Death: The Character of Early Bronze Age Mortuary Mounds in Southern Britain. *World Archaeology* 22(2):179–89.

Bass, William M.
1987 *Human Osteology: A Laboratory and Field Manual of the Human Skeleton*. Columbia: Missouri Archaeological Society.

Beach, Timothy, and Nicholas Dunning
1995 Ancient Maya Terracing and Modern Conservation in the Petén Rainforest of Guatemala. *Journal of Soil & Water Conservation* 50(2):138–45.
1997 An Ancient Maya Reservoir and Dam at Tamarindito, El Petén, Guatemala. *LAA* 8:20–29.

Becker, M. J.
1988 Caches as Burials; Burials as Caches: The Meaning of Ritual Deposits among the Classic Period Lowland Maya. In *Recent Studies in Precolumbian Archaeology*, edited by N. J. Saunders and O. de Montmollin, pp. 117–42. International Series, 421(i). Oxford: British Archaeological Reports.

Beeley, J. G., and D. A. Lunt
1980 The Nature of the Biochemical Changes in Softened Dentine from Archaeological Sites. *JAS* 7:371–77.

Behár, M.
1977 Protein-Calorie Deficits in Developing Countries. *Annals of the New York Academy of Science* 300:176–87.

Benedict, Francis G., and M. Steggerda
1937 *The Food of the Present-day Maya Indians of Yucatan*. Carnegie Institution of Washington, Contributions to American Archaeology, vol. 3, no. 18, pp. 155–88. Washington, D.C.

Bennett, S. L.
1985 *Diet, Health and Status at Tipu.* Unpublished Master's Thesis, State University of New York, Plattsburgh.

Binford, Lewis R.
1971 Mortuary Practices: Their Study and Potential. In *Approaches to the Social Dimensions of Mortuary Practices*, edited by J. A. Brown, pp. 6–29, Memoirs of the Society for American Archaeology No. 25. Washington, D.C.

Bishop, Ronald L., Garman Harbottle, and Edward V. Sayre
1982 Chemical and Mathematical Procedures Employed in the Maya Fine Paste Ceramics Project. In *Excavations at Seibal. Analyses of Fine Paste Ceramics*, edited by Jeremy A. Sabloff, pp. 272–82. Memoirs of the PMAE vol. 15, no. 2.

Blake, Michael, Brian S. Chisholm, John E. Clark, Barbara Voorhies, and Michael W. Love
1992 Prehistoric Subsistence in the Soconusco Region. *Current Anthropology* 33(1):83–94.

Blakely, R. L., and L. A. Beck
1981 Trace Elements, Nutritional Status, and Social Stratification at Etowah, Georgia. *Annals of the New York Academy of Science* 376:417–31.

Blakey, Michael L.
1987 Fetal and Childhood Health in Late 18th and Early 19th Century Afro-Americans: Enamel Hypoplasias and Hypocalcification in the FABC Skeletal Population. *AJPA* 72(2):179.

Blakey, Michael L., Teresa E. Leslie, and Joseph P. Reidy
1994 Frequency and Chronological Distribution of Dental Enamel Hypoplasia in Enslaved African Americans: A Test of the Weaning Hypothesis. *AJPA* 95(4):371–83.

Blitz, Jennifer A.
1995 *Dietary Variability and Social Inequality at Monte Alban, Oaxaca, Mexico.* Unpublished Ph.D. dissertation, University of Wisconsin, Madison.

Bloch, Maurice
1977 The Past and the Present in the Present. *Man* 12:278–92.

Bloch, Maurice, and Jonathan Parry
1982a Introduction: Death and the Regeneration of Life. In *Death and the Regeneration of Life,* edited by Maurice Bloch and Jonathan Parry, pp. 1–44. New York: Cambridge University Press.

Bloch, Maurice, and Jonathan Parry (editors)
1982b *Death and the Regeneration of Life.* New York: Cambridge University Press.

Bogin, Barry
1988 *Patterns of Human Growth.* Cambridge, England: Cambridge University Press.

Bongaarts, John, and Hernan Delgado
1977 *Effects of Nutritional Status on Fertility in Rural Guatemala.* Center for Policy Studies, Working Papers, no. 7. New York: Population Council.

Boutton, T. W., P. D. Klein, M. J. Lynott, and L. L. Tieszen
1984 Stable Carbon Isotope Ratios as Indicators of Prehistoric Human Diet. In *Stable Isotopes in Nutrition*, edited by J. R. Turnlund and P. E. Johnson, pp. 191–204. ACS Symposium Series 258. Washington: American Chemical Society.

Bradley, Richard
1988 Status, Wealth and the Chronological Ordering of Cemeteries. *Proceedings of the Prehistoric Society* 54:327–29.

Brady, James E., Irma Rodas, Lori E. Wright, Kitty Emery, Nora María López, Laura Stiver, and Robert Chatham
1991 Proyecto Arqueológico Regional Cuevas Petexbatun. In *Proyecto Arqueologico Regional Petexbatun. Informe Preliminar 3. Tercera Temporada*, edited by Arthur A. Demarest, Takeshi Inomata, Héctor Escobedo, and Joel Palka, pp. 652–747. Report presented to the Instituto de Antropología e Historia de Guatemala.

Brady, James E., Ann Scott, Allan Cobb, Irma Rodas, John Fogarty, and Monica Urquizú Sánchez
1997 Glimpses of the Dark Side of the Petexbatun Project: The Petexbatun Regional Cave Survey. *AM* 8(2):353–64.

Braun, David P.
1979 Illinois Hopewell Burial Practices and Social Organization: A Reexamination of the

Klunk-Gibson Mound Group. In *Hopewell Archaeology: The Chillicothe Conference*, edited by D. S. Brose and N. Greber, pp. 66–79. Kent, Ohio: Kent State University Press.

1981 A Critique of Some Recent North American Mortuary Studies. *AAnt* 46:398–416.

Bressani, Ricardo, Ramiro Paz y Paz, and Nevin S. Scrimshaw

1958 Chemical Changes in Corn during Preparation of Tortillas. *Agricultural and Food Chemistry* 6(10):770–74.

Bressani, Ricardo, and Nevin Scrimshaw

1958 Effect of Lime Treatment on *in vitro* Availability of Essential Amino Acids and Solubility of Protein Fractions in Corn. *Agricultural and Food Chemistry* 6(10):774–78.

Brewbaker, J. L.

1979 Diseases of Maize in the Wet Lowland Tropics and the Collapse of the Classic Maya Civilization. *Economic Botany* 33:101–18.

Bronson, B.

1966 Roots and the Subsistence of the Ancient Maya. *Southwestern Journal of Anthropology* 22:251–79.

Brown, A. B.

1973 *Bone Strontium Content as a Dietary Indicator in Human Skeletal Populations.* Unpublished Ph.D. dissertation, University of Michigan, Ann Arbor.

Brown, James A.

1971a The Dimensions of Status in the Burials at Spiro. In *Approaches to the Social Dimensions of Mortuary Practices*, edited by James A. Brown, pp. 92–112, Memoirs of the Society for American Archaeology No. 25. Washington, D.C.

1987 Quantitative Burial Analyses as Interassemblage Comparison. In *Quantitative Research in Archaeology: Progress and Prospects*, edited by M. S. Aldenderfer, pp. 294–308. London: Sage Publications.

Brown, James A. (editor)

1971b *Approaches to the Social Dimensions of Mortuary Practices.* Memoirs of the Society for American Archaeology No. 25. Washington, D.C.

Brown, J. S., and J. H. Middlemiss

1956 Bone Changes in Tropical Ulcer. *British Journal of Radiology* 29:213–17.

Buchardt, B., and P. Fritz

1978 Strontium Uptake in Shell Aragonite from the Freshwater Gastropod *Limnaea stagnalis. Science* 199:291–92.

Buikstra, Jane E.

1976 *Hopewell in the Lower Illinois Valley: A Regional Approach to the Study of Human Variability and Prehistoric Behavior.* Northwestern University Archaeological Program Scientific Papers No. 2. Evanston, Illinois.

1992 Diet and Disease in Late Prehistory. In *Disease and Demography in the Americas*, edited by J. Verano and D. H. Ubelaker, pp. 87–101. Washington: Smithsonian Institution Press.

Buikstra, Jane E., William Autry, Emanuel Breitburg, Leslie Eisenberg, and Nikolaas van der Merwe

1988 Diet and Health in the Nashville Basin: Human Adaptation and Maize Agriculture in Middle Tennessee. In *Diet and Subsistence: Current Archaeological Perspectives*, pp. 243–59. Proceedings of the 19th Annual Conference of the Archaeological Association of the University of Calgary. Calgary, Alberta, Canada.

Buikstra, Jane E., and Della C. Cook

1980 Palaeopathology: An American Account. *Annual Review of Anthropology* 9:433–70.

Buikstra, Jane E., S. Frankenberg, Joseph B. Lambert, and L. Xue

1989 Multiple Elements: Multiple Expectations. In *The Chemistry of Prehistoric Human Bone*, edited by T. D. Price, pp. 155–210. Cambridge, England: Cambridge University Press.

Buikstra, Jane E., Lyle W. Konigsberg, and Jill Bullington

1986 Fertility and the Development of Agriculture in the Prehistoric Midwest. *AAnt* 51(3):528–46.

Buikstra, Jane E., and George R. Milner

1991 Isotopic and Archaeological Interpretations of Diet in the Central Mississippi Valley. *JAS* 18:319–29.

Buikstra, Jane E., and Douglas H. Ubelaker
1994 *Standards for Data Collection from Human Skeletal Remains*. Arkansas Archeological Survey No. 44. Fayetteville, Arkansas.

Burko, H., H. Z. Mellins, and J. Watson
1961 Skull Changes in Iron Deficiency Anemia Simulating Congenital Hemolytic Anemia. *American Journal of Roentgenology* 86(447):447–52.

Burton, James H., and T. Douglas Price
1990a Paleodietary Applications of Barium Values in Bone. In *Archaeometry '90: Proceedings of the 27th International Symposium on Archaeometry, Heidelberg*, edited by E. Pericka and G. A. Wagner, pp. 787–95. Basel: Birkhäuser Verlag.
1990b The Ratio of Barium to Strontium as a Paleodietary Indicator of Consumption of Marine Resources. *JAS* 17:547–57.

Burton, James H., T. Douglas Price, and William D. Middleton
1999 Correlation of Bone Ba/Ca and Sr/Ca due to Biological Purification of Calcium. *JAS* 26:609–16.

Burton, James H., and Arleyn W. Simon
1993 Acid Extraction as a Simple and Inexpensive Method for Compositional Characterization of Archaeological Ceramics. *AAnt* 58(1):45–59.

Burton, James H., and Lori E. Wright
1995 Nonlinearity in the Relationship between Bone Sr/Ca and Diet: Paleodietary Implications. *AJPA* 96(3):273–82.

Caffey, John
1937 The Skeletal Changes in the Chronic Hemolytic Anemias (Erythroblastic Anemia, Sickle Cell Anemia and Chronic Hemolytic Icterus). *American Journal of Roentgenology* 37:293–334.

Calloway, D. H., R. D. Giauque, and F. M. Costa
1974 The Superior Mineral Content of Some American Indian Foods in Comparison to Federally Donated Counterpart Commodities. *Ecology of Food and Nutrition* 3:203–11.

Cannon, Aubrey
1989 The Historical Dimension in Mortuary Expressions of Status and Sentiment. *Current Anthropology* 30(4):437–58.

Carlson, D. S., G. J. Armelagos, and D. Van Gerven
1974 Factors Affecting the Etiology of Cribra Orbitalia in Prehistoric Nubia. *Journal of Human Evolution* 3:405–10.

Carr, Christopher
1995 Mortuary Practices: Their Social, Philosophical-Religious, Circumstantial, and Physical Determinants. *Journal of Archaeological Method and Theory* 2(2):105–200.

Chackiel, Juan, Kenneth Hill, and Mario Isaacs
1985 Fertility and Mortality in Guatemala: 1950–1973. In *Fertility and Mortality in Bolivia and Guatemala*, Panel on Latin America, Committee on Population and Demography, National Research Council, Report No. 28. Washington: National Academy Press.

Champion, Sara
1982 Exchange and Ranking: The Case of Coral. In *Ranking, Resource, and Exchange: Aspects of the Archaeology of Early European Society*, edited by C. Renfrew and S. Shennan, pp. 67–72. Cambridge, England: Cambridge University Press.

Chapman, Robert, Ian Kinnes, and Klavs Randsborg
1981 *The Archaeology of Death*. Cambridge, England: Cambridge University Press.

Charles, D. K., K. Condon, J. M. Cheverud, and J. E. Buikstra
1986 Cementum Annulation and Age Determination in *Homo sapiens*. I. Tooth Variability and Observer Error. *AJPA* 71:311–20.

Chase, Arlen F.
1990 Cycles of Time: Caracol in the Maya Realm. In *Sixth Palenque Round Table, 1986*, edited by M. Green Robertson, pp. 32–38. Norman: University of Oklahoma Press.

Chavez, A., and C. Martinez
1982 *Growing Up in a Developing Community*. Guatemala: Instituto de Nutrición de Centro America y Panama.

Chinchilla Mazariegos, Oswaldo
1990 *Estudio nutricional de los restos óseos prehispánicos de Balberta, Escuintla, por medio del análisis de estroncio*. Licenciatura en Químico Biólogo (Unpublished thesis, Department of Biochemistry), Universidad de San Carlos de Guatemala.
1991 Excavaciones en el Grupo N5-6. In *Proyecto Arqueológico Regional Petexbatun: Informe Preliminar 3, Tercera Temporada*, edited by Arthur Demarest, Takeshi Inomata, Héctor Escobedo, and Joel Palka, pp. 69–122. Report presented to the Instituto de Antropología e Historia de Guatemala.

Chinchilla, Oswaldo, Eduardo Morales, Frederic Bove, Marily Baudry, and Magdalena Guamuch
1992 Nutrición prehispánica en la costa sur de Guatemala: Estudio de los restos óseos de Sin Cabezas, Escuintla, por medio del análisis de estroncio. *Apuntes Arqueológicos* 2(2):65–96.

Chisholm, B. S.
1989 Variation in Diet Reconstructions based on Stable Carbon Isotopic Evidence. In *The Chemistry of Prehistoric Human Bone*, edited by T. Douglas Price, pp. 10–37. Cambridge, England: Cambridge University Press.

Chisholm, B. S., D. E. Nelson, and H. P. Schwarcz
1982 Stable-Carbon Isotope Ratios as a Measure of Marine Versus Terrestrial Protein in Ancient Diets. *Science* 216:1131–32.

Coale, A. J., and J. P. Demeny
1983 *Regional Model Life Tables and Stable Populations*. New York: Academic Press.

Coe, Michael D.
1973 *The Maya Scribe and His World*. New York: Grolier Club.
1975 Death and the Ancient Maya. In *Death and the Afterlife in Pre-Columbian America*, edited by E. P. Benson, pp. 87–104. Washington: Dumbarton Oaks.
1988 Ideology of the Maya Tomb. In *Maya Iconography*, edited by E. P. Benson and G. G. Griffin, pp. 222–35. Princeton.: Princeton University Press.

Coe, Sophie D.
1994 *America's First Cuisines*. Austin: University of Texas Press.

Coe, William R.
1990 *Excavations in the Great Plaza, North Terrace, and North Acropolis of Tikal*. Tikal Report, vol. 2, no. 14. Philadelphia: University Museum, University of Pennsylvania.

Coggins, Clemency Chase
1988 Classic Maya Metaphors of Death and Life. *RES Anthropology and Aesthetics* 16:64–84.

Cohen, Mark N., and George J. Armelagos
1984 *Palaeopathology at the Origins of Agriculture*. New York: Academic Press.

Cohen, Mark N., K. O'Connor, M. Danforth, K. Jacobi, and C. Armstrong
1994 Health and Death at Tipu. In *In the Wake of Contact: Biological Responses to Conquest*, edited by C. S. Larsen and G. Milner, pp. 121–33. New York: Wiley-Liss.

Comar, C. L.
1963 Some Over-all Aspects of Strontium-Calcium Discrimination. In *The Transfer of Calcium and Strontium across Biological Membranes*, edited by R. H. Wasserman, pp. 405–18. New York: Academic Press.

Comar, C. L., R. H. Wasserman, S. Ulberg, and G. A. Andrews
1957 Strontium Metabolism and Strontium/Calcium Discrimination in Man. *Proceedings of the Society for Experimental Biology and Medicine* 95:386–91.

Condon, K., D. K. Charles, J. M. Cheverud, and Jane E. Buikstra
1986 Cementum Annulation and Age Determination in *Homo sapiens*. II. Estimates and Accuracy. *AJPA* 71:321–30.

Condon, K. W.
1981 *Correspondence of Developmental Enamel Defects Between the Mandibular Canine and First Premolar*. Unpublished Master's Thesis, University of Arkansas, Fayetteville.

Connor, M., and D. Slaughter
1984 Diachronic Investigation of Inuit Diet Utilizing Trace Element Analysis. *Arctic Anthropology* 21:123–134.

Cook, Della C.
1976 *Pathologic States and Disease Process in Illinois Woodland Populations: An*

Epidemiologic Approach. Unpublished Ph.D. dissertation, University of Chicago.
1981 Mortality, Age Structure, and Status in the Interpretation of Stress Indicators in Prehistoric Skeletons: A Dental Example from the Lower Illinois Valley. In *The Archaeology of Death*, edited by Robert W. Chapman and Klaus R. Randsborg, pp. 133–44. Cambridge, England: Cambridge University Press.
1984 Subsistence and Health in the Lower Illinois Valley: Osteological Evidence. In *Palaeopathology at the Origins of Agriculture*, edited by M. N. Cohen and George J. Armelagos, pp. 237–70. New York: Academic Press.

Cook, Della C., and Jane E. Buikstra
1979 Health and Differential Survival in Prehistoric Populations: Prenatal Dental Defects. *AJPA* 51:649–64.

Cook, O. F.
1921 Milpa Agriculture, a Primitive Tropical System. In *Annual Report of the Smithsonian Institution, 1919*, pp. 307–26. Washington: Smithsonian Institution.

Cooke, C. W.
1931 Why the Mayan Cities of the Peten District, Guatemala, Were Abandoned. *Journal of the Washington Academy of Sciences* 21(13):283–87.

Corruccini, Robert S., Jerome S. Handler, and Keith P. Jacobi
1985 Chronological Distribution of Enamel Hypoplasias and Weaning in a Caribbean Slave Population. *Human Biology* 57(4):699–711.

Costa, J. M. L., K. C. Vale, and F. Franca
1990 Cura espontanea da leishmaiose causada por *Leishmania Viannia braziliensis* em lesoes cutaneas. *Revista da Sociedade Brasileira de Medicina Tropical* (Brasilia, Brazil) 23:205–8. (Abstracted in *Tropical Diseases Bulletin* 89(2):146, 1992).

Cowgill, George L.
1964 The End of Classic Maya Culture: A Review of Recent Evidence. *Southwestern Journal of Anthropology* 20(2):145–59.
1979 Teotihuacan, Internal Militaristic Competition, and the Fall of the Classic Maya. In *Maya Archaeology and Ethnohistory*, edited by N. Hammond and G. R. Willey, pp. 51–62. Austin: University of Texas Press.

Cowgill, Ursula M., and G. E. Hutchinson
1963 El Bajo de Santa Fé. *Transactions of the American Philosophical Society* 53(7):1–50.

Cravioto, R. O., O. Y. Cravioto, G. Massieu H., and J. Guzmán G.
1955 "El pozol" forma indígena de consumir el maíz en el sureste de México y su aporte de nutrientes a la dieta. *Ciencia* (Mexico) 15:27–30.

Culbert, T. Patrick
1977 Maya Development and Collapse: An Economic Perspective. In *Social Process in Maya Prehistory*, edited by N. Hammond, pp. 510–31. London: Academic Press.
1988 The Collapse of Classic Maya Civilization. In *The Collapse of Ancient States and Civilizations*, edited by N. Yoffee and G. L. Cowgill, pp. 69–101. Tucson: University of Arizona Press.
1991a Maya Political History and Elite Interaction: A Summary View. In *Classic Maya Political History: Hieroglyphic and Archaeological Evidence*, edited by T. Patrick Culbert, pp. 311–46. Cambridge, England: Cambridge University Press.

Culbert, T. Patrick (editor)
1973 *The Classic Maya Collapse*. Albuquerque: University of New Mexico Press.
1991b *Classic Maya Political History: Hieroglyphic and Archaeological Evidence*. Cambridge, England: Cambridge University Press.

Dahlin, B. H.
1983 Climate and Prehistory on the Yucatan Peninsula. *Climatic Change* 5:245–63.

Danforth, Marie Elaine
1989 *A Comparison of Childhood Health Patterns in the Late Classic and Colonial Maya Using Enamel Microdefects*. Unpublished Ph.D. dissertation, Indiana University, Bloomington, Indiana.
1994 Stature Change in Prehistoric Maya of the Southern Lowlands. *LAA* 5(3):206–11.

Deevey, E. S., Don S. Rice, Prudence M. Rice, H. H. Vaughan, Mark Brenner, and M. S. Flannery
1979 Mayan Urbanism: Impact on a Tropical Karst Environment. *Science* 206:298–306.

Demarest, Arthur A., Héctor Escobedo, Juan A. Valdés, Stephen Houston, Lori E. Wright, and Kitty F. Emery
1991 Arqueología, epigrafía, y el descubrimiento de una tumba real en el centro ceremonial de Dos Pilas, Petén, Guatemala. *U tz'ib* (Guatemala City) 1(1):14–28.

Demarest, Arthur A.
1978 Interregional Conflict and "Situational Ethics" in Classic Maya Warfare. In *Codex Wauchope: A Tribute Roll*, edited by M. Giardino, B. Edmunson, and W. Creamer, pp. 101–11. New Orleans: Human Mosaic (Tulane University).
1992 Ideology in Ancient Maya Cultural Evolution: The Dynamics of Galactic Polities. In *Ideology and Pre-Columbian Civilizations*, edited by Arthur A. Demarest and G. Conrad, pp. 135–57. School of American Research Seminar. Santa Fe, New Mexico: School of American Research Press.
1996 War, Peace, and the Collapse of a Native American Civilization. In *A Natural History of Peace*, edited by T. Gregor, pp. 215–48. Nashville, Tennessee: Vanderbilt University Press.
1997 The Vanderbilt Petexbatun Regional Archaeological Project 1989–1994: Overview, History, and Major Results of a Multidisciplinary Study of the Classic Maya Collapse. *AM* 8(2):209–27.
2003 Political Disruption, Population Displacement, and Enclave Formation: The Terminal Classic of the Petexbatun and Pasión Regions. In *The Terminal Classic in the Maya Lowlands: Collapse, Transition, and Transformation*, edited by Arthur A. Demarest, Prudence M. Rice, and Don S. Rice. Boulder: University Press of Colorado.
2006 *The Petexbatun Regional Archaeological Project: A Multidisciplinary Study of the Collapse of a Classic Maya Kingdom*. VIMA Series, vol. 1. Vanderbilt University Press, Nashville, Tennessee.

Demarest, Arthur A., and Héctor Escobedo A.
1997a *Proyecto Arqueológico Punta de Chimino, Informe Preliminar*. Report Submitted to the Instituto de Antropología e Historia de Guatemala.
1997b El Proyecto Arqueológico Punta de Chimino: objetivos, descubrimientos e interpretaciones preliminaries de la temporada de campo de 1996. In *X Simposio de Investigaciones Arqueológicas en Guatemala, 1996,* edited by Juan P. Laporte and Héctor Escobedo, pp. 381–84. Museo Nacional de Arqueología e Etnología, Guatemala. Guatemala City: Ministerio de Cultura y Deportes, Instituto de Antropología e Historia, Asociación Tikal.
1998 Acontecimientos, procesos, y movimientos de poblaciones en el Clásico Terminal y el Colapso Maya. In *XI Simposio de Investigaciones Arqueológicas en Guatemala, 1997*, edited by Juan P. Laporte and Héctor Escobedo, pp. 699–712. Museo Nacional de Arqueología e Etnología, Guatemala. Guatemala City: Ministerio de Cultura y Deportes, Instituto de Antropología e Historia, Asociación Tikal.

Demarest, Arthur A., Matt O'Mansky, Claudia Wolley, Dirk Van Tuerenhout, Takeshi Inomata, Joel Palka, and Héctor Escobedo
1997 Classic Maya Defensive Systems and Warfare in the Petexbatun Region: Archaeological Evidence and Interpretations. *AM* 8(2):229–53.

Demirjian, A., and G. Y. Levesque
1980 Sexual Differences in Dental Development and Prediction of Emergence. *Journal of Dental Research* 59(7):1110–22.

DeNiro, Michael J.
1985 Postmortem Preservation and Alteration of *in vivo* Bone Collagen Isotope Ratios in relation to Palaeodietary Reconstruction. *Nature* 317:806–9.
1987 Stable Isotopy and Archaeology. *American Scientist* 75:182–91.

DeNiro, Michael. J., and Samuel Epstein
1978 Influence of Diet on the Distribution of Carbon Isotopes in Animals. *Geochimica et Cosmochimica Acta* 42:495–506.
1981 Influence of Diet on the Distribution of

Nitrogen Isotopes in Animals. *Geochimica et Cosmochimica Acta* 45:341–51.

Ditch, L. E., and J. C. Rose
1972 A Multivariate Dental Sexing Technique. *AJPA* 37:61–64.

Dow, Thomas E.
1977 Breastfeeding and Abstinence among the Yoruba. *Studies in Family Planning* 8(8):208–14.

Drucker, P., and J. W. Fox
1982 Swidden Didn' Make All That Midden: The Search for Ancient Mayan Agronomies. *Journal of Anthropological Research* 38:179–93.

Dunning, Nicholas P., and Timothy Beach
1994 Soil Erosion, Slope Management, and Ancient Terracing in the Maya Lowlands. *LAA* 5:51–69.
n.d. *An Ancient Maya Tropical Landscape: The Environmental Archaeology and Ancient Settlement of the Petexbatun Region, Guatemala.* Monograph in preparation for VIMA Series, Vanderbilt University Press, Nashville, Tennessee.

Dunning, Nicholas P., Timothy Beach, and David Rue
1997 The Paleoecology and Ancient Settlement of the Petexbatun Region, Guatemala. *AM* 8(2):255–66.

Dunning, Nicholas P., David Rue, and Timothy Beach
1991 Ecología y patron de asentamiento prehispánico en la región de Petexbatun: resultados preliminares de la temporada 1991. *Proyecto Arqueológico Regional Petexbatun: Informe Preliminar 3, Tercera Temporada*, edited by Arthur Demarest, Takeshi Inomata, Héctor Escobedo, and Joel Palka, pp. 829–47. Report presented to the Instituto de Antropología e Historia de Guatemala.

Dunning, Nicholas P., David Rue, Timothy Beach, Alan Covich, and Alfred Travers
1998 Human-Environment Interactions in a Tropical Watershed: The Paleoecology of Laguna Tamarindito, El Petén, Guatemala. *Journal of Field Archaeology* 25:139–51.

Early, John D.
1982 *The Demographic Structure and Evolution of a Peasant System: The Guatemalan Population.* Boca Raton: University Presses of Florida.

Edeiken, J., P. J. Hodes, and L. H. Caplan
1966 New Bone Production and Periosteal Reaction. *American Journal of Roentgenology* 97:708–18.

Edwards, G., and D. A. Walker
1983 *C3, C4: Mechanisms, and Cellular and Environmental Regulation, of Photosynthesis.* Berkeley: University of California Press.

El-Najjar, Manmoud Y.
1977 Porotic Hyperostosis in North America: A Theory. In *Porotic Hyperostosis: An Enquiry*, edited by E. Cockburn, pp. 9–10. Paleopathology Association Monograph No. 2. Detroit, Michigan.

El-Najjar, Manmoud Y., Dennis J. Ryan, Christy G. Turner II, and Betsy Lozoff
1976 The Etiology of Porotic Hyperostosis among the Prehistoric and Historic Anasazi Indians of the Southwestern United States. *AJPA* 42:477–88.

Elias, Robert W., Yoshimitsu Hirao, and Clair C. Patterson
1982 The Circumvention of the Natural Biopurification of Calcium along Nutrient Pathways by Atmospheric Inputs of Industrial Lead. *Geochimica et Cosmochimica Acta* 46:2561–80.

Emery, Kitty
1986 *Variation in a Tropical Gastropod Population: Implications for Ancient Maya Subsistence.* Unpublished Honors B.Sc. Thesis, Departments of Biology and Anthropology, Trent University, Peterborough, Ontario, Canada.
1989 *Jute* (*Pachychilus* sp.): A Discussion of the Physical Characteristics, Habitat Preferences, and Available Population. Manuscript on file at Trent University, Peterborough, Ontario, Canada.
1991 Análisis preliminar de los restos oseos de fauna de la región de Petexbatun. In *Proyecto Arqueológico Regional Petexbatun: Informe Preliminar 3, Tercera Temporada*, edited by Arthur Demarest, Takeshi

Inomata, Héctor Escobedo, and Joel Palka, pp. 813–28. Report presented to the Instituto de Antropología e Historia de Guatemala.

Emery, Katherine F.
1997 *The Maya Collapse: A Zooarchaeological Investigation*. Unpublished Ph.D. dissertation, Cornell University, Ithaca, New York.

Emery, Kitty F., Lori E. Wright, and Henry P. Schwarcz
2000 Isotopic Analysis of Ancient Deer Bone: Biotic Stability in Collapse Period Maya Land-Use. *JAS* 27(5):537–50.

Emmons, Louise H.
1990 *Neotropical Rainforest Mammals: A Field Guide*. Chicago: University of Chicago Press.

Ennis, J. T., M. C. Gueri, and G. R. Serjeant
1972 Radiological Changes Associated with Leg Ulcers in the Tropics. *British Journal of Radiology* 45:8–14.

Enwonwu, C. O.
1973 Influence of Socio-Economic Conditions on Dental Development in Nigerian Children. *Archives of Oral Biology* 18:95–107.

Ericson, J. E., M. West, C. H. Sullivan, and H. W. Krueger
1989 The Development of Maize Agriculture in the Viru Valley, Peru. In *The Chemistry of Prehistoric Bone*, edited by T. Douglas Price, pp. 68–104. Cambridge, England: Cambridge University Press.

Escobedo, Héctor L.
1997 Arroyo de Piedra: Sociopolitical Dynamics of a Secondary Center in the Petexbatun Region. *AM* 8(2):307–20.

Ezzo, Joseph A.
1992a Dietary Change and Variability at Grasshopper Pueblo, Arizona. *Journal of Anthropological Archaeology* 11:219–89.
1992b A Test of Diet Versus Diagenesis at Ventana Cave, Arizona. *JAS* 19:23–37.
1994 Zinc as a Paleodietary Indicator: An Issue of Theoretical Validity in Bone-Chemistry Analysis. *AAnt* 59(4):606–21.

Fanning, E. A., and T. Brown
1971 Primary and Permanent Tooth Development. *Australian Dental Journal* (February):41–43.

Farnsworth, P., J. E. Brady, M. J. DeNiro, and R. S. MacNeish
1985 A Reevaluation of the Isotopic and Archaeological Reconstructions of Diet in the Tehuacan Valley. *AAnt* 50:102–16.

Fash, W. L.
1988 A New Look at Maya Statecraft from Copan, Honduras. *Antiquity* 62:157–69.

Fedick, Scott L.
1996 *The Managed Mosaic: Ancient Maya Agriculture and Resource Use*. Salt Lake City: University of Utah Press.

Fedick, Scott L., and Anabel Ford
1990 The Prehistoric Agricultural Landscape of the Central Maya Lowlands: An Examination of Local Variability in a Regional Context. *World Archaeology* 22:18–33.

Flannery, Kent V.
1972 Cultural Evolution of Civilizations. *Annual Review of Ecology and Systematics* 3:399–426.
1982 *Maya Subsistence: Studies in Memory of Dennis E. Puleston*. New York: Academic Press.

Flores, Marina, and Berta Garcia
1966 El estado nutricional de niños de edad preescolar en la población de Amatitlan, Guatemala. 1. Comparación de las dietas de la familia y del niño. *Publicaciones Cientificas del Instituto de Nutrición de Centro America y Panama* no. 136 (Recopilación no. 5):25–36.

Flores, Marina, Berta García, Zoila Flores, and Marta Yolanda Lara
1964 Annual Patterns of Family and Children's Diet in Three Guatemalan Indian Communities. *British Journal of Nutrition* 18:281–93.

Foias, Antonia E.
1992 Excavación de la Estructura L4-2 en la plaza central de Dos Pilas: Operación DP2F. In *Proyecto Arqueológico Regional Petexbatun. Informe Preliminar 4. Cuarta Temporada*, edited by Arthur Demarest, Takeshi Inomata, and Héctor Escobedo, pp. 30–34. Report presented to the Instituto de Antropología e Historia de Guatemala.

1993 Resultados preliminares del análisis ceramico del Proyecto Petexbatun. *Apuntes Arqueológicos* 3(1):37–54.

1996 *Changing Ceramic Production and Exchange Systems and the Classic Maya Collapse in the Petexbatun Region*. Unpublished Ph.D. dissertation, Vanderbilt University, Nashville, Tennessee.

1997 *La Amelia Archaeological Project. Final Report, 1997 Field Season*. Williamstown, Massachusetts: Williams College.

Folan, W. J., L. A. Fletcher, and E. R. Kintz
1979 Fruit, Fiber, Bark, and Resin: Social Organization of a Maya Urban Center. *Science* 204:697–701.

Francalacci, P., and S. Borgognini Tarli
1988 Multielementary Analysis of Trace Elements and Preliminary Results on Stable Isotopes in Two Italian Prehistoric Sites. Methodological aspects. In *Trace Elements in Environmental History*, edited by G. Grupe and B. Herrmann, pp. 41–52. Berlin: Springer-Verlag.

Freidel, David, and Vernon L. Scarborough
1982 Subsistence, Trade, and Development of the Coastal Maya. In *Maya Subsistence: Studies in Memory of Dennis E. Puleston*, edited by K. V. Flannery, pp. 131–55. New York: Academic Press.

Freidel, David A.
1986 Terminal Classic Lowland Maya: Successes, Failures, and Aftermaths. In *Late Lowland Maya Civilization: Classic to Postclassic*, edited by Jeremy A. Sabloff and E. W. Andrews V, pp. 409–30. Albuquerque: University of New Mexico Press.

Fried, Morton H.
1967 *The Evolution of Political Society: An Essay in Political Anthropology*. New York: Random House.

Fry, Brian, Richard S. Scalan, and Patrick L. Parker
1983 $^{13}C/^{12}C$ Ratios in Marine Food Webs of the Torres Striat, Queensland. *Australian Journal of Marine and Freshwater Research* 34:707–15.

Fry, B., and E. B. Sherr
1988 $\delta^{13}C$ Measurements as Indicators of Carbon Flow in Marine and Freshwater Ecosystems. In *Stable Isotopes in Ecological Research*, edited by P. W. Rundel, J. R. Ehlerginger, and K. A. Nagy, pp. 196–229. Berlin: Springer-Verlag.

Fuentes y Guzman, Francisco A.
1932 *Recordación Florida: Discurso Historial y Demostración Natural, Material, Militar y Politica del Reyno de Guatemala.* Vol. 1. Biblioteca "Goathemala" de la Sociedad de Geografía e Historia, Guatemala.

Furst, Jill Leslie McKeever
1995 *The Natural History of the Soul in Ancient Mexico*. New Haven: Yale University Press.

Geertz, Clifford
1980 *Negara: The Theatre State in Nineteenth-Century Bali*. Princeton: Princeton University Press.

Geisler, R., and J. Schneider
1976 The Element Matrix of Amazon Waters and Its Relationship with the Mineral Content of Fishes (Determinations Using Neutron Activation Analysis). *Amazoniana* 6(1):47–65.

Gerry, John Philip
1993 *Diet and Status among the Classic Maya: An Isotopic Perspective*. Unpublished Ph.D. dissertation, Harvard University, Cambridge, Massachusetts.

1997 Bone Isotope Ratios and Their Bearing on Elite Privilege among the Classic Maya. *Geoarchaeology* 12(1):41–69.

Gerry, John P., and H. Krueger
1997 Regional Diversity in Classic Maya Diets. In *Bones of the Maya: Studies of Ancient Skeletons*, edited by S. Whittington and D. Reed, pp. 196–207. Washington: Smithsonian Institution Press.

Gilbert, R. I.
1975 *Trace Element Analysis of Three Skeletal Amerindian Populations at Dickson Mounds*. Unpublished Ph.D. dissertation, University of Massachusetts, Amherst.

Giles, Eugene
1964 Sex Determination by Discriminant Function Analysis of the Mandible. *AJPA* 22:129–36.

1970 Discriminant Function Sexing of the Human

Skeleton. In *Personal Identification in Mass Disasters*, edited by T. D. Stewart, pp. 99–109. Washington: Smithsonian Institution.

Goff, Charles W.
1953 New Evidence of Pre-Columbian Bone Syphilis in Guatemala. In *The Ruins of Zaculeu, Guatemala*, edited by R. B. Woodbury and A. S. Trik, pp. 312–19. Vol. 1. New York: United Fruit Company.
1967 Syphilis. In *Diseases in Antiquity: A Survey of the Diseases, Injuries and Surgery of Early Populations*, edited by D. Brothwell and A. T. Sandison, pp. 279–94. Springfield: C. C. Thomas.

Goldstein, Lynne Gail
1980 *Mississippian Mortuary Practices: A Case Study of Two Cemeteries in the Lower Illinois River Valley*. Northwestern University Archaeological Program Scientific Papers No. 4. Northwestern University, Evanston, Illinois.

Golley, F. B.
1983 Nutrient Cycling and Nutrient Conservation. In *Tropical Rainforest Ecosystems: Structure and Function*, edited by D. W. Goodall, pp. 137–56. Ecosystems of the World, 14A. Amsterdam: Elsevier Scientific Publishing Company.

Golley, Frank B., J. T. McGinnis, R. G. Clements, G. I. Child, and M. J. Duever
1975 *Mineral Cycling in a Tropical Moist Forest Ecosystem*. Athens: University of Georgia Press.

Goodenough, Ward H.
1965 Rethinking 'Status' and 'Role': Toward a General Model of the Cultural Organization of Social Relationships. In *The Relevance of Models for Social Anthropology*, edited by M. Banton. A.S.A. Monographs 1. London: Tavistock.

Goodman, Alan H., Lindsay H. Allen, Gabriela P. Hernandez, Alicia Amador, Luis V. Arriola, Adolfo Chavez, and Gretel H. Pelto
1987 Prevalence and Age at Development of Enamel Hypoplasias in Mexican Children. *AJPA* 72:7–19.

Goodman, Alan H., and George J. Armelagos
1985a The Chronological Distribution of Enamel Hypoplasia in Human Permanent Incisor and Canine Teeth. *Archives of Oral Biology* 30(6):503–7.
1985b Factors Affecting the Distribution of Enamel Hypoplasias within the Human Permanent Dentition. *AJPA* 68:479–93.
1988 Childhood Stress and Decreased Longevity in a Prehistoric Population. *AA* 90:936–44.

Goodman, Alan H., George J. Armelagos, and Jerome C. Rose
1980 Enamel Hypoplasias as Indicators of Stress in Three Prehistoric Populations from Illinois. *Human Biology* 52:515–28.

Goodman, Alan H., C. Martinez, and A. Chavez
1991 Nutritional Supplementation and the Development of Linear Enamel Hypoplasias in Children from Tezonteopan, Mexico. *American Journal of Clinical Nutrition* 53:773–81.

Goodman, Alan H., and Jerome C. Rose
1990 Assessment of Systemic Physiological Perturbations from Dental Enamel Hypoplasias and Associated Histological Structures. *Yearbook of Physical Anthropology* 33:59–110.

Goody, J.
1962 *Death, Property, and the Ancestors*. London: Tavistock.

Gordon, Claire C., and Jane E. Buikstra
1981 Soil pH, Bone Preservation, and Sampling Bias at Mortuary Sites. *AAnt* 46:566–71.

Graham, I.
1967 *Archaeological Explorations in El Peten, Guatemala*. Middle American Research Institute, Tulane University, Pub. 33. New Orleans.

Graham, John A.
1973 Aspects of Non-Classic Presences in the Inscriptions and Sculptural Art of Seibal. In *The Classic Maya Collapse*, edited by T. Patrick Culbert, pp. 207–20. Albuquerque: University of New Mexico Press.

Greenfield, G. B.
1986 *Radiology of Bone Diseases*. Philadelphia: J. B. Lippincott.

Greenfield, G. B., and H. A. Schorsch
1967 The Various Roentgen Appearances of Pulmonary Hypertrophic Osteoarthropathy. *American Journal of Roentgenology* 101:927–31.

Grupe, Gisela
1988 Impact of the Choice of Bone Samples on Trace Element Data in Excavated Human Skeletons. *JAS* 15:123–29.

Grupe, Gisela, and Bernd Herrmann (editors)
1988 *Trace Elements in Environmental History*. Berlin: Springer-Verlag.

Grupe, Gisela, and H. Piepenbrink
1988 Trace Element Contaminations in Excavated Bones by Microorganisms. In *Trace Elements in Environmental History*, edited by Gisela Grupe and Bernd Herrmann, pp. 103–12. Berlin: Springer-Verlag.

Guiteras-Holmes, C.
1961 *Perils of the Soul: The World View of a Tzotzil Indian*. New York: Free Press.

Hackett, Cecil J.
1951 *Bone Lesions of Yaws in Uganda*. Oxford: Basil Blackwell Scientific Publications.
1967 The Human Treponematoses. In *Diseases in Antiquity*, edited by D. Brothwell and A. T. Sandison, pp. 152–69. Springfield, Illinois: Charles C. Thomas.
1976 *Diagnostic Criteria of Syphilis, Yaws and Treponarid (Treponematoses) and of Some Other Diseases in Dry Bones*. Berlin: Springer-Verlag.
1981 Microscopical Focal Destruction (Tunnels) in Exhumed Human Bones. *Medicine Science and the Law* 21(4):243–65.

Hagihara, Y., H. Kaminishi, T. Cho, M. Tanaka, and H. Kaita
1988 Degradation of Human Dentine Collagen by an Enzyme Produced by the Yeast *Candida albicans*. *Archives of Oral Biology*. 33(8):617–19.

Hall, Grant David
1989 *Realm of Death: Royal Mortuary Customs and Polity Interaction in the Classic Maya Lowlands*. Unpublished Ph.D. dissertation, Harvard University, Cambridge, Massachusetts.

Hamblin, Nancy
1984 *Animal Use by the Cozumel Maya*. Tucson: University of Arizona Press.

Hamblin, R. L., and B. L. Pitcher
1980 The Classic Maya Collapse: Testing Class Conflict Hypotheses. *AAnt* 45:246–67.

Hancock, R. G. V., M. D. Grynpas, and K. P. H. Pritzker
1989 The Abuse of Bone Analyses for Archaeological Dietary Studies. *Archaeometry* 31(2):169–79.

Hanson, Douglas B., and Jane E. Buikstra
1987 Histomorphological Alteration in Buried Human Bone from the Lower Illinois Valley: Implications for Palaeodietary Research. *JAS* 14:549–63.

Hare, P. Edgar
1980 Organic Geochemistry of Bone and Its Relation to the Survival of Bone in the Natural Environment. In *Fossils in the Making: Vertebrate Taphonomy and Paleoecology*, edited by A. K. Behrensmeyer and A. P. Hill, pp. 208–19. Chicago: University of Chicago Press.

Hare, P. Edgar, Marilyn L. Fogel, Thomas W. Stafford Jr., Alva D. Mitchell, and Thomas C. Hoering
1991 The Isotopic Composition of Carbon and Nitrogen in Individual Amino Acids Isolated from Modern and Fossil Proteins. *JAS* 18:277–92.

Harris, David R.
1972 Swidden Systems and Settlement. In *Man, Settlement and Urbanism*, edited by P. J. Ucko, R. Tringham, and G. W. Dimbleby. pp. 82–102. London: Duckworth.

Harris, N. H., and W. H. Kirkaldy-Willis
1965 Primary Subacute Pyogenic Osteomyelitis. *Journal of Bone and Joint Surgery* 47B(3):526–32.

Harrison, P. D.
1977 The Rise of the Bajos and the Fall of the Maya. In *Social Process in Maya Prehistory: Studies in Memory of Sir Eric Thompson*, edited by N. Hammond, pp. 469–508. London: Academic Press.

Harrison, P. D., and B. L. Turner
1978 *Pre-Hispanic Maya Agriculture*. Albuquerque: University of New Mexico Press.

Harritt, R. K., and S. C. Radosevich
1992 Results of Instrument Neutron-Activation Trace-Element Analysis of Human Remains from the Naknek Region, Southwest Alaska. *AAnt* 57(2):288–99.

Hastorf, Christine A., and Sissel Johannessen
1993 Pre-Hispanic Political Change and the Role of Maize in the Central Andes of Peru. *AA* 95(1):115–38.

Hatch, J. W., and R. A. Geidel
1985 Status-specific Dietary Variation in Two World Cultures. *Journal of Human Evolution* 14:469–76.

Haviland, William A.
1967 Stature at Tikal, Guatemala: Implications for Classic Maya Demography and Social Organization. *AAnt* 32:316–25.
1969 A New Population Estimate for Tikal, Guatemala. *AAnt* 34:429–33.
1970a *Ancient Lowland Maya Social Organization*. Middle American Research Institute, Tulane University, Pub. 26. New Orleans.
1970b Tikal, Guatemala and Mesoamerican Urbanism. *World Archaeology* 2:186–98.

Haviland, William A., and Hattula Moholy-Nagy
1992 Distinguishing the High and Mighty from the Hoi Polloi at Tikal, Guatemala. In *Mesoamerican Elites: An Archaeological Assessment*, edited by A. Chase and D. Chase, pp. 50–60. Norman: University of Oklahoma Press.

Healy, Paul F., Kitty F. Emery, and Lori E. Wright
1990 Ancient and Modern Maya Exploitation of the Juté Snail (*Pachychilus*). *LAA* 1(2):170–83.

Heaton, T. H. E.
1987 The $^{15}N/^{14}N$ Ratios of Plants in South Africa and Namibia: Relationship to Climate and Coastal/Saline Environments. *Oecologia* 74:236–46.

Heaton, T. H. E., J. C. Vogel, G. von la Chevallerie, and G. Collett
1986 Climatic Influence on the Isotopic Composition of Bone Nitrogen. *Nature* 322:822–23.

Hellmuth, Nicholas M.
1987 *The Surface of the Underwater World: Iconography of the Gods of Early Classic Maya Art in Peten, Guatemala*. Culver City, California: Foundation for Latin American Anthropological Research.

Helms, Mary W.
1979 *Ancient Panama*. Austin: University of Texas Press.
1991 Esoteric Knowledge, Geographical Distance, and the Elaboration of Leadership Status: Dynamics of Resource Control. In *Profiles in Cultural Evolution: Papers from a Conference in Honor of Elman R. Service*, edited by A. T. Rambo and K. Gillogly. Anthropological Papers No. 85, Museum of Anthropology, University of Michigan. Ann Arbor.

Henderson, Helen Hope
1998 *The Organization of Staple Crop Production in Middle Formative, Late Formative, and Classic Period Farming Households at K'axob, Belize*. Unpublished Ph.D. dissertation, University of Pittsburgh.

Hertz, Robert
1907 *Death and the Right Hand*. Translated by Rodney and Claudia Needham. Glencoe, Illinois: Free Press (translation published in 1960).

Hodder, Ian
1979 Economic and Social Stress and Material Culture Patterning. *AAnt* 44:446–54.
1982 The Identification and Interpretation of Ranking in Prehistory: A Contextual Perspective. In *Ranking, Resource and Exchange: Aspects of the Archaeology of Early European Society*, edited by C. Renfrew and S. Shennan, pp. 150–54. Cambridge, England: Cambridge University Press.
1987 The Contribution of the Long Term. In *Archaeology as Long-term History*, edited by I. Hodder, pp. 1–8. Cambridge, England: Cambridge University Press.
1989 *Reading the Past: Current Approaches to*

Interpretation in Archaeology. Cambridge, England: Cambridge University Press.

1992 Symbolism, Meaning and Context. In *Theory and Practice in Archaeology*, edited by I. Hodder, pp. 11–23. London: Routledge.

Hodell, David A., Jason H. Curtis, and Mark Brenner

1995 Possible Role of Climate in the Collapse of Classic Maya Civilization. *Nature* 375:391–94.

Hodges, Denise C.

1987 Health and Agricultural Intensification in the Prehistoric Valley of Oaxaca, Mexico. *AJPA* 73:323–32.

Hodges, Denise C., and Richard G. Wilkinson

1990 Effect of Tooth Size on the Ageing and Chronological Distribution of Enamel Hypoplastic Defects. *American Journal of Human Biology* 2:553–60.

Hodson, F. R.

1970 Cluster Analysis and Archaeology: Some New Developments and Applications. *World Archaeology* 1:289–320.

Holland, Thomas D., and Michael J. O'Brien

1997 Parasites, Porotic Hyperostosis, and the Implications of Changing Perspectives. *AAnt* 62(2):183–93.

Hooton, Earnest A.

1940 Skeletons from the Cenote of Sacrifice at Chichen Itzá. In *The Maya and Their Neighbors*, edited by C. L. Hay, pp. 272–80. New York: D. Appleton-Century.

Hosler, D., Jeremy A. Sabloff, and D. Runge

1977 Situation Model Development: A Case Study of the Classic Maya Collapse. In *Social Process in Maya Prehistory*, edited by N. Hammond, pp. 553–90. London: Academic Press.

Houston, Stephen D.

1987 *The Inscriptions and Monumental Art of Dos Pilas, Guatemala: A Study of Classic Maya History and Politics*. Unpublished Ph.D. dissertation, Yale University, New Haven.

1989 Archaeology and Maya Writing. *Journal of World Prehistory* 3(1):1–31.

1993 *Hieroglyphs and History at Dos Pilas: Dynastic Politics of the Classic Maya*. Austin: University of Texas Press.

Houston, Stephen D., and P. Matthews

1985 *The Dynastic Sequence of Dos Pilas, Guatemala*. Pre-Columbian Art Research Institute Monograph 1. San Francisco.

Houston, Stephen D., David Stuart, and Karl A. Taube

1989 Folk Classification of Classic Maya Pottery. *AA* 91(3):720–26.

Howell, Nancy

1982 Village Composition Implied by a Paleodemographic Life Table: The Libben Site. *AJPA* 59:263–69.

Hudson, E. H.

1965 Treponematosis and Man's Social Evolution. *AA* 67:885–901.

Humphreys, S. C.

1981 Introduction: Comparative Perspectives on Death. In *Mortality and Immortality: The Anthropology and Archaeology of Death*, edited by S. C. Humphreys and H. King, pp. 1–14. London: Academic Press.

Huntington, Ellsworth

1917 Maya Civilization and Climatic Changes. *Proceedings of the 19th International Congress of Americanists*, pp. 150–64. Washington, D.C.

Hutchinson, Dale L., and Clark Spencer Larsen

1988 Determination of Stress Episode Duration from Linear Enamel Hypoplasias: A Case Study from St. Catherines Island, Georgia. *Human Biology* 60(1):93–110.

I.N.C.A.P. (Instituto de Nutrición de Centro America y Panama)

1961 *Food Composition Table for Use in Latin America*. Bethesda, Maryland: National Institutes of Health.

Inomata, Takeshi

1995 *Archaeological Investigations at the Fortified Center of Aguateca, El Peten, Guatemala: Implications for the Study of the Classic Maya Collapse*. Unpublished Ph.D. dissertation, Vanderbilt University, Nashville, Tennessee.

1997 The Last Day of a Fortified Classic Maya Center: Archaeological Investigations at Aguateca, Guatemala. *AM* 8(2):337–51.

2006 *Warfare and the Fall of a Fortified Center: Archaeological Investigations at Aguateca,*

Guatemala. VIMA Series vol. 3. Vanderbilt University Press, Nashville, Tennessee. Forthcoming.

Inomata, Takeshi, Stephen Houston, Kevin Johnston, and Antonia Foias
1989 Registro y rescate en Punta de Chimino. In *Proyecto Arqueológico Regional Petexbatun. Informe Preliminar 1, Primera Temporada,* edited by Arthur Demarest and Stephen Houston, pp. 130–52. Report presented to the Instituto de Antropología e Historia de Guatemala.

Inomata, Takeshi, and Laura R. Stiver
1998 Floor Assemblages from Burned Structures at Aguateca, Guatemala: A Study of Classic Maya Households. *Journal of Field Archaeology* 25(4):431–52.

Jackes, Mary
1992 Paleodemography: Problems and Techniques. In *Skeletal Biology of Past Peoples: Research Methods*, edited by S. R. Saunders and M. A. Katzenberg, pp. 189–224. New York: Wiley-Liss

Janzen, Daniel H.
1983 Food Webs: Who Eats What, Why, How, and with What Effects in a Tropical Forest. In *Tropical Rain Forest Ecosystems: Structure and Function*, edited by F. B. Golley, pp. 167–82. Ecosystems of the World, vol. 14A. Amsterdam: Elsevier Scientific Publishing Company.

Johansson, S. R., and S. Horowitz
1986 Estimating Mortality in Skeletal Populations: Influence of the Growth Rate on the Interpretation of Levels and Trends during the Transition to Agriculture. *AJPA* 71:233–50.

Johnston, Kevin
1994 *The "Invisible" Maya: Late Classic Minimally-Platformed Residential Settlement at Itzán, Petén, Guatemala.* Unpublished Ph.D. dissertation, Yale University, New Haven.

Jones, C.
1977 Inaugural Dates of Three Late Classic Rulers of Tikal, Guatemala. *AAnt* 42:28–60.

Jones, John G.
1994 Pollen Evidence for Early Settlement and Agriculture in Northern Belize. *Palynology* 18:205–11.

Joralemon, Peter David
1974 Ritual Blood-Sacrifice among the Ancient Maya. In *Primera Mesa Redonda de Palenque, Part I*, edited by M. Green Robertson, pp. 59–75. Pebble Beach, California: Robert Louis Stevenson School.

Jordan, Carl F.
1984 Nutrient Regime in the Wet Tropics: Physical Factors. In *Physiological Ecology of Plants of the Wet Tropics*, edited by E. Medina, H. H. Mooney, and C. Vásquez-Yánes, pp. 3–12. The Hague: Dr. W. Junk Publishers.

Jordan, Carl F., Jerry R. Kline, and Donald S. Sasscer
1972 Relative Stability of Mineral Cycles in Forest Ecosystems. *American Naturalist* 106:237–54.

Katz, Darryl, and Judy Myers Suchey
1986 Age Determination of the Male *Os pubis*. *AJPA* 69:427–35.

Katz, S. H., M. L. Hediger, and L. A. Valleroy
1974 Traditional Maize Processing Techniques in the New World. *Science* 184:765–73.

Katzenberg, M. Anne
1984 *Chemical Analysis of Prehistoric Human Bone from Five Temporally Distinct Populations in Southern Ontario*. Mercury Series, Archaeological Survey of Canada, No. 129. Ottawa: National Museums of Canada.
1989 Stable Isotope Analysis of Archaeological Faunal Remains from Southern Ontario. *JAS* 16:319–29.

Katzenberg, M. Anne, D. A. Herring, and S. R. Saunders
1996 Weaning and Infant Mortality: Evaluating the Skeletal Evidence. *Yearbook of Physical Anthropology* 39:177–99.

Keegan, William F., and Michael J. DeNiro
1988 Stable Carbon- and Nitrogen-Isotope Ratios of Bone Collagen Used to Study Coral-Reef and Terrestrial Components of Prehistoric Bahamian Diet. *AAnt* 53(2):320–36.

Kelley, M. A., and M. S. Micozzi
1984 Rib Lesions and Chronic Pulmonary Tuberculosis. *AJPA* 65:381–86.

Kennedy, Brenda V. E.
1988 *Variation in δ^{13}C Values of Post-Medieval Europeans*. Unpublished Ph.D. dissertation, University of Calgary, Alberta, Canada.

Killion, Thomas W.
1992 *Gardens of Prehistory: The Archaeology of Settlement Agriculture in Mesoamerica*. Tuscaloosa: University of Alabama Press.

Killion, Thomas W., Dirk van Turenhout, Daniella Triadan, Inez Verhagen, Matthew McDermott, Lisa Hamerlynck, and Robert Chatham
1991 *Broken Heartland of Cities: Intersite Settlement in the Petexbatun Region, Peten, Guatemala*. 47th International Congress of Americanists, New Orleans.

Kirkpatrick, D. J.
1970 *Donovanosis* (*Granuloma inguinale*): A Rare Cause of Osteolytic Bone Lesions. *Clinical Radiology* 21:101–5.

Klepinger, Linda L.
1984 Nutritional Assessment from Bone. *Annual Review of Anthropology* 13:75–96.
1990 Magnesium Ingestion and Bone Magnesium Concentration in Paleodietary Reconstruction: Cautionary Evidence from an Animal Model. *JAS* 17:513–17.

Klepinger, Linda L., John K. Kuhn, and Wendell S. Williams
1986 An Elemental Analysis of Archaeological Bone from Sicily as a Test of Predictability of Diagenetic Change. *AJPA* 70:325–31.

Kowalski, Jeff Karl
1989 Who Am I Among the Itza? Links between Northern Yucatan and the Western Maya Lowlands and Highlands. In *Mesoamerica After the Decline of Teotihuacan A.D. 700–900*, edited by R. A. Diehl and J. C. Berlo, pp. 173–85. Washington: Dumbarton Oaks.

Krueger, Harold W., and Charles H. Sullivan
1984 Models for Carbon Isotope Fractionation between Diet and Bone. In *Stable Isotopes in Nutrition*. ACS Symposium, edited by J. F. Turnland and P. E. Johnson, pp. 205–20. Washington: American Chemical Society.

Krzanowski, W. J.
1988 *Principles of Multivariate Analysis: A User's Perspective*. Oxford: Oxford Science Publications.

Kuhnlein, Harriet V.
1981 Dietary Mineral Ecology of the Hopi. *Journal of Ethnobiology* 1(1):84–94.

Lainson, R., and J. J. Shaw
1987 Evolution, Classification and Geographical Distribution. In *The Leishmaniases in Biology and Medicine*, edited by Wallace Peters and R. Killick-Kendrick. Vol. 1, *Biology and Epidemiology*, pp. 1–120. London: Academic Press.

Lallo, John W., George J. Armelagos, and Robert P. Mensforth
1977 The Role of Diet, Disease, and Physiology in the Origin of Porotic Hyperostosis. *Human Biology* 49(3):471–83.

Lambert, Joseph B., and Gisela Grupe
1993 *Prehistoric Human Bone: Archaeology at the Molecular Level*. Berlin: Springer-Verlag.

Lambert, Joseph B., Sharon Vlasak Simpson, Jane E. Buikstra, and Douglas K. Charles
1984 Analysis of Soil Associated with Woodland Burials. In *Archaeological Chemistry-III*, edited by JosephB. Lambert, pp. 97–113. Advances in Chemistry Series, 205. Washington: American Chemical Society.

Lambert, Joseph B., S. V. Simpson, Jane E. Buikstra, and D. Hanson
1983 Electron Microprobe Analysis of Elemental Distribution in Excavated Human Femurs. *AJPA* 62:409–23.

Lambert, Joseph B., Sharon Vlasak Simpson, Carole B. Sqpunar, and Jane E. Buikstra
1985 Bone Diagenesis and Dietary Analysis. *Journal of Human Evolution* 14:477–82.

Lambert, Joseph B., S. V. Simpson, C. B. Szpunar, and Jane E. Buikstra
1982 A Comparative Study of the Chemical Analysis of Ribs and Femurs in Woodland Populations. *AJPA* 59:289–94.

Lambert, Joseph B., Jane M. Weydert, Sloan R. Williams, and Jane E. Buikstra
1990 Comparison of Methods for the Removal of Diagenetic Material in Buried Bone. *JAS* 17:453–68.

Lambert, J. D. H., and J. T. Arnason
1982 *Ramón* and Maya Ruins: An Ecological, Not an Economic, Relation. *Science* 216:298–99.

Lange, Frederick W.
1971 Marine Resources: A Viable Subsistence Alternative for the Prehistoric Lowland Maya. *AA* 73:619–39.

Las Casas, Bartolomé de
1909 *Apologética Historia de las Indias*. Madrid: Bailliere e Hijos.

Layrisse, M. J., J. D. Cook, C. Martinez, M. Roch, I. N. Kuhn, R. B. Walker, and C. A. Finch
1969 Food Iron Absorption: A Comparison of Vegetable and Animal Foods. *Blood* 33:430–33.

Lee-Thorp, Julia A., Judith C. Sealy, and Nikolaas J. van der Merwe
1989 Stable Carbon Isotope Ratio Differences between Bone Collagen and Bone Apatite, and Their Relationship to Diet. *JAS* 16:585–99.

Lee-Thorp, Julia A., and Nikolaas J. van der Merwe
1991 Aspects of the Chemistry of Modern and Fossil Biological Apatites. *JAS* 18:343–54.

Lentz, David L.
1990 *Acrocomia mexicana:* Palm of the Ancient Mesoamericans. *Journal of Ethnobiology* 10(2):183–94.
1991 Maya Diets of the Rich and Poor: Paleoethnobotanical Evidence from Copán. *LAA* 2(3):269–87.

Lévi-Strauss, Claude
1976 *Tristes Tropiques*. Harmondsworth: Penguin.

Lindsay, Willard L.
1979 *Chemical Equilibria in Soils*. New York: John Wiley and Sons.

Liniecki, J.
1971 Kinetics of Calcium, Strontium, Barium and Radium in Rabbits. *Health Physics* 21:367–76.

Love, Bruce
1989 Yucatec Sacred Breads through Time. In *Word and Image in Maya Culture: Explorations in Language, Writing and Representation*, edited by W. F. Hanks and Don S. Rice, pp. 336–50. Salt Lake City: University of Utah Press.

Lovejoy, C. Owen, Richard S. Meindl, Thomas R. Pryzbeck, T. S. Barton, K. G. Heiple, and D. Knotting
1977 Paleodemography of the Libben Site, Ottawa County, Ohio. *Science* 198:291–93.

Lovejoy, C. Owen, Richard S. Meindl, Thomas R. Pryzbeck, and Robert P. Mensforth
1985 Chronological Metamorphosis of the Auricular Surface of the Ilium: A New Method for the Determination of Adult Skeletal Age at Death. *AJPA* 68:15–28.

Lowe, J. W. G.
1985 *Dynamics of Apocalypse: A Systems Simulation of the Classic Maya Collapse.* Albuquerque: University of New Mexico Press.

Lundell, Cyrus L.
1939 Plants Probably Utilized by the Old Empire Maya of Petén and Adjacent Lowlands. *Papers of the Michigan Academy of Science, Arts and Letters* 24(1):37–56.

MacKay, R. H.
n.d. *Skeletal Maturation Chart*. Rochester: Eastman Kodak

MacKie, E.
1961 New Light on the End of Classic Maya Culture at Benque Viejo, British Honduras. *AAnt* 27:216–24.

Macko, S. A., M. L. Fogel Estep, M. A. Engel, and P. Edgar Hare
1986 Kinetic Fractionation of Stable Nitrogen Isotopes During Amino Acid Transamination. *Geochimicha et Cosmochimica Acta* 50:2143–46.

Manson-Bahr, P. E. C., and D. J. Winslow
1975 Cutaneous Leishmaniasis. In *Pathology of Protozoal and Helminthic Diseases, with Clinical Correlation*, edited by R.A. Marcial-Rojas, pp. 97–112. Huntington, New York: Robert E. Krieger Publishing.

Marcus, C. S., and R. H. Wasserman
1965 Comparison of Intestinal Discrimination between Calcium 47, Strontium 85, and Barium 133. *American Journal of Physiology* 209:973–77.

Marcus, Joyce
1982 The Plant World of the Sixteenth- and Seventeenth-Century Lowland Maya. In *Maya Subsistence: Studies in Honor of Dennis Puleston*, edited by K. V. Flannery, pp. 239–73. New York: Academic Press.

Marino, Bruno D., and Michael J. DeNiro
1987 Isotopic Analysis of Archaeobotanicals to Reconstruct Past Climates: Effects of Activities Associated with Food Preparation on Carbon, Hydrogen, and Oxygen Isotope Ratios of Plant Cellulose. *JAS* 14:537–48.

Márquez Morfín, L.
1984 Distribución de la estatura en colecciones óseas mayas prehispánicas. In *Estudios de Antropología Biológica* (*II. Colloquio de Antropología Fisica Juan Comas, 1982*), edited by R. Ramos Galvan and R. M. Ramos Rodriguez, pp. 253–71. Instituto de Investigaciones Antropológicas, Serie Antropológica 75. Mexico City: Universidad Nacional Autónoma de México.

Márquez Morfín, Lourdes, and Andrés del Angel
1997 Height among Prehispanic Maya of the Yucatán Peninsula: A Reconsideration. In *Bones of the Maya: Studies of Ancient Skeletons*, edited by S. L. Whittington and D. M. Reed, pp. 51–61. Washington: Smithsonian Institution Press.

Marsden, P. D., R. N. R. Sampaio, R. Rocha, and M. Radke
1977 Mucocutaneous leishmaniasis—an Unsolved Clinical Problem. *Tropical Doctor* 7:7–11.

Massler, M., I. Schour, and H. G. Poncher
1941 Developmental Pattern of the Child as Reflected in the Calcification Pattern of Teeth. *American Journal of Diseases of Children* 62:33–67.

Mathews, Peter, and Gordon R. Willey
1991 Prehistoric Polities of the Pasión Region: Hieroglyphic Texts and Their Archaeological Settings. In *Classic Maya Political History: Hieroglyphic and Archaeological Evidence*, edited by T. Patrick Culbert, pp. 30–71. New York: Cambridge University Press.

May, Richard L., Alan H. Goodman, and Richard S. Meindl
1993 Response of Bone and Enamel Formation to Nutritional Supplementation and Morbidity among Malnourished Guatemalan Children. *AJPA* 92(1):37–51.

McAnany, Patricia A.
1993 The Economics of Social Power and Wealth among Eighth-Century Maya Households. In *Lowland Maya Civilization in the Eighth Century A.D*, edited by Jeremy A. Sabloff and J. S. Henderson, pp. 65–89. Washington: Dumbarton Oaks.

McGee, R. Jon
1990 *Life, Ritual, and Religion among the Lacandón Maya*. Belmont, California: Wadsworth Publishing

Meave del Castillo, Jorge
1990 *Estructura y Composición de la Selva Alta Perennifolia de los Alrededores de Bonampak*. Serie Arquelogía, Colección Científica 185. Mexico City: Instituto Nacional de Antropología e Historia.

Meggers, Betty J.
1954 Environmental Limitation on the Development of Culture. *AA* 56(5):801–24.

Meindl, Richard S., and C. Owen Lovejoy
1985 Ectocranial Suture Closure: A Revised Method for the Determination of Skeletal Age at Death based on the Lateral-Anterior Sutures. *AJPA* 68:57–66.

Meindl, Richard S., C. Owen Lovejoy, Robert P. Mensforth, and Lydia Don Carlos
1985a Accuracy and Direction of Error in the Sexing of the Skeleton: Implications for Paleodemography. *AJPA* 68:79–85.

Meindl, Robert S., C. Owen Lovejoy, Robert P. Mensforth, and Robert A. Walker
1985b A Revised Method of Age Determination Using the Os Pubis, with a Review and Tests of Accuracy of Other Current Methods of Pubic Symphyseal Aging. *AJPA* 68:29–45.

Mensforth, Robert P., C. Owen Lovejoy, John W. Lallo, and George J. Armelagos
1978 The Role of Constitutional Factors, Diet, and Infectious Disease in the Etiology of Porotic Hyperostosis and Periosteal Reactions in Prehistoric Infants and Children. *Medical Anthropology* 2(1):1–57.

Meyers, W. M., and R. C. Neafie
1991 Tropical Phagedenic Ulcer. In *Hunter's Tropical Medicine*, edited by G. T. Strickland, pp. 310–11. Philadelphia: W.B. Saunders.

Miksicek, Charles H.
1983 Macrofloral Remains of the Pulltrouser Area: Settlements and Fields. In *Pulltrouser Swamp: Ancient Maya Habitat, Agriculture, and Settlement in Northern Belize*, edited by B. L. Turner II and P. D. Harrison, pp. 94–104. Austin: University of Texas Press.

Miksicek, Charles H., K. J. Elsesser, I. A. Wuebber, K. O. Bruhns, and N. Hammond
1981 Rethinking Ramón: A comment on Reina and Hill's Lowland Maya Subsistence. *AAnt* 46:916–18.

Miles, S. W.
1957 The Sixteenth-Century Pokom-Maya. *Transactions of the American Philosophical Society* 47:735–81.

Milner, George R., Dorothy A. Humpf, and Henry C. Harpending
1989 Pattern Matching of Age-at-Death Distributions in Paleodemographic Analysis. *AJPA* 80:49–58.

Moholy-Nagy, Hattula
1978 The Utilization of *Pomacea* at Tikal, Guatemala. *AAnt* 43:65–73.
1985 The Social and Ceremonial Uses of Marine Molluscs at Tikal. In *Prehistoric Lowland Maya Environment and Subsistence Economy*, edited by Mary Pohl, pp. 148–58. Papers of the PMAE vol. 77.

Molleson, Theya I., and Percy Cohen
1990 The Progression of Dental Attrition Stages Used for Age Assessment. *JAS* 17:363–71.

Moore, James A., Alan C. Swedlund, and George J. Armelagos
1975 The Use of Life Tables in Paleodemography. In *Population Studies in Archaeology and Biological Anthropology: A Symposium*, edited by Alan C. Swedlund, pp. 57–70. Memoirs of the Society for American Archaeology No. 30. *AAnt* 40(2), pt. 2.

Morgan, M. E., and Margaret J. Schoeninger
1989 Zinc and strontium as dietary indicators in a modern tropical community. *AJPA* 78(2):276.

Morley, S. G.
1937–1938 *The Inscriptions of Peten*. Carnegie Institution of Washington, Pub. 437, 5 vols. Washington D. C.

Morris, Ian
1992 *Death-Ritual and Social Structure in Classical Antiquity*. Cambridge, England: Cambridge University Press.

Mølbak, K., A. Gottschau, P. Aaby, N. Højlyng, L. Ingholt, and A. P. J. da Silva
1994 Prolonged Breast Feeding, Diarrhoeal Disease, and Survival of Children in Guinea-Bissau. *British Medical Journal* 308:1403–6.

Nations, James D.
1979a *Population Ecology of the Lacandon Maya*. Unpublished Ph.D. dissertation, Southern Methodist University, Dallas, Texas.
1979b Snail Shells and Maize Preparation: A Lacandon Maya Analogy. *AAnt* 44:568–71.

Nations, James D., and R. B. Nigh
1980 The Evolutionary Potential of Lacandon Maya Sustained-Yield Tropical Forest Agriculture. *Journal of Anthropological Research* 36:1–30.

Nelson, Dorothy A., and Norman J. Sauer
1984 An Evaluation of Postdepositional Changes in the Trace Element Content of Human Bone. *AAnt* 49(1):144–47.

Nikiforuk, Gordon, and Donald Fraser
1981 The Etiology of Enamel Hypoplasia: A Unifying Concept. *Journal of Pediatrics* 98(6):888–93.

Norr, Lynette C.
1991 *Nutritional Consequences of Prehistoric Subsistence Strategies in Lower Central America*. Unpublished Ph.D. dissertation, University of Illinois, Urbana-Champaign.

Norusis, M. J.
1988 *SPSS/PC+ Advanced Statistics V2.0 for the IBM PC/XT/AT and PS/2*. Chicago: SPSS Inc.

Noss, J. F., G. R. Scott, R. H. Yap Potter, and A. A. Dahlberg
1983 Fluctuating Asymmetry in Molar Dimensions and Discrete Morphological Traits in Pima Indians. *AJPA* 61:437–45.

O'Leary, Marion H.
1983 Carbon Isotopes in Photosynthesis. *Bioscience* 38(5):328–36.

O'Mansky, Matthew, Q. Joshua Hinson, Robert Wheat, and Arthur Demarest
1995 Investigaciones del Transecto 4 oeste de Aguateca. In *Proyecto Arqueológico Petexbatun: Informe Preliminar 6, Sexta Temporada 1994*, edited by Arthur A. Demarest, Juan A. Valdés, and Héctor Escobedo, pp. 447–72.

O'Shea, John M.
1984 *Mortuary Variability*. New York: Academic Press.
1996 *Villagers of the Maros: A Portrait of an Early Bronze Age Society*. New York: Plenum Press.

Ortiz de Montellano, Bernard R.
1990 *Aztec Medicine, Health and Nutrition*. New Brunswick, New Jersey: Rutgers University Press.

Ortner, Donald J., and Walter G. J. Putschar
1985 *Identification of Pathological Conditions in Human Skeletal Remains*. Smithsonian Contributions to Anthropology No. 28. Washington, D.C.: Smithsonian Institution Press.

Ortner, Donald J., N. Tuross, and A. I. Stix
1992 New Approaches to the Study of Disease in Archaeological New World Populations. *Human Biology* 64(6):337–60.

Ortner, Donald J., and Mary Frances Ericksen
1997 Bone Changes in the Human Skull Probably Resulting from Scurvy in Infancy and Childhood. *International Journal of Osteoarchaeology* 7:212–20.

Osborn, J. W.
1973 Variations in Structure and Development of Enamel. *Oral Sciences Review* 3:3–83.

Pader, Ellen-Jane
1982 *Symbolism, Social Relations, and the Interpretation of Mortuary Remains*. BAR International Series 130. Oxford: B.A.R.

Palka, Joel Wade
1995 *Classic Maya Social Inequality and the Collapse at Dos Pilas, Peten, Guatemala*. Unpublished Ph.D. dissertation, Vanderbilt University, Nashville, Tennessee.
1998 Lacandon Maya Culture Change and Survival in the Lowland Frontier of the Expanding Guatemalan and Mexican Republics. In *Studies in Culture Contact: Interaction, Culture Change, and Archaeology*, edited by J. G. Cusick, pp. 457–75. Center for Archaeological Investigations, Occasional Paper No. 25. Carbondale: Southern Illinois University.

Palkovich, A. M.
1987 Endemic Disease Patterns in Paleopathology: Porotic Hyperostosis. *AJPA* 74:527–37.

Parker, Ronald B., and Heinrich Toots
1972 Hollandite-Coronadite in Fossil Bone. *American Mineralogist* 57:1527–30.
1980 Trace Elements in Bones as Paleobiological Indicators. In *Fossils in the Making: Vertebrate Taphonomy and Paleoecology*, edited by A. K. Behrensmeyer and A. P. Hill, pp. 197–207. Chicago: University of Chicago Press.

Pate, Donald, and Kenneth A. Brown
1985 The Stability of Bone Strontium in the Geochemical Environment. *Journal of Human Evolution* 14:483–91.

Pearson, Mike Parker
1999 *Archaeology of Death and Burial*. College Station: Texas A & M University Press.

Peebles, Christopher S., and Susam M. Kus
1977 Some Archaeological Correlates of Ranked Societies. *AAnt* 42(3):421–48.

Pendergast, David M.
1986 Stability through Change: Lamanai, Belize, from the Ninth to the Seventeenth Century. In *Late Lowland Maya Civilization: Classic to Postclassic,* edited by Jeremy Sabloff and

E. W. Andrews V, pp. 223–49. Albuquerque: University of New Mexico Press.

Perine, P. L., D. R. Hopkins, P. L. A. Niemel, R. K. St. John, G. Causse, and G. M. Antal
1984 *Handbook of Endemic Treponematoses: Yaws, Endemic Syphilis, and Pinta*. Geneva, Switzerland: World Health Organization.

Peters, Charles M.
1983 Observations on Maya Subsistence and the Ecology of a Tropical Tree. *AAnt* 48(3):610–15.

Phenice, T. W.
1969 A Newly Developed Visual Method of Sexing the *Os pubis*. *AJPA* 30:297–302.

Pindborg, Jens J.
1982 Aetiology of Developmental Enamel Defects Not Related to Fluorosis. *International Dental Journal* 32(2):123–34.

Pineda, C. J., M. Martinez-Lavin, J. E. Goobar, D. J. Sartoris, P. Clopton, and D. Resnick
1987 Periostitis in Hypertrophic Osteoarthropathy: Relationship to Disease Duration. *American Journal of Roentgenology* 148:773–78.

Pohl, Mary
1985 The Privileges of Maya Elites: Prehistoric Vertebrate Fauna from Seibal. In *Prehistoric Lowland Maya Environment and Subsistence Economy*, edited by Mary Pohl, pp. 133–45. Papers of the PMAE vol. 77.

Pohl, Mary D., Kevin O. Pope, John G. Jones, John S. Jacob, Dolores R Piperno, Susan D. deFrance, David L. Lentz, John A. Gifford, Marie E. Danforth, and J. Kathryn Josserand
1996 Early Agriculture in the Maya Lowlands. *LAA* 7(4):355–72.

Pope, K. O., and B. H. Dahlin
1989 Ancient Maya Wetland Agriculture: New Insights from Ecological and Remote Sensing Research. *Journal of Field Archaeology* 16:87–106.

Powell, Mary Lucas
1988 *Status and Health in Prehistory: A Case Study of the Moundville Chiefdom*. Washington: Smithsonian Institution Press.
1991 Endemic Treponematosis and Tuberculosis in the Prehistoric Southeastern United States: Biological Costs of Chronic Endemic Disease. In *Human Paleopathology: Current Syntheses and Future Options*, edited by D. J. Ortner and A. C. Aufderheide, pp. 173–80. Washington: Smithsonian Institution Press.

Pozo-Ledezma, L. F.
1985 Enfermedades transmitidas por el agua y el colapso de la civilización Maya clásica. *Mesoamérica* 10:391–410.

Price, T. Douglas
1989a Multi-Element Studies of Diagenesis in Prehistoric Bone. In *The Chemistry of Prehistoric Bone,* edited by T. Douglas Price, pp. 126–54. Cambridge, England: Cambridge University Press.

Price, T. Douglas (editor)
1989b *The Chemistry of Prehistoric Human Bone*. Cambridge, England: Cambridge University Press.

Price, T. Douglas, Jennifer Blitz, James Burton, and Joseph A. Ezzo
1992 Diagenesis in Prehistoric Bone: Problems and Solutions. *JAS* 19:513–29.

Price, T. Douglas, and M. Kavanaugh
1982 Bone Composition and the Reconstruction of Diet: Examples from the Midwestern United States. *Mid-Continent Journal of Archaeology* 7:61–79.

Price, T. Douglas, Margaret J. Schoeninger, and George J. Armelagos
1985 Bone Chemistry and Past Behavior: An Overview. *Journal of Human Evolution* 14:419–47.

Puleston, Dennis E.
1968 *Brosimum alicastrum as a Subsistence Alternative for the Classic Maya of the Central Southern Lowlands*. Unpublished Master's Thesis, Department of Anthropology, University of Pennsylvania, Philadelphia.
1971 An Experimental Approach to the Function of Classic Maya Chultuns. *AAnt* 36(3):322–35.
1979 An Epistemological Pathology and the Collapse, or Why the Maya Kept the Short Count. In *Maya Archaeology and Ethnohistory*, edited by N. Hammond and G.

R. Willey, pp. 63–71. Austin: University of Texas Press.

1982 The Role of Ramón in Maya Subsistence. In *Maya Subsistence,* edited by K. Flannery, pp. 353–67. New York: Academic Press.

Pye, Mary Elizabeth

1995 *Settlement and Adaptation in Southern Mesoamerica: Mangrove and Coastal Formative Occupation along the Pacific Coast of Guatemala*. Unpublished Ph.D. dissertation, Vanderbilt University, Nashville, Tennessee.

Quilter, Jeffrey

1989 *Life and Death at Paloma: Society and Mortuary Practices in a Preceramic Peruvian Village*. Iowa City: University of Iowa Press.

Radosevich, Stefan C.

1993 The Six Deadly Sins of Trace Element Analysis: A Case of Wishful Thinking in Science. In *Investigations of Ancient Human Tissue: Chemical Analyses in Anthropology*, edited by M. K. Sandford, pp. 269–332. Amsterdam: Gordon and Breach Science Publishers.

Ragsdale, B. D., J. E. Madewell, and D. E. Sweet

1981 Radiologic and Pathologic Analysis of Solitary Bone Lesions. Part II: Periosteal Reactions. *Radiologic Clinics of North America* 19(4):749–83.

Rands, Robert L., Ronald L. Bishop, and Jeremy A. Sabloff

1982 Maya Fine Paste Ceramics: An Archaeological Perspective. In *Excavations at Seibal. Analyses of Fine Paste Ceramics*, edited by Jeremy A. Sabloff. Memoirs of the PMAE vol. 15, no. 2.

Rathbun, T. A.

1987 Health and Disease at a South Carolina Plantation: 1840–1870. *AJPA* 74:239–53.

Rathje, William L.

1970 Socio-Political Implications of Lowland Maya Burials: Methodology and Tentative Hypotheses. *World Archaeology* 1(3):359–74.

1973 Classic Maya Development and Denouement: A Research Design. In *The Classic Maya Collapse*, edited by T. Patrick Culbert, pp. 405–56. Albuquerque: University of New Mexico Press.

Redfield, Robert, and A. Villa Rojas

1934 *Chan Kom: A Maya Village*. Chicago: University of Chicago Press.

Reed, David M.

1994 Ancient Maya Diet at Copán, Honduras, as Determined through the Analysis of Stable Carbon and Nitrogen Isotopes. In *Paleonutrition: The Diet and Health of Prehistoric Americans,* edited by K. D. Sobolik, pp. 210–21. Center for Archaeological Investigations, Southern Illinois University, Occasional Papers Series No. 22. Carbondale, Illinois.

Reed, David Millard

1998 *Ancient Maya Diet at Copán, Honduras*. Unpublished Ph.D. dissertation, Pennsylvania State University, University Park.

1999 Cuisine from Hun-Nal-Ye. In *Reconstructing Ancient Maya Diet*, edited by C. D. White, pp. 183–96. Salt Lake City: University of Utah Press.

Reeder, M. M., and P. E. S. Palmer

1981 *The Radiology of Tropical Diseases, with Epidemiological, Pathological, and Clinical Correlation*. London: Williams and Wilkins.

Renfrew, Colin

1982 Polity and Power: Interaction, Intensification, and Exploitation. In *An Island Polity: The Archaeology of Exploitation in Melos*, edited by C. Renfrew and M. Wagstaff, pp. 264–90. Cambridge, England: Cambridge University Press.

Resnick, Donald, and Gen Niwayama

1976 Radiographic and Pathological Features of Spinal Involvement in Diffuse Idiopathic Skeletal Hyperostosis (DISH). *Radiology* 119:559–68.

1981 *Diagnosis of Bone and Joint Disorders*. Philadelphia: Saunders.

Rice, Don S.

1993 Eighth-Century Physical Geography, Environment, and Natural Resources in the Maya Lowlands. In *Lowland Maya Civilization in the Eighth Century A.D.*, edited by Jeremy A. Sabloff and J. S. Henderson, pp. 11–63. Washington: Dumbarton Oaks.

Rice, Don S., and P. M. Rice
1984 Lessons from the Maya. *Latin American Research Review* 19:7–34.

Ricketson, Oliver G., and Edith B. Ricketson
1937 *Uaxactun, Guatemala, Group E, 1926–1937.* Carnegie Institution of Washington, Pub. 477. Washington, D.C.

Ridley, D. S.
1987 Pathology. In *The Leishmaniases in Biology and Medicine*, edited by W. Peters and R. Killick-Kendrick. Vol. 2, *Clinical Aspects and Control*, pp. 665–702. London: Academic Press.

Rodríguez Lazcano, Catalina
1991 *Hanal pixan: ceremonia maya de los muertos.* Mexico City: Subdirección de Etnografía, Museo Nacional de Antropología, Instituto Nacional de Antropología e Historia.

Rogan, P. K., and S. E. Lentz
1994 Molecular Genetic Evidence Suggesting Treponematosis in Pre-Columbian, Chilean Mummies. *AJPA Supplement* 18:171–72.

Rojas Lima, Flavio
1988 *La cultura del maíz en Guatemala*. Guatemala City: Ministerio de Cultura y Deportes.

Rosenthal, H. L., M. M. Eves, and O. A. Cochran
1970 Common Strontium Concentration of Mineralized Tissues from Marine and Sweet Water Animals. *Comparative Biochemistry and Physiology* 32:445–50.

Rost, G. S.
1942 Roentgen Manifestations of Bejel ("Endemic Syphilis") as Observed in the Euphrates River Valley. *Radiology* 38:320–25.

Rowton, E. D., M. de Mata, N. Rizzo, C. H. Porter, and T. R. Navin
1992 Isolation of *Leishmania braziliensis* from *Lutzomyia ovallesi* (Diptera: Psychodidae) in Guatemala. *American Journal of Tropical Medicine and Hygiene* 46(4):465–68.

Ruff, Christopher
1992 Biomechanical Analyses of Archaeological Human Skeletal Samples. In *Skeletal Biology of Past Peoples: Research Methods*, edited by S. R. Saunders and M. A. Katzenberg, pp. 37–58. New York: Wiley-Liss

Ruff, C. B., and W. C. Hayes
1983 Cross-Sectional Geometry of Pecos Pueblo Femora and Tibiae: A Biomechanical Investigation. II. Sex, Age, and Side Differences. *AJPA* 60:383–400.

Rundel, P. W., J. R. Ehleringer, and K. A. Nagy
1988 *Stable Isotopes in Ecological Research.* Berlin: Springer-Verlag.

Runia, Lex T.
1987 Strontium and Calcium Distribution in Plants: Effect on Paleodietary Studies. *JAS* 14:599–608.

Ruz Lhuillier, Alberto
1968 *Costumbres funerarias de los antiguos mayas*. Mexico City: Universidad Nacional Autónoma de México, Seminario de Cultura Maya.

Ryan, Alan S.
1997 Iron-Deficiency Anemia in Infant Development: Implications for Growth, Cognitive Development, Resistance to Infection, and Iron Supplementation. *Yearbook of Physical Anthropology* 40:25–62.

Sabloff, Jeremy A.
1973 Continuity and Disruption during Terminal Late Classic Times at Seibal: Ceramic and Other Evidence. In *The Classic Maya Collapse*, edited by T. Patrick Culbert, pp. 107–32. Albuquerque: University of New Mexico Press.
1975 *Excavations at Seibal, Department of Petén, Guatemala. Ceramics.* Memoirs of the PMAE vol. 13, no. 2.

Sabloff, Jeremy A., and G. R. Willey
1967 The Collapse of Maya Civilization in the Southern Lowlands: A Consideration of History and Process. *Southwestern Journal of Anthropology* 23:311–36.

Sahagún, Fray Bernardino de
1950–1963 *Florentine Codex*. Translated by A. J. C. Anderson and Charles E. Dibble. Santa Fe, New Mexico: School of American Research

Salas Cuesta, Maria Elena
1982 *La población de Mexico-Tenochtitlan: estudio de osteología Antropológica.* Colección Científica 126. Mexico City: Instituto

Nacional de Anthropología e Historia, Departamento de Antropología Física.

Salo, Wilmar L., Arthur C. Aufderheide, Jane E. Buikstra, and Todd A. Holcomb
1994 Identification of *Mycobacterium tuberculosis* DNA in a Pre-Columbian Peruvian Mummy. *Proceedings of the National Academy of Sciences* 91:2091–94.

Sanchez, J. L., B. M. Diniega, J. W. Small, R. N. Miller, J. M. Andujar, P. J. Weina, P. G. Lawyer, W. R. Ballou, and J. K. Lovelace
1992 Epidemiologic Investigation of an Outbreak of Cutaneous Leishmaniasis in a Defined Geographic Focus of Tranmission. *American Journal of Tropical Medicine and Hygiene* 47(1):47–54.

Sanders, William T.
1962 Cultural Ecology of the Maya Lowlands (Part I). *Estudios de Cultura Maya* (Mexico City) 2:79–121.
1963 Cultural Ecology of the Maya Lowlands (Part II). *Estudios de Cultura Maya* (Mexico City) 3:203–41.
1973 The Cultural Ecology of the Lowland Maya: A Reevaluation. In *The Classic Maya Collapse*, edited by T. Patrick Culbert, pp. 325–66. Albuquerque: University of New Mexico Press.
1977 Environmental Heterogeneity and the Evolution of Lowland Maya Civilization. In *The Origins of Maya Civilization*, edited by R. E. W. Adams, pp. 287–97. Albuquerque: University of New Mexico Press.

Sandford, Mary K.
1993 *Investigations of Ancient Human Tissue: Chemical Analyses in Anthropology*. Amsterdam: Gordon and Breach Scientific Publishers.

Santley, S. R., T. W. Killion, and M. T. Lycett
1986 On the Maya Collapse. *Journal of Anthropological Research* 42:123–59.

Sattenspiel, L., and H. Harpending
1983 Stable Populations and Skeletal Age. *AAnt* 48:489–98.

Saul, Frank P.
1972 *The Human Skeletal Remains of Altar de Sacrificios: An Osteobiographic Analysis*. Papers of the PMAE vol. 63, no. 2.
1973 Disease in the Maya Area: The Pre-Columbian Evidence. In *The Classic Maya Collapse*, edited by T. Patrick Culbert, pp. 301–24. Albuquerque: University of New Mexico Press.
1977 The Paleopathology of Anemia in Mexico and Guatemala. In *Porotic Hyperostosis: An Enquiry*, edited by E. Cockburn, pp. 10–15, Paleopathology Association Monograph no. 2. Detroit, Michigan.

Saunders, Shelley R., and M. Anne Katzenberg
1992 *Skeletal Biology of Past Peoples: Research Methods*. New York: Wiley-Liss

Sawyer, D. R., and A. L. Nwoku
1985 Malnutrition and the Oral Health of Children in Ogbomosho, Nigeria. *Journal of Dentistry for Children* 52:141–45.

Saxe, Arthur
1970 *Social Dimensions of Mortuary Practices*. Unpublished Ph.D. dissertation, University of Michigan, Ann Arbor.

Schele, Linda, and David Freidel
1990 *A Forest of Kings*. New York: Morrow.

Schele, Linda, and Peter Mathews
1998 *The Code of Kings: The Language of Seven Sacred Maya Temples and Tombs*. New York: Simon and Schuster.

Schele, Linda, and Jeffrey H. Miller
1983 *The Mirror, the Rabbit, and the Bundle: "Accession" Expressions from the Classic Maya Inscriptions*. Studies in Pre-Columbian Art and Archaeology No. 25. Washington: Dumbarton Oaks.

Schele, Linda, and M. Miller
1986 *The Blood of Kings*. Fort Worth: Kimbell Art Museum.

Schimmelman, A.
1985 *Stable Isotopic Studies on Chitin*. Ann Arbor, Michigan: University Microfilms.

Schoeninger, Margaret J.
1979a *Dietary Reconstruction at Chalcatzingo, a Formative Period Site in Morelos, Mexico*. Technical Reports No. 9, Museum of Anthropology, Univeristy of Michigan. Ann Arbor: University of Michigan.
1979b Diet and Status at Chalcatzingo: Some

Empirical and Technical Aspects of Strontium Analysis. *AJPA* 51:295–310.
1985 Trophic Level Effects on $^{15}N/^{14}N$ and $^{13}C/^{12}C$ Ratios in Bone Collagen and Strontium Levels in Bone Mineral. *Journal of Human Evolution* 14:515–25.

Schoeninger, Margaret J., and Michael J. DeNiro
1982 Carbon Isotope Ratios of Apatite from Fossil Bone Cannot Be Used to Reconstruct Diets of Animals. *Nature* 297:577–78.
1983 Reply to "Carbon Isotope Ratios of Bone Apatite and Animal Diet Reconstruction." *Nature* 301:178.
1984 Nitrogen and Carbon Isotopic Composition of Bone Collagen from Marine and Terrestrial Animals. *Geochimica et Cosmochimica Acta* 48:625–39.

Schoeninger, Margaret J., Michael J. DeNiro, and H. Tauber
1983 Stable Nitrogen Isotope Ratios of Bone Collagen Reflect Marine and Terrestrial Components of Prehistoric Human Diet. *Science* 220:1381–83.

Schoeninger, Margaret J., U. T. Iwaniec, K. A. Spielmann, E. W. Treichel, and T. D. Crenshaw
1993 Carbon Stable Isotope Values in Archaeological Populations: Are They Telling Us What We Think They Are? *AJPA Supplement* 16:175.

Schoeninger, Margaret J., K. M. Moore, M. L. Murray, and J. D. Kingston
1989 Detection of Bone Preservation in Archaeological and Fossil Samples. *Applied Geochemistry* 4:281–92.

Schoeninger, Margaret J., and C. S. Peebles
1981 Effect of Mollusc Eating on Human Bone Strontium Levels. *JAS* 8:391–97.

Schroeder, H. A., I. H. Tipton, and A. P. Nason
1972 Trace Metals in Man: Strontium and Barium. *Journal of Chronic Diseases* 25:491–517.

Schwarcz, Henry P.
1991 Some Theoretical Aspects of Isotope Paleodiet Studies. *JAS* 18:261–75.
1994 Some Biochemical Aspects of Carbon Isotopic Paleodiet Studies, or, of Mice and People. Paper presented at the Wenner-Gren Conference on Paleodiet, Banff, Alberta, Canada.

Schwarcz, Henry P., Jerry Melbye, M. Anne Katzenberg, and Martin Knyf
1985 Stable Isotopes in Human Skeletons of Southern Ontario: Reconstructing Palaeodiet. *JAS* 12:187–206.

Schwarcz, Henry P., and Margaret J. Schoeninger
1991 Stable Isotope Analyses in Human Nutritional Ecology. *Yearbook of Physical Anthropology* 34:283–321.

Scrimshaw, Nevin S.
1990 World Nutritional Problems. In *Hunger in History: Food Shortage, Poverty, and Deprivation*, edited by L. F. Newman, pp. 353–73. Oxford: Basil Blackwell.

Scrimshaw, Nevin S., C. E. Taylor, and J. E. Gordon
1968 *Interactions of Nutrition and Infection.* Monograph Series No. 57. Geneva, Switzerland: World Health Organization.

Scrimshaw, Nevin S., and Carlos Tejada
1970 Pathology of Living Indians as seen in Guatemala. In *Handbook of Middle American Indians*, Vol. 9, *Physical Anthropology*, edited by T. D. Stewart, pp. 203–25. Austin: University of Texas Press.

Sealy, Judith C., and Andrew Sillen
1988 Sr and Sr/Ca in Marine and Terrestrial Foodwebs in the Southwestern Cape, South Africa. *JAS* 15:425–38.

Secaira, Estuardo
1992 Estudio agrosocioleconomico de la aldea El Escarbado, occidente de la Laguna Petexbatun, Sayaxche, Peten. In *Proyecto Arqueológico Regional Petexbatun: Informe Preliminar 4, Cuarta Temporada*, edited by Arthur Demarest, Takeshi Inomata, and Héctor Escobedo, pp. 310–69. Report presented to the Instituto de Antropología e Historia de Guatemala.

Sengupta, S.
1985 Musculoskeletal lesions in yaws. *Clinical Orthopaedics* 192:193–98.

Serna-Saldivar, S. O., L. W. Rooney, and L. W. Greene
1991 Effect of Lime Treatment on the Availability of Calcium in Diets of Tortillas and Beans:

Rat Growth and Balance Studies. *Cereal Chemistry* 68(6):565–70.
1992 Effects of Lime Treatment on the Bioavailability of Calcium in Diets of Tortillas and Beans: Bone and Plasma Composition in Rats. *Cereal Chemistry* 69(1):78–81.

Seyle, H.
1956 *The Stress of Life*. New York: McGraw-Hill.

Shanks, Michael, and Christopher Tilley
1982 Ideology, Symbolic Power, and Ritual Communication: A Reinterpretation of Neolithic Mortuary Practices. In *Symbolic and Structural Archaeology*, edited by I. Hodder, pp. 129–54. Cambridge, England: Cambridge University Press.

Sharer, Robert J.
1977 The Maya Collapse Revisited: Internal and External Perspectives, In *Social Process in Maya Prehistory*. edited by N. Hammond, pp. 532–52. London: Academic Press.
1978 Archaeology and History at Quirigua, Guatemala. *Journal of Field Archaeology* 5:51–70.
1994 *The Ancient Maya*. Stanford: Stanford University Press.

Shattuck, George C.
1933 *The Peninsula of Yucatan*. Carnegie Institution of Washington, Pub. 431. Washington, D.C.
1938 *A Medical Survey of the Republic of Guatemala*. Carnegie Institution of Washington, Pub. 499. Washington, D.C.

Shearer, G., and D. H. Kohl
1988 Estimates of N_2 Fixation in Ecosystems: The Need For and Basis of the ^{15}N Natural Abundance Method. In *Stable Isotopes in Ecological Research*, edited by P. W. Rundel, J. R. Ehlerginger, and K. A. Nagy, pp. 342–74. Ecological Studies 68. Berlin: Springer-Verlag.

Sheets, Payson D.
1992 *The Ceren Site: A Prehistoric Village Buried by Volcanic Ash in Central America*. Fort Worth: Harcourt Brace Jovanovich College Publishers.

Shennan, Stephan
1982a Exchange and Ranking: The Role of Amber in the European Early Bronze Age. In *Ranking, Resource, and Exchange*, edited by Colin Renfrew and Stephen Shennan, pp. 33–45. Cambridge, England: Cambridge University Press.

Shennan, Susan
1982b From Minimal to Moderate Ranking. In *Ranking, Resource, and Exchange*, edited by Colin Renfrew and Stephen Shennan, pp. 155–61. Cambridge, England: Cambridge University Press.

Sherman, R. S., and K. Y. Soong
1956 Ewing's Sarcoma: Its Roentgen Classification and Diagnosis. *Radiology* 66:529–39.

Shimkin, Demitri B.
1973 Models for the Downfall: Some Ecological and Culture-Historical Considerations. In *The Classic Maya Collapse*, edited by T. Patrick Culbert, pp. 269–300. Albuquerque: University of New Mexico Press.

Sibrián, Ricardo, and Robert C. Elston
1990 Reciprocal Causal Influences among Malnutrition, Growth Retardation, and Diarrhea in Preschool Children. *American Journal of Human Biology* 2:235–43.

Siemens, A. H., and D. E. Puleston
1972 Ridged Fields and Associated Features in Southern Campeche: New Perspectives on the Lowland Maya. *AAnt* 37:228–39.

Sillen, Andrew
1981 Strontium and Diet at Hayonim Cave. *AJPA* 56:131–37.
1989 Diagenesis of the Inorganic Phase of Cortical Bone. In *The Chemistry of Prehistoric Human Bone*, edited by T. Douglas Price, pp. 211–29. Cambridge, England: Cambridge University Press.
1990 Response to N. Tuross, A. K. Behrensmeyer, and E. D. Eanes. *JAS* 17:595–96.

Sillen, Andrew, and Raquel LeGeros
1991 Solubility Profiles of Synthetic Apatites and of Modern and Fossil Bones. *JAS* 18:385–97.

Sillen, Andrew, Judith C. Sealy, and Nikolaas J. van der Merwe
1989 Chemistry and Paleodietary Research: No More Easy Answers. *AAnt* 54(3):504–12.

Sillen, Andrew, and Patricia Smith
1984 Weaning Patterns Are Reflected in Strontium-Calcium Ratios of Juvenile Skeletons. *Journal of Archaeological Science* 11:237–45.

Skinner, M., and A. H. Goodman
1992 Anthropological Uses of Developmental Defects of Enamel. In *Skeletal Biology of Past Peoples: Research Methods*, edited by S. R. Saunders and M. A. Katzenberg, pp. 153–74. New York: Wiley-Liss.

Sminia, T., N. D. De With, J. L. Bos, M. E. van Nieuwmegen, M. P. Witter, and J. Wondergem
1977 Structure and Function of the Calcium Cells of the Freshwater Pulmonate Snail *Lymnaea stagnalis*. *Netherlands Journal of Zoology* 27(2):195–208.

Smith, A. L.
1972 *Excavations at Altar de Sacrificios. Architecture, Settlement, Burials, and Caches.* Papers of the PMAE vol. 62, no. 2.

Spielmann, K. A.
1989 A Review: Dietary Restrictions on Hunter-Gatherer Women and the Implications for Fertility and Infant Mortality. *Human Ecology* 17:321–45.

Spielmann, K. A., Margaret J. Schoeninger, and K. Moore
1990 Plains-Pueblo Interdependence and Human Diet at Pecos Pueblo, New Mexico. *AAnt* 55:745–65.

Spinden, Herbert J.
1928 *The Ancient Civilizations of Mexico and Central America.* Handbook Series No. 3. New York: American Museum of Natural History.

Spjut, H. J., H. D. Dorfman, R. E. Fechner, and L. V. Ackerman
1971 *Atlas of Tumor Pathology*. Second Series, Fascicle 5, *Tumors of Bone and Cartilage*. Washington, D. C.: Armed Forces Institute of Pathology.

Sponheimer, Matt, and Julia A. Lee-Thorp
1999 Alteration of Enamel Carbonate Environments during Fossilization. *JAS* 26(2):143–50.

Spross Hansen, Barbara C.
1990 Pollen Stratigraphy of Laguna de Cocos. In *Ancient Maya Wetland Agriculture: Excavations on Albion Island, Northern Belize*, edited by Mary D. Pohl, pp. 155–86. Boulder, Colorado: Westview Press.

Steele, D. G., and C. A. Bramblett
1988 *The Anatomy and Biology of the Human Skeleton*. College Station: Texas A & M University Press.

Steggerda, Morris, and Thomas J. Hill
1942 Eruption Time of Teeth among Whites, Negroes, and Indians. *American Journal of Orthodontics and Oral Surgery* 28:361–70.

Steinbock, R. Ted
1976 *Paleopathological Diagnosis and Interpretation: Bone Diseases in Ancient Human Populations*. Springfield, Illinois: Charles C. Thomas.

Stevens, Rayfred L.
1964 The Soils of Middle America and Their Relation to Indian Peoples and Cultures. In *Handbook of Middle American Indians.* Vol. 1, *Natural Environment and Early Cultures*, edited by R. C. West, pp. 265–315. Austin: University of Texas Press.

Stewart, T. D., and Alexander Spoehr
1952 Evidence on the Paleopathology of Yaws. *Bulletin of the History of Medicine* 26:538–53.

Storey, Rebecca
1985 An Estimate of Mortality in a Pre-Columbian Urban Population. *AA* 87:519–35.
1992a The Children of Copan: Issues in Paleopathology and Paleodemography. *AM* 3:161–67.
1992b Patterns of Susceptibility to Dental Defects in the Deciduous Dentition of a Precolumbian Skeletal Population. In *Recent Contributions to the Study of Enamel Developmental Defects*, edited by Alan L. Goodman and Luigi Capasso, pp. 171–83. Journal of Paleopathology, Monographic

Publications 2. Chieti, Italy: Edigrafital Teramo.

Strauss, R. G.
1978 Iron deficiency, Infections, and Immune Function: A Reassessment. *American Journal of Clinical Nutrition* 31:660–66.

Stuart, David
1984 Royal Auto-Sacrifice among the Maya: A Study of Image and Meaning. *RES Anthropology and Aesthetics* 7/8:6–20.
1985 The "Count of Captives" Epithet in Classic Maya Writing. In *Fifth Palenque Round Table*,1983, vol. 7, edited by M. G. Robertson and V. M. Fields, pp. 97–102. San Francisco: Pre-Columbian Art Research Institute.
1988a Blood Symbolism in Maya Iconography. In *Maya Iconography*, edited by E. P. Benson and G. G. Griffin, pp. 175–221. Princeton,: Princeton University Press.
1988b The Rio Azul Cacao Pot: Epigraphic Observations on the Function of a Maya Ceramic Vessel. *Antiquity* 62:153–57.
1993 Historical Inscriptions and the Maya Collapse. In *Lowland Maya Civilization in the Eighth Century A.D.*, edited by Jeremy A. Sabloff and J. S. Henderson, pp. 321–54. Washington: Dumbarton Oaks.

Stuart-Macadam, Patty
1985 Porotic Hyperostosis: Representative of a Childhood Condition. *AJPA* 66:391–98.
1987a Porotic Hyperostosis: New Evidence to Support the Anemia Theory. *AJPA* 74:521–26.
1987b A Radiographic Study of Porotic Hyperostosis. *AJPA* 74:511–20.
1989 Porotic Hyperostosis: Relationship between Orbital and Vault Lesions. *AJPA* 80:187–93.
1991 Porotic Hyperostosis: Changing Interpretations. In *Human Paleopathology: Current Syntheses and Future Options*, edited by D. J. Ortner and A. C. Aufderheide, pp. 36–39. Washington: Smithsonian Institution Press.
1992 Porotic Hyperostosis: A New Perspective. *AJPA* 87(1):39–47.

Subira, M. E., and A. Malgosa
1991 Alkaline Earth Metal Content of Human Bones at the Site of «S'Illot des Porros» (Iron Age, Mallorca, Spain). *International Journal of Anthropology* 6(4):225–31.

Suchey, Judy Myers, S. T. Brooks, and D. Katz
1988 *Instructional Materials Accompanying Female Pubic Symphyseal Models of the Suchey-Brooks System*. Distributed by France Casting (Diane France, 2190 West Drake Road, Suite 259, Fort Collins, Colorado 80526).

Suchey, Judy Myers, Dean V. Wisely, Richard F. Green, and Thomas T Noguchi
1979 Analysis of Dorsal Pitting in the *Os Pubis* in an Extensive Sample of Modern American Females. *AJPA* 51(4):517–40.

Suckling, G.
1989 Developmental Defects of Enamel: Historical and Present-day Perspectives of Their Pathogenesis. *Advances in Dental Research* 3:87–94.

Sullivan, Charles H., and Harold W. Krueger
1981 Carbon Isotope Analysis of Separate Chemical Phases in Modern and Fossil Bone. *Nature* 292:333–35.
1983 Carbon Isotope Ratios of Bone Apatite and Animal Diet Reconstruction. *Nature* 301:177–78.

Swärdstedt, T.
1966 *Odontological Aspects of a Medieval Population in the Province of Jamtland/Mid-Sweden*. Stockholm: Tiden-Barnangen AB.

Sweeney, Edward A., and Romeo de Leon
1971 Linear Hypoplasia of Deciduous Incisor Teeth in Malnourished Children. *American Journal of Clinical Nutrition* 24:29–31.

Szpunar, C. B.
1977 *Atomic Absorption Analysis of Archaeological Remains: Human Ribs from Woodland Mortuary Sites*. Unpublished Ph.D. dissertation, Northwestern University, Evanston, Illinois.

Tainter, Joseph A.
1975 Social Inference and Mortuary Practices: An Experiment in Numerical Classification. *World Archaeology* 7(1):1–15.
1978 Mortuary Practices and the Study of Prehistoric Social Systems. In *Advances in Archaeological Method and Theory*, edited

by M. B. Schiffer, pp. 105–41, New York: Academic Press.

1981 Reply to "A Critique of Some Recent North American Mortuary Studies." *AAnt* 46(2):416–20.

1988 *The Collapse of Complex Societies*. Cambridge, England: Cambridge University Press.

Tatsuoka, M. M.

1971 *Multivariate Analysis*. New York: John Wiley and Sons.

Taube, Karl A.

1989 The Maize Tamale in Classic Maya Diet, Epigraphy, and Art. *AAnt* 54(1):31–51.

Tedlock, Dennis

1985 *Popol Vuh*. New York: Simon and Schuster

Thompson, J. Eric S.

1954 *The Rise and Fall of Maya Civilization*. Norman: University of Oklahoma Press.

1970 *Maya History and Religion*. Norman: University of Oklahoma Press.

Tieszen, Larry L.

1991 Natural Variations in the Carbon Isotope Values of Plants: Implications for Archaeology, Ecology, and Paleoecology. *JAS* 18:227–48.

Tieszen, Larry L., and T. W. Boutton

1988 Stable Carbon Isotopes in Terrestrial Ecosystem Research. In *Stable Isotopes in Ecological Research*, edited by P. W. Rundel, J. R. Ehlerginger, and K. A. Nagy, pp. 167–95. Ecological Studies 68. Berlin: Springer-Verlag.

Tieszen, Larry L., and Tim Fagre

1993a Carbon Isotopic Variability in Modern and Archaeological Maize. *JAS* 20:25–40.

1993b Effect of Diet Quality and Composition on the Isotopic Composition of Respiratory CO_2, Bone Collagen, Bioapatite, and Soft Tissues. In *Prehistoric Human Bone: Archaeology at the Molecular Level*, edited by Joseph B. Lambert and Gisela Grupe, pp. 121–55. Berlin: Springer-Verlag.

Tieszen, Larry L., M. M. Senyimba, S. K. Imbamba, and J. H. Troughton

1983 Fractionation and Turnover of Stable Carbon Isotopes in Animal Tissues: Implications for the $\delta^{13}C$ Analysis of Diet. *Oecologia* 57:32–37.

Tourtellot, Gair, III

1970 The Peripheries of Seibal: An Interim Report. In *Monographs and Papers in Maya Archaeology*, edited by W. R. Bullard, pp. 405–15. Papers of the PMAE vol. 61.

1988 *Excavations at Seibal, Department of Peten, Guatemala. Peripheral Survey and Excavation, Settlement and Community Patterns*. Memoirs of the PMAE vol. 16.

1990 *Excavations at Seibal, Department of Peten, Guatemala. Burials: A Cultural Analysis*. Memoirs of the PMAE vol. 17, no. 2.

Tourtellot, Gair, III, and Jason J. González

2004 The Last Hurrah: Continuity and Transformation at Seibal. In *The Terminal Classic in the Maya Lowlands: Collapse, Transition, and Transformation*, edited by Arthur A. Demarest, Prudence M. Rice, and Don S. Rice. pp. 60–82. Boulder: University Press of Colorado.

Tourtellot, Gair, III, Norman Hammond, and Richard Rose

1978 *Excavations at Seibal, Department of Peten, Guatemala. A Brief Reconnaissance of Itzan*. Memoirs of the PMAE vol. 14, no. 3.

Tozzer, Alfred M.

1907 *A Comparative Study of the Maya and the Lacandon*. New York: MacMillan.

1941 *Landa's Relación de las Cosas de Yucatan*. Papers of the PMAE vol. 18.

Turner, B. L., II

1974 Prehistoric Intensive Agriculture in the Maya Lowlands. *Science* 185:118–24.

1983 *Once Beneath the Forest: Prehistoric Terracing in the Rio Bec Region of the Maya Lowlands*. Latin American Studies No. 13. Boulder, Colorado: Westview Press.

1990 The Rise and Fall of Population and Agriculture in the Central Maya Lowlands: 300 B.C. to Present. In *Hunger in History: Food Shortage, Poverty, and Deprivation*, edited by L. F. Newman, pp. 178–211. Oxford: Basil Blackwell.

Tuross, Noreen, Anna K. Behrensmeyer, and E. D. Eanes
1989 Strontium Increases and Crystallinity Changes in Taphonomic and Archaeological Bone. *JAS* 16:661–72.

Tykot, Robert H., Nikolaas J. van der Merwe, and Norman Hammond
1996 Stable Isotope Analysis of Bone Collagen and Apatite in the Reconstruction of Human Diet: A Case Study from Cuello, Belize. In *Archaeological Chemistry: Organic, Inorganic, and Biochemical Analysis*, edited by M. V. Orna, pp. 355–65. ACS Symposium Series 625. Washington: American Chemical Society.

Ubelaker, D. H.
1978 *Human Skeletal Remains: Excavation, Analysis, Interpretation*. Washington: Taraxacum.

Ucko, Peter J.
1969 Ethnography and Archaeological Interpretation of Funerary Remains. *World Archaeology* 1:262–81.

Ulloa, M., and T. Herrera
1986 Fermented Corn Products of Mexico. In *Indigenous Fermented Food of Non-Western Origin*, edited by C. W. Hesseltine and H. L. Wang, pp. 151–67. Mycologia Memoir No. 11. Berlin: J. Cramer.

Urteaga-Ballon, Oscar
1991 Medical Ceramic Representation of Nasal Leishmaniasis and Surgical Amputation in Ancient Peruvian Civilization. In *Human Paleopathology: Current Syntheses and Future Options*, edited by D. J. Ortner and A. C. Aufderheide, pp. 95–101. Washington: Smithsonian Institution Press.

Valdés, Juan Antonio
1997 Tamarindito: Archaeology and Regional Politics in the Petexbatun Region. *AM* 8(2):321–35.

Valdés, Juan Antonio, and José Suasnávar
1991 Estudio preliminar de la arquitectura en la región de Petexbatun. In *Proyecto Arqueologico Regional Petexbatun. Informe Preliminar 3. Tercera Temporada*, edited by Arthur A. Demarest, Takeshi Inomata, Héctor Escobedo, and Joel Palka, pp. 785–806. Report presented to the Instituto de Antropología e Historia de Guatemala.

van der Borght, O., and S. van Puymbroeck
1966 Calcium Metabolism in a Freshwater Mollusc: Quantitative Importance of Water and Food as Supply for Calcium during Growth. *Nature* 210:791–93.

van der Merwe, Nikolaas J.
1982 Carbon Isotopes, Photosynthesis, and Archaeology. *American Scientist* 70(6):596–606.

van der Merwe, Nikolaas J., and Ernesto Medina
1991 The Canopy Effect, Carbon Isotope Ratios, and Foodwebs in Amazonia. *JAS* 18:249–59.

van der Merwe, Nikolaas J., and J. C. Vogel
1978 ^{13}C Content of Human Collagen as a Measure of Prehistoric Diet in Woodland North America. *Nature* 276:815–16.

Van Gennep, Arnold
1909 *The Rites of Passage.* Translated by Monika B. Vizedom and Gabrielle L. Caffe. Chicago: Phoenix Books, University of Chicago (translation published in 1960).

van Vark, G. N., and W. Schaafsma
1992 Advances in the Quantitative Analysis of Skeletal Morphology. In *Skeletal Biology of Past Peoples: Research Methods*, edited by S. R. Saunders and M. A. Katzenberg, pp. 225–57. New York: Wiley-Liss.

Vargas, Luis A.
1990 Old and New Transitions and Nutrition in Mexico. In *Disease in Populations in Transition*, edited by A. C. Swedlund and George J. Armelagos, pp. 145–60. New York: Bergin and Garvey.

Vaughan, Hague H., Edward S. Deevey Jr., and S. E. Garrett-Jones
1985 Pollen Stratigraphy of Two Cores from the Petén Lake District, with an Appendix on Two Deep-Water Cores. In *Prehistoric Lowland Maya Environment and Subsistence Economy*, edited by Mary Pohl, pp. 73–89. Papers of the PMAE vol. 77.

Vaupel, J. W., and A. I. Yashin
1985 Heterogeneity's Ruses: Some Surprising Effects of Selection on Population Dynamics. *American Statistician* 39:176–85.

Vinson, G. L.
1960 Las ruinas mayas de Petexbatun. *Antropología e Historia de Guatemala* (Guatemala City) 12(2):3–9.

Virginia, R. A., W. M. Jarrell, P. W. Rundel, G. Shearer, and D. H. Kohl
1988 The Use of Variation in the Natural Abundance of ^{15}N to Assess Symbiotic Nitrogen Fixation by Woody Plants. In *Stable Isotopes in Ecological Research*, edited by P. W. Rundel, J. R. Ehlerginger, and K. A. Nagy, pp. 375–94. Ecological Studies 68. Berlin: Springer-Verlag.

Vogel, J. C., and Nikolaas J. van der Merwe
1977 Isotopic Evidence for Early Maize Cultivation in New York State. *AAnt* 42:238–42.

Wagner, Philip L.
1964 Natural Vegetation of Middle America. In *Handbook of Middle American Indians*. Vol. 1, *Natural Environment and Early Cultures*, edited by R.C. West, pp. 216–64. Austin: University of Texas Press.

Waldvogel, F. A., G. Medoff, and M. N. Swartz
1970 Osteomyelitis: A Review of Clinical Features, Therapeutic Considerations and Unusual Aspects. *New England Journal of Medicine* 282:198–206, 260–6, 316–22.

Walker, Phillip L.
1986 Porotic Hyperostosis in a Marine-Dependent California Indian Population. *AJPA* 69:345–54.

Walter, Tomás, Manuel Olivares, Fernando Pizarro, and Carlos Muñoz
1997 Iron, Anemia, and Infection. *Nutritional Reviews* 55(4):111–24.

Waterlow, J. C., and P. R. Payne
1975 The Protein Gap. *Nature* 258:113–17.

Webb, Malcolm C.
1973 The Peten Maya Decline Viewed in the Perspective of State Formation. In *The Classic Maya Collapse*, edited by T. Patrick Culbert, pp. 367–404. Albuquerque: University of New Mexico Press.

Webster, David
1985 Surplus, Labor, and Stress in Late Classic Maya Society. *Journal of Anthropological Research* 41(4):375–99.

Webster, David, William T. Sanders, and Peter van Rossum
1992 A Simulation of Copan Population History and Its Implications. *AM* 3:185–97.

Weinberg, Eugene D.
1992 Iron Withholding in Prevention of Disease. In *Diet, Demography, and Disease: Changing Perspectives on Anemia*, edited by S. Kent and P. Stuart-Macadam, pp. 105–50. New York: Aldine de Gruyter.

Weiss, K. M.
1972 On the Systematic Bias in Skeletal Sexing. *AJPA* 37:239–50.
1973 *Demographic Models for Anthropology*. Memoirs of the Society for American Archaeology No. 27. Washington, D.C.

Welsh, W. B. M.
1988 *An Analysis of Classic Lowland Maya Burials*. International Series 409. Oxford: British Archaeological Reports.

White, Christine D.
1986 *Paleodiet and Nutrition of the Ancient Maya at Lamanai, Belize: A Study of Trace Elements, Stable Isotopes, Nutritional and Dental Pathologies*. Unpublished Master's Thesis, Trent University, Peterborough, Ontario, Canada.
1988 The Ancient Maya from Lamanai, Belize: Diet and Health over 2,000 Years. *Canadian Review of Physical Anthropology* 6(2):1–21.
1990 *Isotopic Analysis of Multiple Human Tissues from Three Ancient Nubian Populations*. Unpublished Ph.D. dissertation, University of Toronto, Ontario, Canada.
1997 Ancient Diet at Lamanai and Pacbitun: Implications for the Ecological Model of Collapse. In *Bones of the Maya: Studies of Ancient Skeletons*, edited by S. L. Whittington and D. M. Reed, pp. 171–80. Washington: Smithsonian Institution Press.

White, Christine D., Paul F. Healy, and Henry P. Schwarcz
1993 Intensive Agriculture, Social Status, and Maya Diet at Pacbitun, Belize. *Journal of Anthropological Research* 49:347–75.

White, Christine D., Mary E. D. Pohl, Henry P. Schwarcz, and Fred J. Longstaffe
2001 Isotopic Evidence for Maya Patterns of Deer and Dog Use at Preclassic Colha. *JAS* 28:89–107.

White, Christine D., and Henry P. Schwarcz
1989 Ancient Maya Diet: As Inferred from Isotopic and Chemical Analysis of Human Bone. *JAS* 16:451–74.
1994 Temporal Trends in Stable Isotopes for Nubian Mummy Tissues. *AJPA* 93:165–87.

White, Christine D., Lori E. Wright, and David M. Pendergast
1994 Biological Disruption in the Early Colonial Period at Lamanai. In *In the Wake of Contact: Biological Responses to Conquest*, edited by C. S. Larsen and G. Milner, pp. 135–45. New York: Wiley-Liss.

White, E. M., and L. A. Hannus
1983 Chemical Weathering of Bone in Archaeological Soils. *AAnt* 48:316–22.

Whittington, S. L.
1989 *Characteristics of Demography and Disease in Low Status Maya from Classic Period Copan, Honduras*. Unpublished Ph.D. dissertation, Pennsylvania State University, University Park.
1991 Detection of Significant Demographic Differences between Subpopulations of Prehispanic Maya from Copan, Honduras, by Survival Analysis. *AJPA* 85:167–84.

Willey, Gordon R.
1973 *The Altar de Sacrificios Excavations: General Summary and Conclusions*. Papers of the PMAE vol. 64, no. 3.
1982 Maya Archaeology. *Science* 215:260–67.
1986 The Classic Maya Sociopolitical Order: A Study in Coherence and Instability. In *Research and Reflections in Archaeology and History. Essays in Honor of Doris Stone*, edited by E. W. Andrews V, pp. 189–98. Middle American Research Institute, Tulane University, Pub. 57. New Orleans.
1990 *Excavations at Seibal. No. 4. General Summary and Conclusions*. Memoirs of the PMAE vol. 17, no. 4.

Willey, Gordon R., W. R. Bullard, J. B. Glass, and J. C. Gifford
1965 *Prehistoric Maya Settlements in the Belize Valley*. Papers of the PMAE vol. 54.

Willey, Gordon R., and Dimitri B. Shimkin
1973 The Maya Collapse: A Summary View. In *The Classic Maya Collapse*, edited by T. Patrick Culbert, pp. 457–502. Albuquerque: University of New Mexico Press.

Willey, Gordon R., and A. L. Smith
1969 *The Ruins of Altar de Sacrificios, Department of Peten, Guatemala: An Introduction*. Papers of the PMAE vol. 62, no. 1.

Willey, Gordon R., A. L. Smith, G. Tourtellot, and I. Graham
1975 *Excavations at Seibal: Introduction, the Site, and Its Setting*. Memoirs of the PMAE vol. 13, no. 1.

Wiseman, Fred
1985 Agriculture and Vegetation Dynamics of the Maya Collapse in Central Peten, Guatemala. In *Prehistoric Lowland Maya Environment and Subsistence Economy*, edited by Mary D. Pohl, pp. 63–71. Papers of the PMAE vol. 77.

Wiseman, Frederick M.
1983 Analysis of Pollen from the Fields at Pulltrouser Swamp. In *Pulltrouser Swamp: Ancient Maya Habitat, Agriculture, and Settlement in Northern Belize*, edited by B. L. Turner II and P. D. Harrison, pp. 105–119. Austin: University of Texas Press.

Wolley, Claudia, and Lori Wright
1990a Punta de Chimino: Sondeos en el sistema defensivo. In *Proyecto Arqueológico Regional Petexbatun: Informe Preliminar 2, Segunda Temporada*, edited by Arthur Demarest and Stephen Houston, pp. 423–37. Report presented to the Instituto de Antropología e Historia de Guatemala.
1990b Operación DP7: Investigaciones en el Grupo L4-4. In *Proyecto Arqueológico Regional Petexbatun: Informe Preliminar 2, Segunda Temporada*, edited by Arthur Demarest and Stephen Houston, pp. 44–65. Report presented to the Instituto de Antropología e Historia de Guatemala.

Wood, James W., George R. Milner, Henry C. Harpending, and Kenneth M. Weiss

1992 The Osteological Paradox: Problems of Inferring Prehistoric Health from Skeletal Samples. *Current Anthropology* 33(4):343–70.

Wright, Lori E.

1989 *Cemental Annulation: A Test of Its Application to the Colonial Maya of Tipu, Belize*. Unpublished Master's Thesis, University of Chicago.

1990 Stresses of Conquest: A Study of Wilson Bands and Enamel Hypoplasias in the Maya of Lamanai, Belize. *American Journal of Human Biology* 2:25–35.

1994 *The Sacrifice of the Earth? Diet, Health, and Inequality in the Pasión Maya Lowlands*. Unpublished Ph.D. dissertation, University of Chicago.

1997a Biological Perspectives on the Collapse of the Pasión Maya. *AM* 8(2):267–73.

1997b Intertooth Patterns of Hypoplasia Expression: Implications for Childhood Health in the Classic Maya Collapse. *AJPA* 102(2):233–47.

1999 The Elements of Maya Diets: Alkaline Earth Baselines and Paleodietary Reconstruction in the Pasión Zone. In *Reconstructing Ancient Maya Diet*, edited by C. D. White, pp. 197–219. Salt Lake City: University of Utah Press.

Wright, Lori E., and Francisco Chew

1998 Porotic Hyperostosis and Paleoepidemiology: A Forensic Perspective on Anemia among the Ancient Maya. *AA* 100(4):924–39.

Wright, Lori E., and Henry P. Schwarcz

1996 Infrared and Isotopic Evidence for Diagenesis of Bone Apatite at Dos Pilas, Guatemala: Paleodietary Implications. *JAS* 23(6):933–44.

1998 Stable Carbon and Oxygen Isotopes in Human Tooth Enamel: Identifying Breastfeeding and Weaning in Prehistory. *AJPA* 106(1):1–18.

Wright, Lori E., and Christine D. White

1996 Human Biology in the Classic Maya Collapse: Evidence from Paleopathology and Paleodiet. *Journal of World Prehistory* 10(2):147–98.

Wright, Lori E., and A. M. Witte

1998 Observaciones sobre la osteologia humana en Piedras Negras: Reporte Preliminar 2. In *Proyecto Arqueologico Piedras Negras, Informe preliminar 2,* edited by Stephen Houston and Héctor Escobedo, pp. 393–97. Report submitted to the Instituto de Antropología e Historia de Guatemala.